Neurology of Bladder, Bowel, and Sexual Dysfunction

Blue Books of Practical Neurology
(Volumes 1–14 published as BIMR Neurology)

1   **Clinical Neurophysiology**
    Erik Stålberg and Robert R. Young

2   **Movement Disorders** (reissued in Blue Books of Practical Neurology)
    C. David Marsden and Stanley Fahn

3   **Cerebral Vascular Disease**
    Michael J. G. Harrison and Mark L. Dyken

4   **Peripheral Nerve Disorders**
    Arthur K. Asbury and R. W. Gilliatt

5   **The Epilepsies**
    Roger J. Porter and Paolo I. Morselli

6   **Multiple Sclerosis**
    W. I. McDonald and Donald H. Silberberg

7   **Movement Disorders 2** (reissued in Blue Books of Practical Neurology)
    C. David Marsden and Stanley Fahn

8   **Infections of the Nervous System**
    Peter G. E. Kennedy and Richard T. Johnson

9   **The Molecular Biology of Neurological Disease**
    Roger N. Rosenberg and Anita E. Harding

10 **Pain Syndromes in Neurology**
    Howard L. Fields

11 **Principles and Practice of Restorative Neurology**
    Robert R. Young and Paul J. Delwaide

12 **Stroke: Populations, Cohorts, and Clinical Trials**
    Jack P. Whisnant

13 **Movement Disorders 3**
    C. David Marsden and Stanley Fahn

14 **Mitochondrial Disorders in Neurology**
    Anthony H. V. Schapira and Salvatore DiMauro

15 **Peripheral Nerve Disorders 2**
    Arthur K. Asbury and P. K. Thomas

16 **Contemporary Behavioral Neurology**
    Michael R. Trimble and Jeffrey L. Cummings

17 **Headache**
    Peter J. Goadsby and Stephen D. Silberstein

18 **The Epilepsies 2**
    Roger J. Porter and David Chadwick

19 **The Dementias**
    John H. Growdon and Martin N. Rossor

20 **Hospitalist Neurology**
    Martin A. Samuels

21 **Neurologic Complications in Organ Transplant Recipients**
    Eelco F. M. Wijdicks

22 **Critical Care Neurology**
    David H. Miller and Eric C. Raps

23 **Neurology of Bladder, Bowel, and Sexual Dysfunction**
    Clare J. Fowler

Neurology of Bladder, Bowel, and Sexual Dysfunction

Edited by

Clare J. Fowler, M.Sc., F.R.C.P.
Reader in Clinical Neurology, Institute of Neurology, University College London; Consultant in Uro-Neurology, The National Hospital for Neurology and Neurosurgery, University College London Hospitals Trust

with 25 contributors

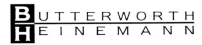

Boston   Oxford   Auckland   Johannesburg   Melbourne   New Delhi

Every effort has been made to ensure that the drug dosage schedules within this text are accurate and conform to standards accepted at time of publication. However, as treatment recommendations vary in the light of continuing research and clinical experience, the reader is advised to verify drug dosage schedules herein with information found on product information sheets. This is especially true in cases of new or infrequently used drugs.

 Recognizing the importance of preserving what has been written, Butterworth–Heinemann prints its books on acid-free paper whenever possible.

 Butterworth–Heinemann supports the efforts of American Forests and the Global ReLeaf program in its campaign for the betterment of trees, forests, and our environment.

Library of Congress Cataloging-in-Publication Data

Neurology of bladder, bowel, and sexual dysfunction / edited by Clare
   J. Fowler
          p.   cm. -- (Blue books of practical neurology ; 23)
     Includes bibliographical references and index.
     ISBN 0-7506-9959-0
     1. Neurogenic bladder. 2. Intestines--Diseases. 3. Sexual
disorders. 4. Pelvis--Innervation. 5. Nervous system--Diseases-
-Complications. I. Fowler, Clare J. II. Series.
     [DNLM: 1. Bladder, Neurogenic--etiology. 2. Colonic Diseases-
-etiology. 3. Nervous System Diseases--complications. 4. Sex
Disorders--etiology. W1 BU9749 v.23 1999 / WJ 500 N4943 1999]
RC921.N4N48 1999
616.8--dc21
DNLM/DLC
for Library of Congress   99-20093
                                                                CIP

British Library Cataloguing-in-Publication Data
A catalogue record for this book is available from the British Library.

The publisher offers special discounts on bulk orders of this book.
For more information, please contact:
Manager of Special Sales
Butterworth–Heinemann
225 Wildwood Avenue
Woburn, MA 01801-2041
Tel: 781-904-2500
Fax: 781-904-2620

For information on all Butterworth–Heinemann publications available,
contact our World Wide Web home page at: http://www.bh.com

10 9 8 7 6 5 4 3 2 1

Printed in the United States of America

*To Alice and Ben, and William,
who sometimes might have wished their mother had
had different medical interests*

Contents

Contributing Authors   xi
Series Preface   xv
In Memory of C. David Marsden   xvii
Preface   xix
Acknowledgments   xxi

Part I   Neurologic Control   **1**

1 Introduction   3
   William C. de Groat and Clare J. Fowler

2 Lumbosacral Plexus and Innervation of the Pelvic Floor
   in Humans and Their Comparative Anatomy   5
   P. K. Thomas

3 Neurophysiology of the Bladder and Bowel   19
   Michael D. Craggs and Carolynne Jane Vaizey

4 Physiology of Female Sexual Function and Effect
   of Neurologic Disease   33
   Per Olov Lundberg

5 Physiology of Male Sexual Function and Dysfunction
   in Neurologic Disease   47
   Rupert O. Beck

6 Consequences of the Neuropathic Bladder and Bowel for Patients   57
   Scott Glickman and Julia Segal

7 Impact of Neurologic Disability on Sex and Relationships   69
   Barbara J. Chandler

Part II   Investigations   **95**

8 Urodynamics   97
   Michael J. Swinn

9 Clinical Neurophysiology 109
David B. Vodušek and Clare J. Fowler

10 Investigation of Male Erectile Dysfunction 145
Rupert O. Beck

Part III Treatments **161**

11 Treatment of Neurogenic Bladder Dysfunction 163
Prokar Dasgupta and Collette Haslam

12 Investigation and Treatment of Bowel Problems 185
Christine Norton and Michael Henry

13 Treatment of Sexual Dysfunction and Infertility
in Patients with Neurologic Diseases 209
Dimitrios G. Hatzichristou

Part IV Specific Conditions **227**

14 Cerebral Control of Bladder, Bowel, and Sexual Function
and Effects of Brain Disease 229
Ryuji Sakakibara and Clare J. Fowler

15 Urogenital Disorders in Parkinson's Disease
and Multiple System Atrophy 245
Vijay A. Chandiramani and Clare J. Fowler

16 Disorders of Bowel Function in Parkinsonism 255
Fabrizio Stocchi

17 Urinary Incontinence in the Elderly 265
Derek J. Griffiths

18 Spinal Cord Injury 275
E. P. Arnold

19 Bladder and Sexual Dysfunction in Multiple Sclerosis 289
Christopher D. Betts

20 Bowel Dysfunction in Multiple Sclerosis 309
Clare J. Fowler and Michael Henry

21 Tropical Spastic Paraparesis 315
Prokar Dasgupta and Iqbal F. Hussain

22 Cauda Equina Damage and Its Management 325
Iqbal F. Hussain

23 Peripheral Neuropathy 339
Prokar Dasgupta and P. K. Thomas

24 Spina Bifida 353
Matgorzata Borzyskowski

25 Nonpsychogenic Urinary Retention in Young Women 367
Michael J. Swinn and Clare J. Fowler

Index 373

Contributing Authors

E. P. Arnold, M.B.Ch.B. (NZ), Ph.D. (London), F.R.C.S. (Eng), F.R.A.C.S.
Associate Professor of Urology, Christchurch School of Medicine, Christchurch, New Zealand; Consultant Urologist, Christchurch Hospital

Rupert O. Beck, M.B.B.S., F.R.C.S. (Urol)
Consultant Urologist, Princess Margaret Hospital, Swindon, United Kingdom

Christopher D. Betts, M.B.Ch.B., F.R.C.S. (Urol)
Consultant Urological Surgeon, Hope Hospital, Salford, Greater Manchester, United Kingdom

Matgorzata Borzyskowski, M.B., B.S., F.R.C.P., F.R.C.P.C.H.
Consultant Neurodevelopmental Paediatrician, Guys' and St. Thomas' Hospital Trust, London

Vijay A. Chandiramani, M.B.B.S., M.S., F.R.C.S., F.R.C.S. (Urol)
Consultant Urologist, University Hospital of South Manchester, Manchester, United Kingdom

Barbara J. Chandler, B.Med.Sci., M.D., M.R.C.P.
Honorary Clinical Lecturer in Neuroscience, University of Newcastle Upon Tyne, United Kingdom; Consultant in Rehabilitation Medicine, Hunters Moor Regional Rehabilitation Centre, Newcastle City Health Trust, Newcastle Upon Tyne

Michael D. Craggs, Ph.D., B.Sc., C.Biol., M.I.P.E.M.
Reader in Neurophysiology and Nephrology, Royal Free and University College Medical School, Institute of Urology, London; Honorary Consultant Clinical Scientist, University College London Hospitals Trust

Prokar Dasgupta, M.Sc. (Urol), F.R.C.S.
Honorary Lecturer in Uro-Neurology, Institute of Neurology, London; Specialist Registrar in Urology, Edith Cavell Hospital, Peterborough, United Kingdom

William C. de Groat, Ph.D.
Professor of Pharmacology, University of Pittsburgh School of Medicine

Clare J. Fowler, M.Sc., F.R.C.P.
Reader in Clinical Neurology, Institute of Neurology, University College London; Consultant in Uro-Neurology, The National Hospital for Neurology and Neurosurgery, University College London Hospitals Trust

Scott Glickman, F.R.C.S.
Senior Lecturer in Rehabilitation Medicine, Imperial College School of Medicine, London; Consultant in Neuroscience, The Hammersmith Hospitals National Health Service Trust, London

Derek J. Griffiths, Ph.D.
Griffiths Urodynamics and Pro-Continence Consulting, Edmonton, Alberta, Canada

Collette Haslam, R.G.N.
Clinical Nurse Specialist in Uro-Neurology, The National Hospital for Neurology and Neurosurgery, University College London Hospitals Trust

Dimitrios G. Hatzichristou, M.D., Ph.D.
Assistant Professor of Urology and Director, Center for Sexual Dysfunction, Aristotle University of Thessaloniki, Thessaloniki, Greece

Michael Henry, M.B., F.R.C.S.
Consultant Surgeon, Chelsea and Westminster Hospital and Royal Marsden Hospital, London

Iqbal F. Hussain, B.Sc., M.B.B.S., F.R.C.S. (Eng)
Research Fellow in Uro-Neurology, The National Hospital for Neurology and Neurosurgery, University College London Hospitals Trust, London; Higher Surgical Trainee in Urology, Institute of Urology and Nephrology, London

Per Olov Lundberg, M.D., Ph.D.
Professor of Neurology, Uppsala University, Uppsala, Sweden; Consultant in Sexology, University Hospital, Uppsala

Christine Norton, M.A. (Cantab), R.G.N.
Nurse Specialist in Continence, St. Mark's Hospital, Middlesex, United Kingdom

Ryuji Sakakibara, M.D.
Instructor in Neurology, Chiba University, Chiba, Japan

Julia Segal, M.A. (Cantab)
Senior Counsellor, Multiple Sclerosis Unit, North West London Hospitals National Health Service Trust

Fabrizio Stocchi, M.D., Ph.D.
Reader, Department of Neurosciences, University La Sapienza, Rome; Consultant in Neurology, San Raffaele Hospital, Rome

Michael J. Swinn, M.B.B.S., B.Sc., F.R.C.S.
Registrar in Uro-Neurology, The National Hospital for Neurology and Neurosurgery, University College London Hospitals Trust

P. K. Thomas, C.B.E., D.Sc., M.D., F.R.C.P.
Emeritus Professor of Neurology, Royal Free and University College Medical School and Institute of Neurology, London; Honorary Consultant Neurologist, Royal Free Hospital and National Hospital for Neurology and Neurosurgery, University College London Hospitals Trust; Editor, *Journal of Anatomy*, London

Carolynne Jane Vaizey, F.R.C.S., F.C.S.
Consultant Surgeon in Colorectal Surgery, University College London Hospitals Trust; Honorary Senior Research Fellow, St. Mark's Hospital, Middlesex, United Kingdom

David B. Vodušek, M.D., D.Sc.
Medical Director, Division of Neurology, University Medical Centre, Ljubljana, Slovenia; Professor of Neurology, University of Ljubljana

Series Preface

The *Blue Books of Practical Neurology* denotes the series of monographs previously named the *BIMR Neurology* series, which was itself the successor to the *Modern Trends in Neurology* series. As before, the volumes are intended for use by physicians who grapple with the problems of neurologic disorders on a daily basis, be they neurologists, neurologists in training, or those in related fields such as neurosurgery, internal medicine, psychiatry, and rehabilitation medicine.

Our purpose is to produce monographs on topics in clinical neurology in which progress through research has brought about new concepts of patient management. The subject of each book is selected by the Series Editors using two criteria: first, that there has been significant advance in knowledge in that area and, second, that such advances have been incorporated into new ways of managing patients with the disorders in question. This has been the guiding spirit behind each volume, and we expect it to continue. In effect, we emphasize research, both in the clinic and in the experimental laboratory, but principally to the extent that it changes our collective attitudes and practices in caring for those who are neurologically afflicted.

C. David Marsden
Arthur K. Asbury
Series Editors

In Memory of C. David Marsden

David Marsden was the first Series Editor for these monographs; he was asked by Butterworths in 1982 to take on this duty. Shortly thereafter, he recruited one of us (A. K. A.) to join him. The principle that evolved for the Series was that each volume should feature practical aspects of neurology, with emphasis on those areas in which the fruits of research had improved and expanded the management of the neurologic disorders in question. This principle is the guiding spirit for the *Blue Books of Practical Neurology* and will remain so as long as these volumes are published. It is one of the many legacies that David Marsden bequeathed to the fields of neurology and neuroscience, and it will serve as a living commemoration of this extraordinary man and his manifold accomplishments.

Arthur K. Asbury
Anthony H. V. Schapira
Series Editors

Preface

This book was written primarily for neurologists and other physicians; however, I hope that surgeons, too, will be interested. It considers function of the pelvic organs from an electrician's point of view rather than a plumber's. Many non-surgical treatments are now possible for urogenital problems and are more suitable than surgical interventions for patients with progressive neurologic disease.

This book is being published at a propitious time: Neurologists have become increasingly concerned about their patients' neurogenic pelvic organ dysfunctions and are often able to suggest successful treatments for these problems. Formerly a somewhat neglected field of neuroscience, work on the neurologic control of bladder, bowel, and sexual function is in an explosive phase in basic science and pharmaceutical laboratories, which can only be of benefit to patients with problems in these areas.

Clare J. Fowler

Acknowledgments

Thanks go to my authors, who managed to produce their contributions while carrying on busy full-time jobs. I enjoyed working with those who spent time in my department and learning about the neurology of the pelvic organs with them. Other authors are friends, whether long-standing or of more recent acquaintance, and I am indebted to them for the time and effort they have taken to contribute to this book. I learned a lot from their texts.

Particular thanks go to Professor Ian McDonald, who early in my career recognized the importance of treating problems of bladder and sexual dysfunction in patients with multiple sclerosis and therefore made it easier for me to establish a department of uro-neurology.

It is with thanks to the late Professor David Marsden that I am editor of this volume in the prestigious series of which he and Doctor Arthur K. Asbury were editors-in-chief. At times, I questioned whether I was happy about the various writing tasks that David volunteered me for, but I know the real answer is "yes." I shall always be grateful to him for his invaluable support of both my academic and clinical activities.

Dr. Peter Nathan was the first uro-neurologist, in the early 1960s, and I hope he thinks this book's review of his work does him justice. Miss Enid Halsey was there when the specialty of uro-neurology was first beginning as a clinical service, and she always insisted it was a good idea. In producing this book, I must also thank Mrs. Lizzie Boal, who helped work on edited manuscripts and other things. As with so many of my activities, the whole enterprise would not have been possible without the patient and unfailing secretarial assistance of Mrs. Katia Matthews. Thanks also go to Leslie Kramer and Susan Pioli at Butterworth–Heinemann, who were efficient and encouraging throughout production of this book.

I join other editors and authors who are thankful for word processing, and I would also like to express my deep gratitude to the inventors of e-mail. The speed with which electronic text can be exchanged has, I suspect, transformed the job of a book editor—very little time has had to be spent in tedious text housekeeping. Receiving the chapters, putting in the edits, and passing them on to the publisher has been an interesting and rewarding experience.

Clare J. Fowler

I
NEUROLOGIC CONTROL

1
Introduction

William C. de Groat and Clare J. Fowler

Interest in the neurologic aspects of pelvic organ dysfunction, formerly a somewhat neglected area, has increased considerably. Neurologists had been disinterested for several reasons: (1) The range of symptoms produced by the organs is limited. For example, the bladder in its bimodal existence of storing or eliminating urine can fail in either (or both) modes, resulting in incontinence or retention irrespective of the wide range of possible underlying pathophysiologies. (2) Few pertinent neurologic signs can be elicited in the context of pelvic organ disorders, and the laboratory investigations are mostly non-neurologic. (3) Physicians and patients alike have been reluctant to discuss highly personal complaints. However, that reservation has now changed, and in a society in which people generally feel more comfortable discussing intimate matters, patient-doctor relationships can be less inhibited. (4) Few effective treatments were available for pelvic organ dysfunction. Now, however, because of the growing scientific understanding of the neurologic control of bladder, bowel, and sexual functions, many valuable therapies can be offered to patients for symptom management. The appropriate questions are being asked of patients, and treatments are being given to relieve the embarrassing and socially incapacitating symptoms that affect so many neurologic patients as part of their illness.

On reflection, it is not surprising that any text that attempts to cover aspects of bladder, bowel, and sexual dysfunction should be considering the topics from a neurologic perspective. A number of common features are seen in the peripheral neural control of the pelvic organs. On the other hand, traditionally little overlap has existed when each organ is considered functionally, because medical care of each has developed its own specialty. Thus, although moves have been made to reduce the barriers between urologists, urogynecologists, andrologists, and coloproctologists, a tendency remains for the function of each of the pelvic organs to be considered separately.

The pelvic organs receive an innervation from the same sacral spinal segments; therefore, a neurologic lesion affecting their common nerve roots or peripheral nerve supply can cause bladder, bowel, and sexual dysfunction. Clinically, a cauda equina lesion affecting S2–S4 produces a deficit of all three functions. A severe generalized peripheral neuropathy can do the same, but lesions to the peripheral innervation within the pelvis, such as damage to the pelvic nerves without damage to the pudendal nerves, are likely to produce a partial deficit.

More proximally located lesions, however, have a variable effect on the function of these organs, and much can be deduced about the neurologic abnormality from considering the combination of symptoms. The pelvic organ dysfunctions that appear after spinal cord lesions are more complicated and demonstrate the extent to which some pelvic functions are dependent on central nervous control, whereas others are subserved by peripheral neural mechanisms.

According to current concepts, micturition is regulated by neural circuitry in the pons, which coordinates the activity of the bladder and urethral outlet. This circuitry is in turn modulated by neural activity arising in the forebrain. Supraspinal influences on voiding are mediated by spinal tracts that convey information between the pons and the lumbosacral spinal cord. Spinal segmental reflex arcs also play an important role, particularly after spinal cord injury; however, pontine-spinal connections are critical for full voluntary control of voiding.

Supraspinal circuitry is less critical for bowel control. This is attributable in part to the relative infrequency of bowel excretory activity under physiologic circumstances and the nonfluid nature of fecal matter. In addition, the bowel has a rich intrinsic innervation that can mediate an effective reflex control independent of connections with the spinal cord. Thus, although voluntary control of defecation is lost after spinal cord injury, distal bowel function is less severely affected than bladder function.

Sexual function is dependent on spinal and supraspinal neural mechanisms. Responses, such as penile erection, that are mediated to a large extent by intrinsic spinal reflexes persist after injury to the rostral spinal cord, whereas those requiring supraspinal control are markedly suppressed.

Lesions in the brain stem may interfere with urogenital and distal bowel function by damaging specific nuclei involved in supraspinal reflex circuits or by interrupting long fiber tracts connecting the lumbosacral spinal cord to higher centers. The lesions can therefore alter sensory and motor pathways.

Although the cortical control of bladder, bowel, and sexual function has been little studied, frontal lobe influences are known to be important. Because excretory activity involves social planning, urinary and fecal incontinence resulting from frontal lobe damage is likely to be due in part to an effect on behavior as well as to an alteration of reflex mechanisms. Modesty, which deeply shrouds all human activities of the pelvic organs—an aspect of behavior other animals and even higher primates do not exhibit—probably relates to frontal lobe influences.

This book describes the nervous control of the pelvic organs and the investigations that can be performed to evaluate neurogenic disorders of these organs. It also covers in some detail various diseases and neurologic lesions that are known to disrupt bladder, bowel, and sexual function.

2

Lumbosacral Plexus and Innervation of the Pelvic Floor in Humans and Their Comparative Anatomy

P. K. Thomas

The limb girdle plexuses are complex anatomic networks in which nerve fibers derived from the dorsal and ventral roots, together with others from the sympathetic chain and the preganglionic parasympathetic pathways, are sorted into the complicated system of peripheral nerves that supplies the limbs and the adjacent parts of the trunk. With regard to the lower limb plexuses, for descriptive purposes it is convenient to separate lumbar, sacral, and coccygeal plexuses, although they are closely linked anatomically. The present discussion is restricted to the innervation of the pelvic and perineal musculature and viscera, and the cutaneous nerve supply to the pubic and perineal regions. Before the disposition and distribution of these plexuses are considered, a brief survey of the muscles of the pelvic floor and perineum may be helpful.

MUSCLES OF THE PELVIC FLOOR

The paired levator ani and coccygeus muscles together constitute the basinlike pelvic diaphragm that spans the true pelvis and supports the pelvic viscera (Figure 2.1). The levator ani is a broad sheet of muscle attached to the inner walls of the true pelvis. It is composed of two portions, the medial pubococcygeus and the more lateral iliococcygeus. The coccygeus is the outermost component of the diaphragm.

The pubococcygeus arises from the posterior aspect of the pubis and extends backward almost horizontally to terminate in a tendinous plate that is attached to the anterior surface of the coccyx. Anteriorly, the most medial fibers of the pubococcygeus blend with those of the sphincter urethrae and, in the male, form the levator prostatae. More posteriorly, in the female, some fibers are inserted into the walls of the vagina as the *pubovaginalis*, and into the perineal body and the walls of the rectum in both sexes. Those that are inserted into the rectum, referred to as the *puboanalis*, join with the longitudinal rectal muscle and fascia to form the conjoint coat of the anal canal. Posterior to the rectum, most of the fibers of the pubococcygeus form a tendinous plate that is attached to the coccyx. A thick puborectalis muscle separates from the pubococcygeus and, passing inferiorly and

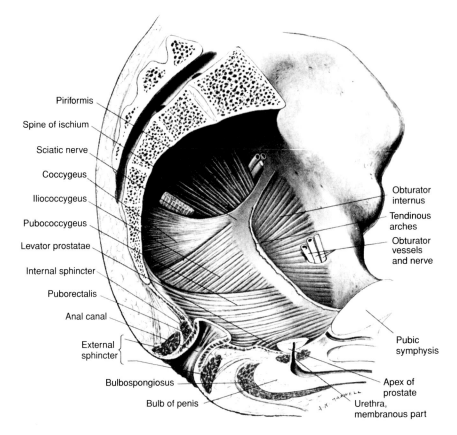

Labels on figure:
Piriformis
Spine of ischium
Sciatic nerve
Coccygeus
Iliococcygeus
Pubococcygeus
Levator prostatae
Internal sphincter
Puborectalis
Anal canal
External sphincter
Bulbospongiosus
Bulb of penis
Obturator internus
Tendinous arches
Obturator vessels and nerve
Pubic symphysis
Apex of prostate
Urethra, membranous part

Figure 2.1   Left pelvic floor showing the pelvic diaphragm made up of the levator ani (ilio-coccygeus, pubococcygeus, and puborectalis) and coccygeus muscles. It is penetrated by the anal canal, the urethra, and the obturator vessels and nerves. (Reprinted with permission from PL Williams [ed], Gray's Anatomy. Edinburgh, UK: Churchill Livingstone, 1995.)

posteriorly, fuses with the opposite puborectalis and with the external anal sphincter to form a sling behind the anorectal junction.

Lateral to the pubococcygeal part of the levator ani, the iliococcygeus is thin and aponeurotic. It arises from the obturator fascia on the pelvic surface of the obtura-tor internus muscle and extends posteriorly to join with its fellow from the oppo-site side in a midline raphe that contributes to the anococcygeal ligament and that is attached posteriorly to the terminal two segments of the coccyx. An accessory slip in its posterior portion attaching to the sacrum is referred to as the *iliosacralis*.

The coccygeus constitutes the most posterolateral part of the pelvic diaphragm and consists of an approximately triangular fibromuscular sheet. At its apex, it arises from the internal aspect of the pelvis and the tip of the ischial spine. Its posterolateral mar-gin is fused with the sacrospinous ligament; posteriorly, it is attached to the lateral margins of the coccyx and the fifth sacral segment.

Rudimentary anterior and posterior sacrococcygeal muscles may be present. These extend from the sacrum to the coccyx, anterior and posterior to the sacroiliac joints.

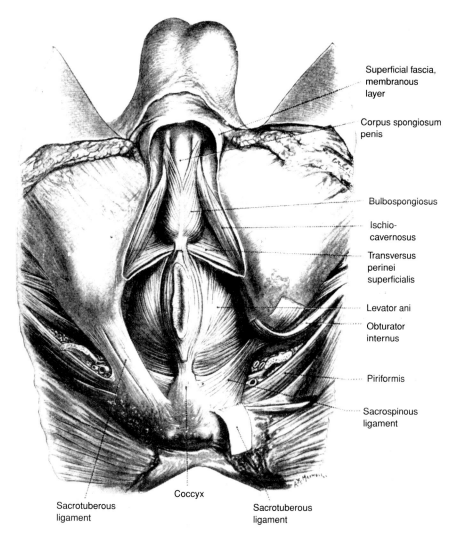

Superficial fascia, membranous layer

Corpus spongiosum penis

Bulbospongiosus

Ischio-cavernosus

Transversus perinei superficialis

Levator ani

Obturator internus

Piriformis

Sacrospinous ligament

Sacrotuberous ligament

Coccyx

Sacrotuberous ligament

Figure 2.2   Muscles of the male perineum. (Reprinted with permission from PL Williams [ed], Gray's Anatomy. Edinburgh, UK: Churchill Livingstone, 1995.)

The homologies of the muscles of the pelvic floor with those in tailed mammals are considered later.

Perineal Musculature

The perineum consists of a trapezoidal region inferior to the pelvic diaphragm. A transverse line anterior to the ischial tuberosities divides the perineum into posterior anal and anterior urogenital triangles. The male perineal musculature is shown in Figure 2.2.

The anal triangle includes the central anus with its internal and external sphincters. The anal canal is bounded on either side by the ischiorectal fossae and linked to the coccyx posteriorly by an anococcygeal ligament.

The urogenital triangle is bounded superficially by the superficial perineal fascia with its deep membranous layer. Laterally, this layer is attached to the margins of the pubic rami and the ischium; posteriorly, the layer blends with the fascial perineal membrane and perineal body. The perineal membrane stretches across the pubic arch. It is penetrated by the urethra and by vessels and nerves destined for the penis in men or for the vagina in women. The perineal body is a fibromuscular structure located in the midline between the anal canal and the urogenital apparatus, immediately inferior to the rectovesical or rectovaginal septum. The urogenital triangle is divided into the superficial and deep perineal spaces. The superficial space lies between the perineal fascia and the perineal membrane, and the deep space lies between the perineal membrane and the pelvic diaphragm.

Anal Musculature

The external anal sphincter encircles the anal canal (see Figure 2.1). It is composed of skeletal-type striated muscle and overlaps the internal anal sphincter, which is comprised of nonstriated muscle. Its organization has been disputed [1]. Milligan and Morgan [2] separated it into three parts, and this organization is accepted in standard descriptions [3]. The proposed subdivisions are as follows: (1) A subcutaneous part lies between the skin of the anal orifice around the lower anal canal, inferior to the lowest part of the internal anal sphincter. Some of its anterior fibers are described as joining the perineal body, and some of the posterior ones as attaching to the anococcygeal ligament. (2) A superficial part is situated superior to the subcutaneous part and surrounds the lowermost part of the internal sphincter. Posteriorly it is attached to the terminal segment of the coccyx by the median anococcygeal raphe, and anteriorly it is attached to the anococcygeal body. (3) The deep part is described as lying internally and surrounding the upper part of the internal sphincter. Some fibers are attached to the anococcygeal raphe, and anterior fibers, especially in females, intermingle with the superficial transverse perineal muscles. The fibers of its deeper part blend with those of the puborectalis. Golligher et al. [4] and Ayoub [5], on the other hand, were unable to detect any division into separate segments; rather, the muscle appeared as a single sheet. A two-component organization was proposed by Oh and Kark [6]. These studies used dissection or relied on surgical experience [1]. One report correlated endoanal magnetic resonance imaging with histologic sections [7]. No separation of the external anal sphincter into separate components was identified.

The anococcygeal ligament is a musculotendinous complex in the midline between the anorectum and the coccyx. Together with the superimposed presacral fascia, it forms the postnatal plate [8], on which is situated the terminal rectum. This plate, from above down, consists of the presacral fascia, the tendinous plate of the pubococcygeus, the raphe of the iliococcygeus, and the posterior attachments of the puborectalis and the external anal sphincter.

Male Urogenital Musculature

The urogenital muscles are separable into superficial and deep groups, situated in the superficial and deep perineal spaces, respectively (see Figure 2.2). They are separated by the perineal membrane, which provides a base for these muscles. The superficial group comprises the median bulbospongiosus muscle, the paired ischiocavernosus muscles, and the variable superficial transverse perineal muscles. The bulbospongiosus muscle has complex actions and is involved in emptying the urethra after micturition, in ejaculation, and in assisting penile erection. The ischiocavernosus muscle maintains erection by compressing the crus penis. The deep group of perineal muscles consists of the sphincter urethrae and the deep transverse perineal muscles. The latter extend between the ischial rami laterally and the perineal body centrally and hence are involved in tightening the perineum and visceral canals.

The urogenital muscles and their related fasciae are sometimes referred to as the *urogenital diaphragm,* situated below the pelvic diaphragm, although they do not in fact form a continuous sheet [9].

Female Urogenital Musculature

The female urogenital triangle is generally similar to that of men, but its organization is affected by the presence of the vagina and the female external genitalia. The bulbospongiosus partially encloses the vestibular bulb and the greater vestibular glands, and extends forward on either side of the vagina to reach the corpora cavernosa of the clitoris. Posteriorly, it is attached to the perineal body. It is involved in contraction of the vaginal orifice and in compression of the vestibular glands, and contributes to erection of the clitoris by compression of its deep dorsal vein. A sphincter urethrae surrounds the urethra and is contiguous superiorly with the muscles of the bladder neck. The compressores urethrae arise from the ischiopubic rami on either side and join in the midline ventral to the urethra. Only rarely do they reach the perineal body to form deep transverse perineal muscles as in men. The sphincter urethrovaginalis arises from the perineal body and encircles the lower vagina and lower urethra inferior to the compressores urethrae.

LUMBAR PLEXUS

Derivation from Ventral Rami

The dorsal and ventral spinal roots join to form spinal nerves that divide into dorsal and ventral primary rami. The lumbar plexus (Figure 2.3) originates from the first three lumbar ventral rami together with the major part of the fourth lumbar ramus and a contribution from the last thoracic ventral ramus. These emerge from the intervertebral foramina and lie between the anterior and posterior paravertebral masses of psoas major, the posterior mass being attached to the transverse processes of the vertebrae and the anterior to the vertebral bodies, intervertebral disks, and tendinous arches.

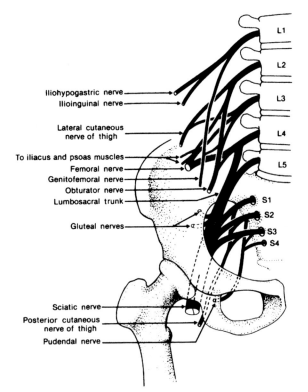

Figure 2.3   Diagram of the lumbosacral plexus shows the main nerves derived from it. (Reprinted from JD Stewart. Clinical Examination in Neurology. Philadelphia: Saunders, 1963;181. By permission of Mayo Foundation.)

The precise arrangements in the lumbar plexus may vary from one individual to another. Most commonly, the first lumbar ramus is joined by a contribution from the twelfth thoracic ramus. The combined rami divide into a larger upper part that gives rise to the iliohypogastric and ilioinguinal nerves. The lower part is joined by a branch from the second lumbar ramus to form the genitofemoral nerve. The remainder of the second lumbar ramus, the third, and part of the fourth divide into dorsal and ventral branches. The ventral branches join and become the obturator nerve. The dorsal branches give rise to the cutaneous nerve of the thigh (lateral femoral cutaneous nerve) and the femoral nerve. An accessory obturator nerve derived from the third and fourth rami is occasionally present.

The lumbar and sacral plexuses are linked in the formation of the lumbosacral trunk (Figure 2.4; see Figure 2.3), which is derived by union of the central branches of the fourth and fifth lumbar rami. The lumbosacral trunk joins the sacral plexus (see Figure 2.4). As occurs with the brachial plexus, the lumbar plexus can be prefixed or postfixed. The fourth lumbar ventral ramus is sometimes termed the *nervus furcalis*, because it is divided between the two plexuses. If the lumbosacral trunk is formed from the third and fourth rami, the plexus is said to be *prefixed*. A more common variation is for the fifth ramus to be furcal, in which case the plexus is said to be *postfixed*.

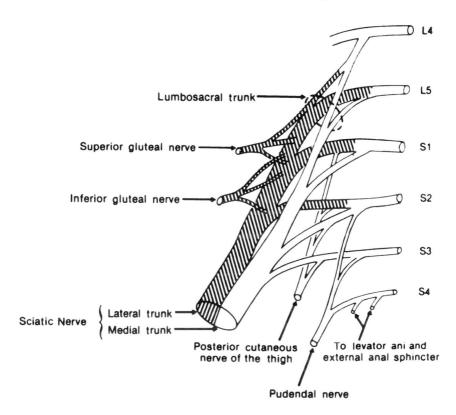

Figure 2.4 Diagram of the sacral plexus and the main nerves derived from it. The ventral rami from the L4–S2 spinal nerves divide into dorsal and ventral branches that give rise to the lateral and medial trunks of the sciatic nerve. (Reprinted with permission from JD Stewart. Focal Peripheral Neuropathies [2nd ed]. Philadelphia: Lippincott–Raven, 1993.)

Branches of the Lumbar Plexus

Only branches of the lumbar plexus of direct relevance to bladder, bowel, and sexual function are considered here (see Figure 2.3).

Iliohypogastric Nerve

After emerging from the lateral border of the psoas major and crossing anterior to the quadratus lumborum, the iliohypogastric nerve pierces the transverse abdominis and internal oblique muscles that it supplies, dividing into lateral and anterior cutaneous branches. The former emerges above the iliac crest and is distributed to the skin of the posterolateral gluteal region. The anterior cutaneous branch emerges medial to the superior iliac spine and supplies the skin of the suprapubic region.

Ilioinguinal Nerve

The ilioinguinal nerve initially follows a course similar to that of the iliohypo-gastric nerve, but then descends into the upper part of the pelvis, crosses the ili-acus, traverses the inguinal canal, and emerges with the spermatic cord through the superficial inguinal ring to supply the skin of the upper inner aspect of the thigh and either the penile root and upper scrotum, or the mons pubis and adja-cent labia majora.

Genitofemoral Nerve

After traversing the psoas major and emerging close to its medial border, the genitofemoral nerve descends beneath the peritoneum, crosses behind the ureter, and divides into the genital and femoral branches. The former enters the inguinal canal and emerges to supply the cremaster and the skin of the scrotum in men. In women, it accompanies the round ligament and supplies the skin of the mons pubis and the labia majora. The femoral branch passes posterior to the inguinal ligament, enters the femoral sheath lateral to the femoral artery, and surfaces to supply the skin over the femoral triangle.

SACRAL AND COCCYGEAL PLEXUSES

The upper four sacral ventral rami reach the pelvis through the anterior sacral foramina, and the fifth ventral ramus reaches the pelvis between the sacrum and the coccyx. Their size decreases from proximal to distal; the first and second rami are large. Each ramus receives gray rami communicantes from the pelvic part of the sympathetic chain. Visceral efferent rami emerge from the second to the fourth rami to reach the pelvic viscera as the pelvic splanchnic nerves. They con-tain parasympathetic efferent fibers derived from the sacral autonomic nucleus, a column of cells in the lateral part of Rexed's lamina VII in the second, third, and fourth segments of the spinal cord.

Sacral Plexus

The sacral plexus is derived from the lumbosacral trunk and the first to third sacral ventral rami as well as part of the fourth (see Figure 2.3). The remainder of the fourth ramus joins the coccygeal plexus. The first, second, and third sacral ventral rami split into dorsal and ventral divisions. The lumbosacral trunk emerges from the medial border of the psoas major, crosses over the pelvic brim in front of the sacroiliac joint, and unites with the ventral division of the first sacral ramus. Together with the ventral divisions of the second and third ventral rami, it descends toward the greater sciatic foramen, where it is joined by the dorsal divisions of the fifth lumbar and first and second sacral ventral rami, together with a contribution from the third ramus, to form the sciatic nerve (see

Figure 2.4). A branch from the ventral division of the second sacral ventral ramus joins with branches from the third and fourth sacral ventral rami to give rise to the pudendal nerve.

Onuf's Nucleus

The cells of origin for the motor fibers that innervate the muscles of the pelvic floor and perineum lie in Onuf's nucleus [10, 11]. This nucleus is situated in Rexed's lamina IX, in the ventrolateral part of the anterior horns in the first and second sacral segments, with a variable extension into the third [12–14]. It is larger in male than in female rats [15] and dogs [16]. Forger and Breedlove [16] reported that the numbers of neurons in this nucleus were greater in the male than in the female human. Pullen et al. [14] were unable to confirm this statistically in a smaller number of cases. They found that the nucleus was cigar-shaped and 4–7 mm long. The upper limit was in the rostral S1 segment in three of their cases and in midcaudal S1 in the other three. Sexual dimorphism for length was also not detectable. Proximally, the nucleus was located in the ventral horn, midway between the ventrolateral and ventromedial motor nuclei. At the S2 level it was located more ventrally, immediately adjacent to the boundary between gray and white matter.

The neurons on Onuf's nucleus have the distinction of being resistant to degeneration in motor neuron disease (amyotrophic lateral sclerosis) [17–19]. Observations in humans and in other species, including studies of its presynaptic input [20], suggest that this nucleus has autonomic-like features or properties hybrid with those of somatic motor neurons. Support for this view is provided by the observation that the nucleus codegenerates with autonomic neurons in the Shy-Drager form of multisystem atrophy [17, 21–23].

Pudendal Nerve

The pudendal nerve leaves the pelvis through the greater sciatic foramen to reach the gluteal region by passing between the coccygeus and piriformis muscles (Figure 2.5). It then crosses the sacrospinous ligament to enter the ischiorectal fossa where, accompanied by the pudendal vessels, it lies in the pudendal canal. This canal runs along the lateral wall of the fossa, which consists of the obturator internus and its overlying fascia. In the posterior part of the canal, the pudendal nerve gives rise to the dorsal nerve of the penis or clitoris and then to the inferior rectal nerve, and continues as the perineal nerve. In the female, it supplies sensory branches to the lower part of the vagina.

The dorsal nerve of the penis supplies the corpus cavernosum and terminates in the glans. The inferior rectal nerve crosses the ischiorectal fossa to supply the external anal sphincter, the lower anal canal, and the perianal skin. The perineal nerve runs anteriorly, providing muscular branches to the superficial and deep transverse perineal muscles, the sphincter urethrae, the bulbospongiosus, the ischiocavernosus, and the corpus spongiosum of the penis. It also gives rise to the posterior scrotal or labial nerves, which reach their destination by passing through the urogenital triangle. In

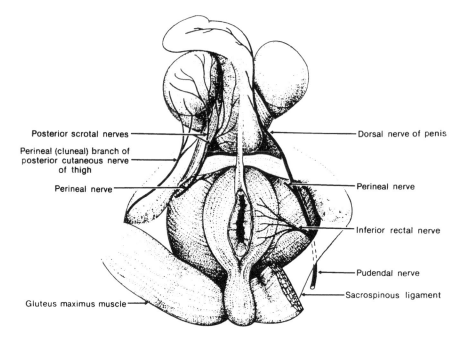

Figure 2.5   Male perineum showing the course and branches of the pudendal nerve. For clarity, the course of the perineal nerve has been shown only on one side. (Reprinted with permission from JD Stewart. Focal Peripheral Neuropathies [2nd ed]. Philadelphia: Lippincott–Raven, 1993.)

addition, the scrotal or labial skin receives a perineal branch from the posterior femoral cutaneous nerve (posterior cutaneous nerve of the thigh; see Figure 2.5).

Coccygeal Plexus

The descending branch from the fourth sacral ventral ramus joins the fifth sacral ventral ramus that emerges from the sacral hiatus (the inferior opening of the sacral canal) and runs over the pelvic surface of the coccygeus. Before the two join, the branch from the fourth sacral ventral ramus gives rise to muscular branches that innervate the levator ani and coccygeus and, after entering the ischiorectal fossa by piercing the coccygeus or passing between it and the levator ani, also supply the external anal sphincter. In addition, it gives rise to cutaneous branches that supply the skin between the anus and the coccyx. The combined fourth and fifth sacral ventral rami are joined by the single small coccygeal ventral ramus, which also exits from the sacral hiatus and pierces the coccygeus. It gives rise to the anococcygeal nerves, some branches of which pierce the coccygeus and the sacrotuberous ligament to reach the skin over the coccyx.

THE LUMBAR, SACRAL, AND COCCYGEAL DORSAL SPINAL RAMI

The lumbar dorsal (or posterior primary) rami, after separating from the ventral rami, divide into medial and lateral branches. The medial branches run posteriorly close to the vertebral articular processes to supply the multifidus muscle. The lateral branches innervate the erector spinae muscles, and the upper three give rise to cutaneous branches that supply the gluteal region.

The sacral dorsal spinal rami are small. The first four emerge through the dorsal sacral foramina; the fifth dorsal spinal ramus and the single coccygeal dorsal ramus leave through the sacral hiatus. The normal anatomy of the dorsal sacral foramina has been investigated in recent years both radiologically [24] and by dissection [25]. The medial branches of the first three sacral dorsal rami end in the multifidus muscle; their lateral branches join with lateral branches from the fifth lumbar and fourth sacral dorsal rami to form two series of loops, the deeper lying on the sacrotuberous ligament and the more superficial beneath the gluteus maximus. From the latter, cutaneous branches reach the gluteal area. The fourth and fifth sacral dorsal rami and the coccygeal ramus join together to form loops dorsal to the sacrum. They give rise to branches that supply the skin over the coccyx.

A study on the upper three dorsal foramina by dissection [25] was prompted by the recent interest in sacral nerve neuromodulation, which requires an electrode to be passed through the third sacral foramina in a needle cannula. It showed that the foramina were covered posteriorly by a fibrous membrane, probably equivalent to the ligamenta flava in the mobile regions of the vertebral column. The second, third, and fourth dorsal spinal rami had an oblique course, superiorly to inferiorly, during their course through the foramen before emerging through the covering membrane where they were surrounded by fat. A foraminal arterial branch was constantly present, situated close to the inferolateral margins of the foramina. A venous plexus was not detected in the foramina, but one was present around the proximal part of the dorsal root ganglia that communicated with the presacral venous plexus. To minimize the chance of nerve root or vascular damage, it was advised that needle insertion for neuromodulation should be made at the upper lateral edge of the foramen.

LUMBAR AND PELVIC SYMPATHETIC SYSTEM

The lumbar segment of the sympathetic chain usually possesses four interconnected ganglia. It lies anterior to the vertebral column and medial to the psoas major behind the peritoneum. The first, second, and occasionally the third ventral rami are linked to the lumbar sympathetic chain by white rami communicantes transmitting small myelinated preganglionic nerve fibers derived from the intermediolateral cell column of the spinal cord. The lumbar ventral rami receive gray rami communicantes from the last four lumbar sympathetic ganglia. They accompany the lumbar arteries around the vertebral bodies deep to the psoas major and contain unmyelinated postganglionic axons. Lumbar splanchnic nerves, usually four in number and derived from the ganglia of the lumbar sympathetic chain, join the coeliac, renal, intermesenteric, and superior hypogastric plexuses to supply abdominal viscera. Vascular branches from the lumbar sympathetic ganglia join the aortic plexus.

The pelvic sympathetic chain, which is continuous with the lumbar chain, possesses four or five ganglia. Inferiorly, it terminates in the midline ganglion on the anterior aspect of the coccyx. Gray rami communicantes join the sacral and coccygeal spinal nerves. Branches that pass medially from the ganglia form the inferior hypogastric (or pelvic) plexus, which is connected with the superior hypogastric plexus. Fibers from the inferior hypogastric plexus innervate the pelvic viscera.

COMPARATIVE ANATOMY

The organization of the pelvic floors in quadrupedal mammals differs considerably from that in the bipedal human [26]. The pelvic diaphragm is at a higher level in quadrupeds and is less complete, there being less necessity to support the abdominal viscera. The pelvic diaphragm forms a vertical partition to separate the pelvic and abdominal cavities. As in the human, it comprises the levator ani and coccygeus, but these muscles arise at a higher (i.e., more anterior) level. The levator ani arises from the pelvic brim, from the symphysis pubis and pubic rami, and from the shaft of the ilium. It fans out vertically and then condenses into a tendon that is inserted into the coccygeal vertebrae. The coccygeus lies in a more posterior (i.e., caudal) plane to the levator ani; it arises by a tendon from the ischial spine, spreads out in a fanlike manner, and is inserted into the transverse processes of the coccygeal vertebrae in the tail. The levator ani and coccygeus are thus depressors of the tail when they act together. When they act unilaterally, the coccygeus and the iliococcygeus component of the levator ani are lateral flexors of the tail. In the human, loss of the tail frees these muscles so that they are able to produce a more complete pelvic diaphragm.

In the human, the levator ani and coccygeus are supplied via the pudendal nerve. In tailed animals, in conformity with the different anatomic organization of the pelvic diaphragm, these muscles are innervated directly by ventral branches from the third sacral and first coccygeal nerves. Otherwise, the pudendal nerve has the same distribution in tailed mammals as in humans. The organization of the motor neurons innervating the perineal muscles has been analyzed in the male rat by Schroder [27], in the cat by Sato et al. [28], and in the monkey by Roppolo et al. [29].

Apart from the coccygeus and levator ani, in tailed mammals, muscles inserting into the coccygeal vertebrae arise from the sacrum and sometimes from the lumbar vertebrae. The sacrococcygeus dorsalis arises from the dorsal aspect of the lowest sacral spines (and some coccygeal spines) and is inserted onto the dorsal surfaces of the coccygeal vertebrae. It is an extensor of the tail. The sacrococcygeus ventralis, a tail flexor, arises from the ventral surface of the sacrum and sometimes also from lumbar vertebrae, and is inserted into the transverse process and central surfaces of the coccygeal vertebrae. The sacrococcygeus lateralis, a lateral flexor, arises on both sides from the lateral aspect of the sacral spines and the transverse processes of the upper coccygeal vertebrae, and is inserted into the lateral aspects of the coccygeal vertebrae. The intertransversalis caudae muscles are intrinsic muscles of the tail and lie in the intervals between the coccygeal transverse processes, to which they are attached. The number of coccygeal nerves varies across species, but the dorsal and ventral primary rami unite on each side to form dorsal and ventral trunks that run the full length of the tail and supply the sacrococcygeus and intrinsic tail muscles.

The rudimentary dorsal and ventral sacrococcygeal muscles in the human are probably equivalent to the well-developed muscles of the same name in tailed mammals.

REFERENCES

1. Dalley AF II. The riddle of the sphincters: the morphophysiology of the anorectal mechanism reviewed. Am Surg 1987;53:298-306.
2. Milligan ETC, Morgan CN. Surgical anatomy of the anal canal. Lancet 1934;11:1150–1156.
3. Williams PL (ed). Gray's Anatomy. Edinburgh, UK: Churchill Livingstone, 1995.
4. Golligher JC, Leacock AG, Brossy JJ. The surgical anatomy of the anal canal. Br J Surg 1955;43: 51–61.
5. Ayoub SF. Anatomy of the external anal sphincter in man. Acta Anat 1979;105:25–36.
6. Oh C, Kark AE. Anatomy of the external anal sphincter. Br J Surg 1972;59:717–723.
7. Hussain SM, Stoker J, Zwamborn AW, et al. Endoanal MRI of the anal sphincter complex: correlation with cross-sectional anatomy and histology. J Anat 1996;189:677–682.
8. Wendell-Smith CP, Wilson PM. Musculature of the Pelvic Floor. In EE Philipp, J Barnes, M Newton (eds), Scientific Foundations of Obstetrics and Gynaecology (2nd ed). London: Heinemann, 1977; 78–84.
9. Oelrich TM. The striated urogenital sphincter muscle in the female. Anat Rec 1983;205:223–232.
10. Onufrowicz B. Notes on the arrangement and function of the cell groups in the sacral region of the spinal cord. J Nerv Ment Dis 1889;26:498–504.
11. Onufrowicz B. On the arrangement and function of the cell groups in the sacral region of the sacral spinal cord in man. Arch Neurol Psychopathol 1890;3:387–411.
12. Holstege G, Tan J. Supraspinal control of motoneurons innervating the striatal muscles of the pelvic floor including urethral and anal sphincters in the cat. Brain 1987;110:1323–1344.
13. Schroder HD. Onuf's nucleus X: a morphological study of a human spinal nucleus. Anat Embryol 1981;162:443–453.
14. Pullen AH, Tucker D, Martin JE. Morphological and morphometric characterization of Onuf's nucleus in the spinal cord in man. J Anat 1997;191:201–213.
15. Breedlove SM, Arnold AP. Sexually dimorphic motor nucleus in the rat lumbar spinal cord: response to adult hormone manipulation, absence in androgen insensitive rats. Brain Res 1981;225:297–307.
16. Forger N, Breedlove S. Sexual dimorphism in human and canine spinal cord: role of early androgen. Proc Natl Acad Sci U S A 1986;83:7527–7531.
17. Iwata M, Hirano A. Sparing of the Onufrowicz nucleus in sacral anterior horn lesions. Ann Neurol 1978;4:245–249.
18. Mannen T, Iwata M, Toyokura Y, Nagashima K. Preservation of a certain motoneurone group of the sacral cord in amyotrophic lateral sclerosis: its clinical significance. J Neurol Neurosurg Psychiatry 1982;40:464–469.
19. Toyokura Y. Amyotrophic lateral sclerosis: a clinical and pathological study of the "negative features" of the disease. Jpn J Med 1977;16:269–273.
20. Pullen AH, Martin JE, Swash M. Ultrastructure of pre-synaptic input to motor neurons in Onuf's nucleus: controls and motor neuron disease. J Neurol Neurosurg Psychiatry 1992;18:213–231.
21. Sung JH, Mastri AE, Segal E. Pathology of Shy-Drager syndrome. J Neuropathol Exp Neurol 1979;38:353–368.
22. Konno H, Yamamoto T, Iwashi Y, Iizuku H. Shy-Drager syndrome and amyotrophic lateral sclerosis: cytoarchitectonic and morphometric studies of sacral autonomic neurones. J Neurol Sci 1986;73:193–204.
23. Chalmers D, Swash M. Selective vulnerability of urinary Onuf motoneurons in Shy-Drager syndrome. J Neurol 1987;234:259–260.
24. Jackson H, Burke JT. The sacral foramina. Skeletal Radiol 1984;1:282–288.
25. Liguoro D, Viejo-Fuertes D, Midy D, Guerin J. An anatomical study of the posterior sacral foramina. J Anat 1999; in press.
26. Sisson S, Grossman JD. The Anatomy of Domestic Animals (4th ed). Philadelphia: Saunders, 1975.

27. Schroder HD. Organization of the motoneurons innervating pelvic muscles of the male rat. J Comp Neurol 1980;192:567–587.
28. Sato M, Mizuno M, Konishi I. A localization of motoneurons innervating perineal muscles: a HRP study in cat. Brain Res 1978;140:149–154.
29. Roppolo JR, Nadelhaft I, DeGroat WC. The organization of pudendal motoneurons and primary afferent projections in the spinal cord of the rhesus monkey revealed by horseradish peroxidase. J Comp Neurol 1985;243:475–488.

3
Neurophysiology of the Bladder and Bowel

Michael D. Craggs and Carolynne Jane Vaizey

Micturition, defecation, and maintenance of continence are daily functions that develop into socially acceptable behaviors during early childhood, so that bowel and bladder emptying can be voluntarily postponed until circumstances are appropriate. Mature toilet behavior requires the closest possible integration between the autonomic and somatic nervous systems at both the conscious and subconscious levels of neural control. When pathways in these systems are disrupted, as in traumatic injury or neurologic disease, storage and voiding functions may be so seriously compromised that the ability to postpone or initiate voiding is lost. Invariably, the result is incontinence of urine or feces, and sometimes of both.

BOWEL

Constipation is often found in neurologic disease, and to some extent this protects against incontinence even in the presence of a poorly functioning sphincter muscle. Severe constipation, however, can lead to impaction and to overflow incontinence, a problem in which only liquid can seep past a bolus of fecal material that is blocking all normal passage of stool. Poor emptying may be a factor leading to constipation in neurologic disease, but more important may be the disruption of normal gut transit secondary to autonomic dysfunction, which can be exacerbated by certain drug therapies.

Fecal incontinence may be multifactorial. The external anal sphincter is a striated muscle that is weakened by any disease process affecting the somatic sacral nerves. The internal anal sphincter is a smooth muscle that may be rendered "unstable" and may exhibit abnormal spontaneous relaxations after lesions of the autonomic nerves in the region of the pelvic-hypogastric plexus. Deficient sensory innervation of the anorectum affects the ability to distinguish solid from liquid stool or gas and the storage capabilities of the rectum.

BLADDER

Retention of urine is sometimes found in neurologic disease, but intermittent obstruction to the passage of urine during voiding is more common. This obstruction is attributable to dyssynergic function of the urethral sphincters, particularly the rhabdosphincter muscle. Incontinence, on the other hand, usually results from uninhibited reflex contractions of the detrusor smooth muscle, with incompetent sphincter function also playing a part. Genuine stress incontinence occurs when the sphincters do not reflexively respond to sudden rises in intra-abdominal pressure. The combination of detrusor hyperreflexia and sphincter dyssynergia can lead to dangerously high bladder pressures that, if left untreated, may seriously compromise renal function. Treatment always aims to restore low reservoir pressure and large capacity, usually through the use of drugs, while providing a means of emptying the bladder completely—as, for example, through the use of intermittent catheterization.

NEUROLOGIC LESIONS

Suprasacral lesions in the central nervous system may cause incontinence by interruption of both the descending and ascending pathways that normally modulate pelvic sphincter function and coordinate micturition and defecation. Such lesions (e.g., traumatic spinal cord injury, multiple sclerosis) are conventionally termed *upper motor neuron lesions*. Lumbosacral lesions, on the other hand (e.g., myelodysplasia, cauda equina injury), involve disconnection from the lower motor neurons and can result in loss of reflex control of the bladder, bowel, and sphincters, again leading to serious problems of storage and voiding. Finally, patients with neurologic lesions above the spinal cord (e.g., stroke, Parkinson's disease) can be at risk for developing both bladder and bowel problems.

Through a comprehensive knowledge of the physiologic mechanisms controlling the pelvic organs, we can hope to develop more reliable diagnostic techniques and treatments for managing people with bladder and bowel problems caused by specific neurologic disorders. This chapter reviews that knowledge and puts it in the general context of neurologic disease.

NEUROANATOMIC SPECIALIZATION
OF THE BLADDER AND BOWEL

The bladder and colorectum, together with their respective outlet sphincters, show many similarities in muscular organization and extrinsic nerve supply; however, their functions are very different and depend on neuroanatomic specialization. The colorectum has a well-developed enteric (intrinsic) nervous system that coordinates motility of its smooth muscle, secretion, and absorption and is modulated by extrinsic nerves. The bladder, on the other hand, is controlled almost exclusively by extrinsic nerves, so that contraction of its smooth muscle is a coordinated event for efficient voiding but remains quiescent at all other times.

The intrinsic nerve supply to the colorectum is derived from the myenteric and submucosal plexuses. These plexuses have a complex structural organization and involve the interactions of many different neurotransmitter pathways, including the modulating influences of sympathetic and parasympathetic nerves [1]. The plexuses in the rectum and distal colon are dense and irregular compared to those in the more proximal colon. Sacral parasympathetic innervation of the rectum and distal colon is clearly an important aspect of extrinsic control for defecation.

Outlet function is also very specialized [2]. The anorectum is able to distinguish solid, liquid, and gas by a complex sampling mechanism and to facilitate selective passage of gas when appropriate; urethrovesical muscle function is very well coordinated, so that even the smallest leakage of urine is prevented at socially inconvenient times [3]. Interestingly, evidence exists that retrograde contractions of the rectum may propel stool cephalad from the rectum to the colon for storage after sampling has occurred [4]. Both the bladder and colorectum have important roles as storage organs; however, whereas the entry of feces into the rectum is usually fairly rapid and pulsatile, urine flow into the bladder is a slow and continuous process. Both organs can accommodate relatively large volumes before the need to evacuate. Both have extrinsic parasympathetically innervated smooth muscle walls that contract to cause evacuation, and both have extrinsic sympathetically innervated smooth muscle regions at their outlets to help maintain continence. The parasympathetic system appears to be inhibitory to these muscles.

Unlike the urethra, which does not have a clearly defined internal sphincter, the smooth muscle of the internal anal sphincter has both an intrinsic and extrinsic nerve supply. The intrinsic supply, which comes from the gut wall plexuses, mediates the anorectal inhibitory reflex. The outlets also have external striated sphincters under voluntary control linked functionally to the muscles of the pelvic floor. The urethral wall also possesses a special type of additional intrinsic striated muscle known as the *rhabdosphincter*, which possesses tone and the ability to respond rapidly to rises in intra-abdominal pressures to preserve continence.

The close reciprocal relationship between the smooth muscles of the bladder and rectum and the sphincteric muscles of their outlets is of special interest in the maintenance of continence and voiding. This relationship is also reflected in the similarity of the peripheral lumbosacral innervation to these organs and the way in which the autonomic and somatic motor pathways interact at the spinal and supraspinal levels to coordinate bladder and bowel function.

The bladder detrusor smooth muscle and smooth muscles of the distal rectal wall receive parasympathetic innervation from motor neurons in the intermediolateral part of the S2–S4 sacral segments of the spinal cord via postganglionic neurons originating in ganglia of the pelvic plexus or the viscus wall itself [1]. Interacting at the peripheral ganglia are sympathetic motor fibers of the hypogastric nerve plexus, which have their origin in the lumbar spinal cord between T9 and L2 and synapse first in the prevertebral ganglia [5].

Electrical stimulation of the parasympathetic nerves at the sacral anterior root level contracts both bladder and rectal smooth muscle, giving reliable emptying of the bladder and bowel [6]. Postganglionic parasympathetic motor pathways in humans are almost exclusively cholinergic; for example, detrusor muscle contraction caused by electrical stimulation is completely abolished by low doses of anticholinergic drugs [7]. Putative noncholinergic nonadrenergic parasympathetic pathways found in many animals—for example, those involving purinergic neurotransmission [1]—may also exist in humans, but probably only in the presence of specific pathologies of the bladder [8].

The modulatory effects of extrinsic sympathetic nerve activity (via α-adreno-ceptors) on the parasympathetic pathway at the ganglia are said to be mainly inhibitory to the detrusor and large bowel [9] but excitatory to the bladder neck [10] and smooth muscle of the anal canal [11]. In humans, little is known about either direct sympathetic β-adrenergic effects on smooth muscle function of the bladder and rectum, but beta receptors have been found in both organs, and they are said to be relaxant [12].

Smooth muscles of the bladder neck, urethra, and internal anal sphincter are innervated by excitatory sympathetic α-adrenergic and β-adrenergic inhibitory nerves. A number of other neurotransmitters, including nitric oxide, have been implicated in the modulation of both urethral and anal smooth muscle [10, 11], but little is known about their importance for intrinsic anorectal reflex function. Analogous urethrovesical reflexes have not been demonstrated in humans, but evidence exists that nitric oxide may play a role in relaxing the detrusor at the level of the bladder neck [3].

The striated urethral and anal sphincter muscles receive their innervation via the somatic pelvic and pudendal nerves, respectively, from motor neurons in Onuf's nucleus, a specialized group of anterior horn cells spanning the second and third sacral spinal segments. Unlike the anal canal, the urethral wall also contains a peculiar but predominantly slow-twitch striated muscle sphincter (rhabdosphinc-ter), which is innervated by small motor neurons in Onuf's nucleus and closely related to the intermediolateral motor neurons of the parasympathetic pathway. This close anatomic relationship may be of significance for somaticovisceral functional integration. The rhabdosphincter is said to have no muscle spindles and is therefore quite distinct from other striated muscles of the pelvic floor, but the presence of spindles in the external anal sphincter is uncertain [13, 14].

The other pelvic floor muscles are innervated by either pelvic or pudendal branches of the sacral anterior roots. Of these muscles, the levator ani group comprises a mixture of slow-twitch and fast-twitch fibers that functionally provide sustained tone and phasic antistress contractions, respectively, to give periurethral and perianal occlusion.

Pelvic visceral nerves are the main sensory pathways from the bladder and rectum, but some sensory information is also conveyed in the sympathetic hypogastric nerves to the thoracolumbar spinal cord, especially from the colorectum, bladder, and proximal urethra [15]. Sensory information from the distal urethra, anal canal, and perineum is carried almost exclusively by the pudendal nerves.

Normal micturition or defecation is initiated voluntarily at an appropriate and socially convenient time when this sensory information signals fullness in the bladder or rectum. Although the sensations of fullness are sometimes difficult to suppress, both micturition and defecation can be suspended for some length of time and continence controlled even when the bladder and rectum are very full. The mechanisms of control in humans are likely to be a balance of modulatory mechanisms at many levels in the neuraxis from brain to pelvic floor (Figure 3.1).

Many of these mechanisms take place automatically at the subconscious level, but when micturition or defecation becomes urgent, more direct corticospinal pathways mediate voluntary control over the striated sphincter muscles to enhance urethral or anal closure and prevent leaking. Lesions in any of these cen-

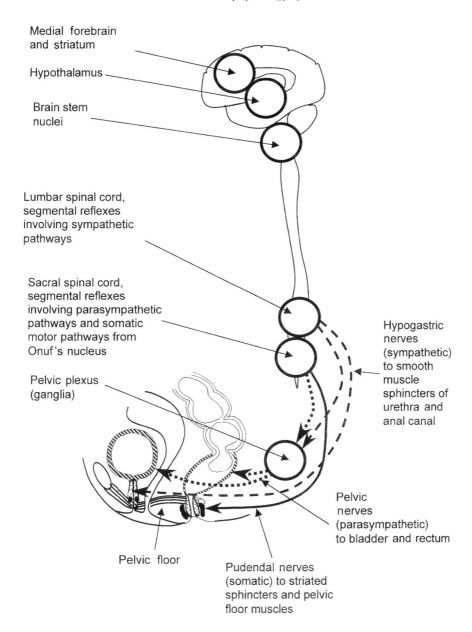

Medial forebrain and striatum

Hypothalamus

Brain stem nuclei

Lumbar spinal cord, segmental reflexes involving sympathetic pathways

Sacral spinal cord, segmental reflexes involving parasympathetic pathways and somatic motor pathways from Onuf's nucleus

Pelvic plexus (ganglia)

Hypogastric nerves (sympathetic) to smooth muscle sphincters of urethra and anal canal

Pelvic nerves (parasympathetic) to bladder and rectum

Pelvic floor

Pudendal nerves (somatic) to striated sphincters and pelvic floor muscles

Figure 3.1   Principal neuroanatomic sites (*circled*) concerned with the modulation of bladder, bowel, and sphincter function.

tral nervous pathways are likely to cause disturbance in the normal control of micturition or defecation, or sometimes both, in the case of traumatic spinal injury or lesions of the frontal lobes in the brain [16].

CONTROL OF URINARY CONTINENCE AND VOIDING

Coordinated function of the urinary bladder and its sphincters depends on the complete integrity of central and peripheral nervous pathways in a complex neural control system located in the brain and spinal cord. This control system is believed to act like a switching circuit to maintain a reciprocal relationship between the reservoir function of the bladder and sphincteric outlet function in the urethra [17]. As the bladder slowly fills, any tendency for spontaneous reflex contractions of the detrusor smooth muscle in the bladder wall are inhibited, while urethral smooth and striated muscle sphincters are contracted to prevent leakage. Voiding requires a complete relaxation of the sphincters and the reciprocal action of a powerful but sustained detrusor contraction so that urine is expelled quickly and efficiently from the bladder. This synergistic relationship between the muscles of the bladder wall and the urethra is essential for maintaining continence on the one hand and unobstructed voiding on the other. Damage or disease in any of the nervous pathways controlling the lower urinary tract can cause serious disruption to this relationship, leading to uncoordinated somaticovisceral reflexes, impairment of normal vesicourethral function, voiding dysfunction, and incontinence [18].

Normal voiding is preceded by sphincter relaxation and detrusor smooth muscle contraction mediated through the "sacral micturition center" via parasympathetic pathways. Actual voiding begins when the bladder pressure rises sufficiently to exceed the residual urethral pressure (micturition threshold). These initial actions rely essentially on the integrity of the brain stem pathways—in particular, those traversing and connecting with the pontine nuclei. Complete emptying of the bladder depends on consistent sphincter relaxation and a sustainable detrusor contraction driven reflexively by pelvic afferent activity from the bladder wall. After micturition, activity from these same afferents is then probably switched back to facilitate bladder inhibition via lumbar sympathetic pathways as the bladder begins to refill [19] and store urine again.

During normal bladder filling, high wall compliance helps to keep intravesical pressure low (<10 cm H_2O), and reflex inhibition of the detrusor muscle probably is not needed until the bladder is quite full. When the first sensations of the urge to void are reached (often at a functional bladder volume of approximately 300 ml), then reflex control of detrusor contractions invokes various supraspinal, spinal, and peripheral modulatory mechanisms to suppress unwanted bladder contractions while maintaining a closed urethra (Figure 3.2).

Our knowledge of supraspinal mechanisms in humans is sparse and, until recently, has derived mainly from observations in patients undergoing cranial surgery for a variety of neurologic disorders [20] or those with stroke [21]. Much of our understanding of the role that different brain structures play in the control of urinary continence and voiding has been extrapolated from animal experiments. For example, specific areas in the brain stem and the diencephalon of the cat, including the dorsomedial pontine tegmentum, periaqueductal gray substance, and

STORAGE PHASE   VOIDING PHASE

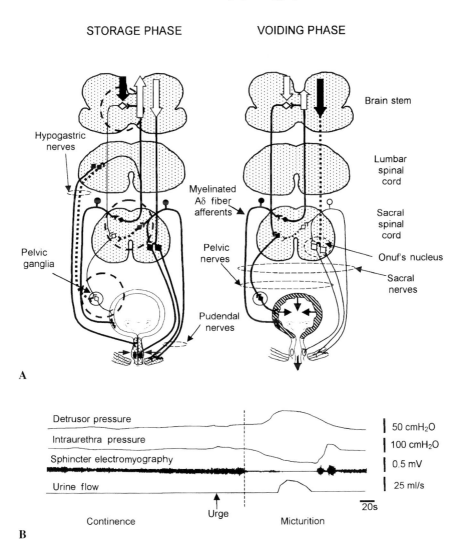

Figure 3.2 (**A**) Neural control of the bladder and its sphincters during the storage and voiding of urine. Large arrows at the brain stem level represent inhibitory (*black arrows*) and excitatory (*white arrows*) effects that involve more rostral brain structures. The principal sites for these inhibitory effects are shown in the dashed ovals. The dotted pathways represent inhibitory pathways. (**B**) Example of normal urodynamic measurements recorded with bladder and urethral pressure catheters and sphincter electromyographic electrodes shows that an appropriate and reciprocal relationship exists between the bladder and sphincter activity during both the storage and voiding phases of the micturition cycle.

preoptic area of the hypothalamus, are known to be closely involved in the control of micturition. Important among the mechanisms revealed in animal experiments has been the cerebral control of the micturition reflex (spino-bulbo-spinal or SBS reflex) itself, a reflex involving afferents from the bladder impinging on the periaqueductal gray substance, which in turn projects to the pontine nuclei of the brain stem [22]. These nuclei then give rise to descending excitatory and inhibitory pathways that influence the excitability of lumbosacral segmental reflexes to coordinate bladder and sphincter function [23]. Modern imaging techniques, such as positron emission tomography of the brain, show that some important parallels exist between the roles of these structures in animals and in humans [24].

At the lumbosacral spinal level, converging somaticovisceral reflexes involving pudendal (somatic) to hypogastric (sympathetic) and pudendal to pelvic (parasympathetic) pathways [19] probably play a significant part in local control of the lower urinary tract. Reflexes mediated via the hypogastric nerves begin to operate at low bladder pressures (<5 cm H_2O), whereas pudendal-pelvic interaction is believed to be more important for detrusor inhibition at higher pressures (>15 cm H_2O) during the storage of urine.

In the dorsal horn of the sacral spinal cord, bladder afferent activity may be inhibited through interneurons activated by somatic sensory pathways originating in the external genitalia, perineum, and some muscles of the pelvic floor via the pudendal nerves. This inhibitory interaction between larger somatic sensory fibers and small bladder afferents (Aδ or unmyelinated C fibers) could operate in a way similar to that hypothesized in the "gate control" theory of pain [25]. However, whereas small myelinated Aδ fibers from the bladder wall sense bladder filling by mechanoreceptors, the C fibers in healthy individuals are probably "silent" for most of the time, responding only to the presence of noxious stimuli in the bladder. Although the Aδ fibers may have a role in local segmental reflexes, in the normal adult animal, their main projection is probably to brain stem sites [19], especially the periaqueductal gray substance [26]. Both types of sensory activity can be modulated at the sacral segmental level by descending pathways; this modulation includes inhibitory effects on C fiber activity via enkephalin and serotonergic pathways originating in the brain stem, and facilitatory effects on the Aδ mediated pelvic reflex by noradrenergic pathways from Barrington's nucleus [27]. It is this nucleus, near the locus coeruleus in the pontine region of the brain stem, that is of major importance in the normal micturition reflex.

The firing of detrusor preganglionic parasympathetic motor neurons in the intermediolateral parts of the sacral cord may be directly inhibited by both somatic efferent and nonspecific afferent pathways controlling the striated sphincters during the continence phase. These sphincters are innervated by specialized anterior horn motor neurons in Onuf's nucleus. Interestingly, local recurrent inhibition may help to modulate the frequency and duration of efferent discharge in the detrusor motor neurons [28], but the sphincter motor neurons of Onuf's nucleus do not appear to have such inhibition.

Some controversy exists as to whether the sympathetic system has an important effect on the activity of the human bladder. An argument against such an effect is based on the minimal effects of adrenergic-stimulating drugs during filling in the healthy human bladder. However, little doubt exists that, in animals, transmission of impulses to the postganglionic parasympathetic nerves is controllable at the level of the autonomic ganglia in or near the bladder by sympathetic nerves [29, 30]. Hypogastric nerve stimulation profoundly inhibits neurotransmission at these ganglia through α-adrenergic mechanisms acting perhaps through small intermediary cells on both the preganglionic and postganglionic parasympathetic pathway. In the cat, this mechanism can be elicited reflexively by pudendal stimulation to give prolonged bladder relaxation [31]. Another pathway that appears to depress detrusor activity in animals by actions both centrally and at the level of the pelvic ganglia involves the neurotransmitters γ-aminobutyric acid and leu-enkephalin [32], but what role such a pathway would play in normal micturition and whether it would be reflexively active to pudendal stimulation is unclear.

At a terminal level of sympathetic modulation of bladder activity, β_3-adrenergic relaxant effects on both normal and neurogenic human detrusor smooth muscle strips have been demonstrated [33], but little evidence is found to suggest that such inhibitory mechanisms are important in either normal or pathologic bladders.

CONTROL OF FECAL CONTINENCE AND DEFECATION

The maintenance of fecal continence is a product of stool consistency, colorectal activity, and the synchronous relationship between the external and internal anal sphincters [34]. The internal sphincter maintains a constant tone and prevents stool leakage during everyday activities. The external sphincter acts as an "emergency brake," being used maximally when there is a feeling of impending defecation, thus allowing time to organize a suitable situation for defecation.

The internal sphincter is a smooth muscle that is maintained at near maximal contraction and is modulated by a balance of α-adrenergic and β-adrenergic effects via the hypogastric nerves. A common response associated with the internal anal sphincter is the rectoanal inhibitory reflex. This effect is a locally mediated response to distension of the rectum that results in relaxation of the internal sphincter and a reduction of the resting pressure. As the internal anal sphincter is a continuation of the circular muscle of the gut, this response can be equated with the relaxation that occurs in the segment of gut immediately distal to a distended portion [35]. The function of this seemingly "antisocial" reflex is to allow rectal contents to come into contact with the mucosa of the upper anal canal so that solid, liquid, and gas can be distinguished. Maintenance of continence at this time is dependent on contraction of the external sphincter. In contrast to the internal sphincter muscle, the external sphincter is a striated muscle under voluntary control. It has a predominance of type I (slow) fibers, but the tonic contraction of the external sphincter is not at a level of maximum contraction, and its major activity is a contraction response. This response can be both voluntary and involuntary. Maximum contraction can only be sustained for periods of approximately 60 seconds, which is usually long enough for the peristaltic contractions of the rectum, and the associated urge to defecate, to pass. Coordinated reflexes of the external sphincter are dependent on perianal cutaneous sensation transmitted by afferent fibers in the inferior hemorrhoidal nerves.

The longitudinal smooth muscle is a direct continuation of the outer or longitudinal muscle coat of the rectum, which runs outside the internal sphincter. The anal canal is therefore surrounded by two layers of smooth muscle, which appear to be physiologically distinct. Little agreement is found as to the anatomy of the longitudinal muscle, and especially its medial, lateral, and inferior extensions [36]. The intricate association of this structure with the external and internal sphincters suggests an essential role in the sphincter mechanism, and opinion so far has favored a possible role in defecation and minimal involvement in the maintenance of continence.

Both rectal and colonic factors are important in the maintenance of continence. Increased bowel frequency and loose bowel actions are found in patients with fecal incontinence [37]; widespread gut dysfunction is demonstrated in some patients [4].

A combination of propulsive contractions and removal of the barriers maintaining continence is necessary for the efficient passage of stool from the colorectum through the anal canal. Most commonly, the colon is emptied from descending colon to rectum, but the proportion of colon emptied can be very variable [38]. Propulsive contractions passing along the colon have been shown to create pressures of up to 500 cm H_2O within the colon [4]. The anorectal angle is straightened by adoption of the squatting position and by inhibition of tonic puborectalis contraction to allow descent of the pelvic floor. As stool enters the rectum, the rectoanal inhibitory reflex is triggered and the internal anal sphincter relaxes. Usually, a voluntary relaxation of the external sphincter occurs, and when the rectal pressure exceeds that of the anal canal, then actual defecation begins and the expulsion of stool commences (Figure 3.3). The exact role of rectal motor activity remains unquantified.

Defecation is an organized sequence of responses that can occur in patients with paraplegia because it is organized in the lumbosacral spinal cord largely independently of input from the brain. However, a major voluntary input from the brain takes place in normal subjects. When the urge to defecate is experienced, a decision follows as to whether to respond to this urge immediately or to defer the activity to a more appropriate time. Voluntary contraction of the external sphincter muscle holds back the stool until rectal relaxation has occurred and the urge passes. A combination of external sphincter contraction and retrograde contractile movements propel the stool cephalad [4], and this action is combined with an overall slowing of colonic transit. The feeling of urgency and rectal filling may occur independently, and the sensation may be experienced in the lower abdomen or in the perineum. When convenient, defecation can be initiated by the performance of Valsalva's maneuver, with contraction of the abdominal muscles and splinting of the diaphragm. This maneuver raises intra-abdominal pressure and may cause movement of the stool, triggering contractions in the sigmoid colon and proximal rectum.

The perception of stool in the rectum may be based partly on sensation transmitted from the rectal wall; however, it must also have an extrinsic element, because it is maintained after removal of the rectum, such as in patients who have undergone a restorative proctocolectomy or "pouch" operation, in which the rectum is removed and a neorectum is created from the terminal ileum. First sensations of rectal filling occur at low volumes of approximately 45 ml, and the feeling of urgency to defecate occurs from a volume of approximately 90 ml; the maximum tolerated rectal volumes are around 200 ml [39].

Although we have developing knowledge of the neural control of the urinary bladder and its sphincters (see Figure 3.2), less is known about the precise role of spinal reflex mechanisms and central modulatory effects on bowel function. Similarities are likely to exist, however. Whereas the enteric nervous system plays the major role in coordinating anorectal function, the extrinsic autonomic influences of the sacral parasympathetic pathway through the pelvic nerves and lumbar sympathetic pathways via the inferior mesenteric plexus and hypogastric nerves, together with their central connections via the brain stem, do play an important part in the modulation of these intrinsic effects in the normal bowel. Direct sympathetic stimulation decreases contractility and motility of the colorectum and constriction of the internal anal sphincter, whereas parasympathetic stimulation has the opposite effects.

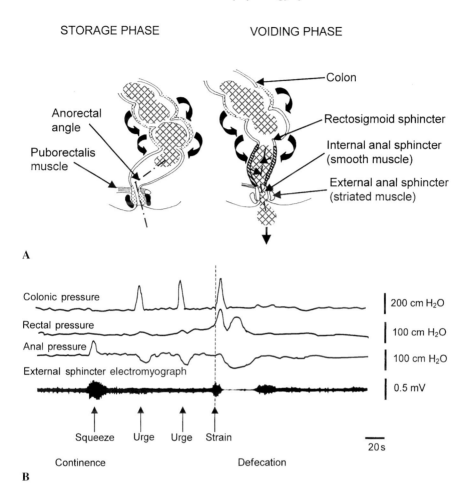

Figure 3.3 (**A**) Control of the anorectum during continence and defecation. Fecal matter does not normally pass beyond the rectosigmoid sphincter until the act of defecation begins. Until then, continence is maintained by a combination of the acute anorectal angle caused by puborectalis contraction, internal anal sphincter tone, and voluntary squeezes of the external anal sphincter to suppress the sensations of urge. Accumulation of stool in the rectum stretches the rectal wall, which causes local reflex relaxation of the internal anal sphincter, allowing feces to enter the anal canal. Sampling of the canal contents and sensation then determines the need to adopt a defecating posture, relax the puborectalis sling to make the anorectal angle obtuse, and strain abdominally to assist the passage of feces out of the anal canal. Reflex contraction of the rectum under sacral parasympathetic control assists in this evacuation process. Defecation can be terminated voluntarily by further contractions of the external anal sphincter. (**B**) Anorectal dynamics. Study of the various pressures in the colon, rectum, and anal canal, together with sphincter electromyography, shows the normal sequence of physiologic events associated with the maintenance of continence through to successful defecation.

CONCLUSIONS

The lower urinary tract, comprising the bladder, urethra, and associated sphincters, has only two functions in humans: to store urine and to eliminate it from the body at socially convenient times. By contrast, the bowel, comprising the colon, rectum, and anal canal with its sphincters, has a more sophisticated role, depending on the consistency of its contents. Like micturition, however, defecation (of feces or wind) also must be performed consistent with socially acceptable behavior. Normal functions of the bladder and bowel depend on the total integrity of the nervous system, from pelvic floor to brain. Many different neurotransmitter pathways are involved, modulating proper voluntary control over the reciprocal relationship between the storage function of these organs and their outlet sphincters. When voluntary control is lost or disrupted through neurologic disease or damage, then aberrant reflexes can take over; the result can be uncoordinated function of the bladder and bowel, causing a mixture of symptoms including incontinence, constipation, and voiding dysfunction (Figure 3.4) [40–42]. Through our increasing knowledge of the physiology of some of the normal mechanisms in the nervous system controlling the bladder, bowel, and sphincters of the pelvic floor, we are now

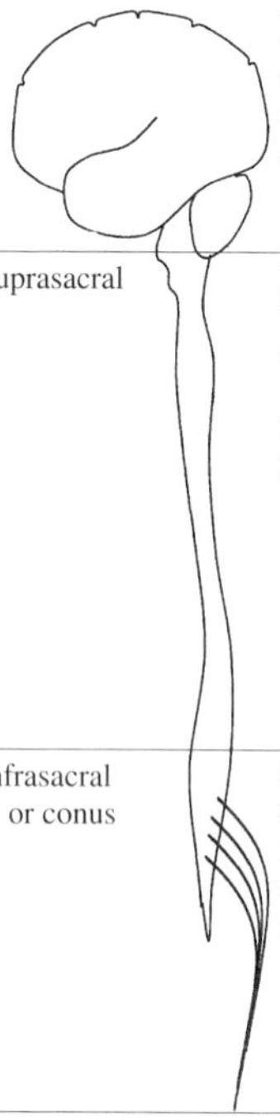

Level of lesion	Neurologic disease	Bladder dysfunction	Bowel dysfunction
Suprapontine	Dementia Parkinson's disease Cerebral vascular accident Cerebral tumor Cerebral palsy Shy-Drager syndrome	Inappropriate toilet behavior Detrusor hyper-reflexia with coordinated external sphincter and bladder neck activity Incontinence	Inappropriate toilet behavior Incontinence Fecal impaction following immobility
Suprasacral	Multiple sclerosis Traumatic injury Compression (e.g., tumors, cervical spondylosis) Myelitis Spina bifida	Hyperreflexic with uncoordinated external sphincter and uncoordinated bladder neck if above T6 Sensory impairment Incontinence	High cord lesions—colonic mobility reduced and delayed colonic transit Low cord lesions—colonic mobility increased, reduced compliance, instability in rectum Loss of voluntary control over sphincters, pelvic floor, and abdominal muscles Rectal prolapse Mixed incontinence
Infrasacral or conus	Sacral agenesis Cauda equina disease Pelvic surgery Childbirth injury Diabetes mellitus	Areflexic/underactive with denervated/underactive external sphincter but coordinated bladder neck Sensory impairment Incontinence	Weakness or loss of pelvic floor and sphincter muscle, voluntary control, and spinal reflexes Rectal prolapse Impaired pelvic sensation Areflexic rectum Mixed incontinence

Figure 3.4   Pathophysiology of bladder and bowel function associated with neurologic disease at different neuroanatomic sites.

developing new strategies for making clearer diagnoses and improving treatments and management of patients with a wide range of neurologic disease.

REFERENCES

1. Burnstock G. Innervation of Bladder and Bowel. In G Block, J Whelan (eds), Neurobiology of Incontinence. Chichester, UK: Wiley, 1990;2–26. Ciba Foundation Symposium 151.
2. Mathers S. Neural Control of the Pelvic Sphincters. In MM Henry, M Swash (eds), Coloproctology and the Pelvic Floor. Oxford, UK: Butterworth–Heinemann, 1992;61–71.
3. Mundy AR, Thomas PJ. Clinical Physiology of the Bladder, Urethra and Pelvic Floor. In AR Mundy, TP Stephenson, AJ Wein (eds). Urodynamics—Principles, Practice and Application. Edinburgh, UK: Churchill Livingstone, 1994;15–27.
4. Herbst F, Kamm MA, Morris GP, et al. Gastro-intestinal transit and prolonged ambulatory colonic motility in health and faecal incontinence. Gut 1997;42:381–389
5. De Groat WC. Central Nervous System Control of Micturition. In P O'Donnell (ed). Urinary Incontinence. St Louis: Mosby, 1997;33–47.
6. Brindley GS, Rushton DN. Long-term follow-up of patients with sacral anterior root stimulator implants. Paraplegia 1990;28:469–475.
7. Craggs MD, Rushton DN, Stephenson JD. A putative non-cholinergic mechanism in urinary bladders of new but not old world primates. J Urol 1986;136:1348–1350.
8. Ruggieri MR, Whitmore KE, Levin RM. Bladder purinergic receptors. J Urol 1990;144:176–181.
9. De Groat WC, Nadelhaft I, Milne RJ, et al. Organisation of the sacral parasympathetic reflex pathways to the urinary bladder and large intestine. J Auton Nerv Syst 1981;3:135–160.
10. Levin RM, Wein AJ, Longhurst PA. Neuropharmacology of the Lower Urinary Tract. In AR Mundy, TP Stephenson, AJ Wein (eds), Urodynamics—Principles, Practice and Application. Edinburgh, UK: Churchill Livingstone, 1994;29–42.
11. Burleigh DE. Pharmacology of the Internal Anal Sphincter. In MM Henry, M Swash (eds), Coloproctology and the Pelvic Floor. Oxford, UK: Butterworth–Heinemann, 1992;37–53.
12. Igawa Y, Yamazaki Y, Takeda H, et al. The role of β_3-adrenoceptors in normal and neurogenic detrusors. Neurourol Urodyn 1997;16:363–365.
13. Gould RP. Sensory innervation of the anal canal. Nature 1960;187:337–338.
14. Schröder HD, Reske-Nielsen E. Fiber S types in the striated urethral and anal sphincters. Acta Neuropathol (Berl) 1983;60:278–282.
15. Jänig W, Morrison JFB. Functional Properties of Spinal Visceral Afferents Supplying Abdominal and Pelvic Organs with Special Emphasis on Visceral Nociception. In F Cervero, JFB Morrison (eds), Visceral Sensation. Amsterdam, the Netherlands: Elsevier, 1986;87–114. Progress in Brain Research; vol 69.
16. Andrew J, Nathan PW. Lesions of the frontal lobes and disturbances of micturition and defaecation. Brain 1964;87:233–262.
17. De Groat WC, Booth AM, Yoshimura N. Neurophysiology of Micturition and Its Modification in Animal Models of Human Disease. In CA Maggi (ed), Nervous Control of the Urogenital System. London: Harwood, 1993. The Autonomic Nervous System; vol 3.
18. Blaivas JG, Chancellor MB. Classification of Neurogenic Bladder Disease. In MB Chancellor, JG Blaivas (eds), Practical Neurourology—Genitourinary Complications in Neurologic Disease. Boston: Butterworth–Heinemann,1995;25–32.
19. De Groat WC. Central Neural Control of the Lower Urinary Tract. In G Block, J Whelan (eds), Neurobiology of Incontinence. Chichester, UK: Wiley, 1990;27–56. Ciba Foundation Symposium 151.
20. Nathan PW. The Central Nervous Connections of the Bladder. In DI Williams, GD Chisholm (eds), Scientific Foundations of Urology (Vol 2). St Louis: Mosby, 1976;51–58.
21. Burney TL, Senapati M, Desai S, et al. Effects of cerebrovascular accident on micturition. Urol Clin North Am 1996;23:483–490.
22. Blok BFM, Holstege G. Ultrastructural evidence for a paucity of projections from the lumbosacral cord to the pontine micturition center or M-region in the cat: a new concept for the organization of the micturition reflex with the periaqueductal gray as central relay. J Comp Neurol 1995;359:300–309.
23. Morrison JB. Bladder Control: Role of Higher Levels of the Central Nervous System. In M Torrens, JB Morrison (eds), Physiology of the Lower Urinary Tract. London: Springer, 1987;237–274.
24. Blok BFM, Willemsen ATM, Holstege G. A PET study on brain control of micturition in humans. Brain 1997;120:111–121.

25. Melzack R, Wall P. Pain mechanisms: a new theory. Science 1965;150:971–979.
26. Noto H, Roppolo JR, Steers WD, de Groat WC. Electrophysiological analysis of the ascending and descending components of the micturition reflex pathway in the rat. Brain Res 1991;549:95–105.
27. Barrington FJF. The effect of lesions of the hind and midbrain on micturition in the cat. Q J Exp Physiol 1925;15:181–202.
28. De Groat WC, Ryall RW. Recurrent inhibition in sacral parasympathetic pathways to the bladder. J Physiol 1968;196:579–591.
29. De Groat WC, Saum W. Sympathetic inhibition of the urinary bladder and of pelvic ganglionic transmission in the cat. J Physiol 1972;214:297–314.
30. Vaughan CW, Satchell PM. Urine storage mechanisms. Prog Neurobiol 1995;46:215–237.
31. Lindström S, Fall M, Carlsson CA, Erlandson BE. The neurophysiological basis of bladder inhibition in response to intravaginal electrical stimulation. J Urol 1983;129:405–410.
32. Simmonds WF, Booth AM, Thor KB, et al. Parasympathetic ganglia: naloxone antagonises inhibition by leucine-enkephalin and GABA. Brain Res 1983;271:365–370.
33. Igawa Y, Yamazaki Y, Takeda H, et al. The role of β_3-adrenoceptors in normal and neurogenic detrusors. Neurourol Urodyn 1997;16:363–365.
34. Engel AF, Kamm MA, Bartram CI, Nicholls RJ. Relationship of symptoms in faecal incontinence to specific sphincter abnormalities. Int J Colorectal Dis 1995;10:152–155.
35. Dalley AF. The riddle of the sphincters: the morphophysiology of the anorectal mechanism reviewed. Am Surg 1987;53:298–306.
36. Lunniss PJ, Phillips RKS. Anatomy and function of the anal longitudinal muscle. Br J Surg 1992;79:882–884.
37. Talley NJ, O'Keefe EA, Zinsmeister AR, Melton LJ. Prevalence of gastrointestinal symptoms in the elderly: a population based study. Gastroenterology 1992;102:895–901.
38. Lubowski DZ, Nicholls RJ, Swash M, Jordan MJ. Neural control of internal sphincter function. Br J Surg 1987;74:668–670.
39. Jameson JS, Chia YW, Kamm MA. Effect of age, sex and parity on anorectal function. Br J Surg 1994;81:1689–1692.
40. Swash M, Henry MM. Neurological Disease and Coloproctology. In MM Henry, M Swash (eds), Coloproctology and the Pelvic Floor. Oxford, UK: Butterworth–Heinemann, 1992;455–458.
41. Norris JP, Staskin DR. History, physical examination, and classification of neurogenic voiding dysfunction. Urol Clin North Am 1996;23:337–343.
42. Longo WF, Ballantyne GH, Modlin IM. The colon, anorectum, and spinal cord patient. Dis Colon Rectum 1989;32:261–267.

4
Physiology of Female Sexual Function and Effect of Neurologic Disease

Per Olov Lundberg

PHYSIOLOGY OF FEMALE SEXUAL FUNCTION IN HEALTH

Sexual Response Phases

Based on observations in a laboratory setting, Masters and Johnson [1] constructed a model of the sexual response cycle comprising four different phases: excitement, plateau, orgasm, and resolution (EPOR). The EPOR model achieved wide publicity and is used in most textbooks about sexual physiology [2]. However, the observations of Masters and Johnson, although pioneering, were not well controlled or quantified, and their four-phase model has been criticized. According to their model, sexual desire is not a phase. Kaplan [3] simplified the sexual response model into three phases: desire, excitement, and orgasm. Most therapists find this model very helpful in their work with patients.

Role of the Brain in Sexual Desire and Sexual Reactions

The full role of the human brain in regulating sexual functions is poorly understood, but four areas are known to be of particular importance.

1. The hypothalamus is the part of the human brain that directly controls the gonadotrophic functions of the pituitary. Hypothalamic activity determines both prenatal development of the genital organs, pubertal development, and the menstrual cycle. The basal hypothalamus is known to be a center for sexual desire. In this area, the sex steroid hormones—testosterone, dihydrotestosterone, and estradiol—regulate desire. Destruction of the hypothalamus by a tumor or surgery leads to loss of sexual desire. Animal experiments have shown that a dopaminergic stimulating and serotoninergic inhibiting mechanism within the hypothalamus effects sexual desire. A series of observations on humans supports the existence of a similar mechanism in humans. Sexually dimorphic nuclei are localized in the anterior hypothalamus–preoptic region, but their importance is uncertain.

Patient studies indicate that, among female patients with hypothalamopituitary disorders, two-thirds noticed loss of sexual desire. Women with hyperprolactinemia more commonly complain of this problem than do those with normal serum prolactin levels. Most women with hypothalamopituitary disorders have amenorrhea. Those with normal sexual desire and function are more likely to show normal menstrual pattern, young age, and small tumor size [4]. For further details, see Lundberg [5].

2. The center for sensory input from the genitalia is the primary sensory cortex in the parasagittal region of the brain. This conclusion is based mainly on observations from a limited number of cases of parasagittal tumors.

3. The rhinencephalon, including the limbic cortex, is important for sexual behavior as well as sexual desire. Evidence for this role of the rhinencephalon comes from a large number of clinical observations.

4. Lesions of the frontal lobes, the basal medial part in particular, may lead to loss of social control, which may affect sexual behavior.

Brain Stem and Spinal Cord

Efferent nerve impulses are conveyed from the brain stem through the spinal cord mainly via the periependymal tract. Afferent and efferent nerve pathways connect the spinal cord with the genital region via the sympathetic and parasympathetic nervous system and through the somatic nerves.

A number of observations support the theory that a significant center for orgasm and ejaculation is in the cervical spinal cord. A center of emission and ejaculation is thought to exist at the low thoracic level (spinal cord segments T10–T12). The impulses are conveyed via the sympathetic nervous system. Cerebral (psychogenic) erection, as well as the inhibition of erection in a stressful situation, is also effected through the sympathetic nervous system. A center with parasympathetic nerve outflow is found at the sacral level (S2–S4). The innervation arising at this level regulates reflex erection, lubrication, and changes in blood flow in the genital area. Sensory nerve impulses from the sex organs reach this center through both parasympathetic and somatic nerves.

Onuf's nucleus, which contains the alpha motor neurons that innervate the pelvic floor muscles [6], lies in the sacral spinal cord. These anterior horn cells have special properties that prevent them from degenerating in motor neuron disease [7] or poliomyelitis [8]. This nucleus also contains nerve cells belonging to the parasympathetic nervous system.

Innervation of the Internal Sex Organs

The neurologic control of the internal sex organs in women is less well understood than it is in men. However, from the macroanatomic point of view, female innervation is similar to that of the male. Thus, there is predominantly sympathetic innervation from the hypogastric nerves and hypogastric plexus, mainly parasympathetic innervation from the pelvic nerves and pelvic plexus, and bilateral somatic innervation from the pudendal nerves.

The hypogastric plexus is continuous with the pelvic plexus (sometimes called the inferior hypogastric plexus) situated in the region beneath the cervix of the uterus and the superior part of the vagina and rectum. The pelvic nerves enter this plexus from sacral segments S2–S4 [9]. Within this plexus are many nerve cells, jointly called the *hypogastric ganglion* or *Frankenhäuser's ganglion*, which receive the sensory innervation from the uterus. Extirpation of the pelvic plexus and the ganglion of Frankenhäuser alleviates pain of uterine origin. These nerve structures may be damaged during surgery to the uterus or the rectum.

The vagina is densely innervated by adrenergic nerves [10] that are sympathetic in origin and arise partly from short hypogastric neurons and partly from long sympathetic neurons. The finding of acetylcholinesterase-positive nerves around blood vessels in the vagina provides evidence for the parasympathetic control of vaginal vasodilation secretomotor function. Paracervical ganglia contain reduced nicotinamide-adenine dinucleotide phosphate diaphorase-reactive nerve fibers that appear to play an important role in the regulation of uterine vascular tone by liberating nitric oxide [11].

That stimulation of the vagina and cervix results in a series of physiologic reactions is well known from animal experiments. Mechanical stimulation of the anterior wall of the vagina in women leads to a pronounced increase of the thresholds for pain detection and pain tolerance in the whole body [12]. Mechanical stimulation of this part of the vagina may also result in sexual arousal. Thus, this type of stimulation brings about a hyperalgesia but not a hyperesthesia. Such a hyperalgesia cannot be achieved by stimulation of the posterior wall of the vagina or the clitoris. This analgesic function occurs naturally during labor in women [13]. The anatomic correlates of this physiologic control mechanism are not known; the afferent pathways go through the pelvic nerves in rats [14] but probably also through somatic nerve fibers to S3–S4 above the pelvic floor.

Increased vaginal blood flow, erection of the cavernous tissue both in the clitoris and around the outer part of the vagina, and lubrication are thought to be brought about through neural mechanisms similar to those mediating erection in males, although this has not yet been proved. Sensory receptors are localized at several places in the vaginal walls and its surroundings; the vaginal wall muscles have been demonstrated to contain muscle spindles that are sensitive to changes in the length of the muscle and to the velocity of such changes [15]. Temperature sensitivity in this part of the human body is of particular importance, and probably this quality of sensation makes possible the differentiation between gas, fluid, and solid contents in the rectum. The discriminative quality of touch is less developed within the internal pelvic organs, and discrimination among different sizes and forms of objects inserted into the vagina has been shown to be difficult—a fact that has forensic significance. It is common knowledge that a smooth object, such as the penis, inserted in the vagina gives less discomfort and more sexual arousal than an asymmetrical object, and vaginal dilatation or deep thrusts provide more intense sexual arousal. The mechanisms behind these phenomena are not well studied.

Innervation of the Clitoris

The clitoris is the most densely innervated part of the human body surface. The number of nerve fibers in the dorsal clitoral nerve is twice that in the dorsal penile nerve. The sensory thresholds of the clitoral area are also lower than those of the glans penis. A young woman can feel a vibration amplitude of 0.2–0.4 μm, which is similar to the sensitivity threshold for vibration of the hand of a young person [16], whereas the corresponding figure for the glans penis is significantly higher. The sensitivity threshold increases with normal aging to approximately double the value given here.

The regenerative capacity of the innervation is good, so that a woman who has undergone pharaonic circumcision with extirpation of the clitoris in early childhood may well have a threshold for vibration in this area of 0.4–1.0 μm in adult life (PO Lundberg, B Hulter, unpublished observations).

Our knowledge of the neurophysiology of the clitoris is partly based on observations on the ewe [17]. Three types of nerve endings are found in the clitoral area that respond to exteroceptive stimuli [18]. These nerve endings are localized not only in the clitoris proper, but also in the inner labia and around the urethral orifice. The most superficial layer of skin and mucosa contains free nerve endings that respond to painful stimuli. Signals elicited by such stimuli are conveyed through small-diameter nerve fibers in the somatic peripheral nerves and then within the spinal cord at a conduction velocity of 1–2 m per second.

Beneath the skin and mucosal layer lie the genital nerve corpuscles. These nerve endings look like balls of yarn and have a central nucleus. They react to both pressure and movement, and the impulses are conveyed via medium-diameter, myelinated nerve fibers with a relatively high velocity (40–60 m per second) to the cerebral cortex. Finally, arranged along the nerves and the tendons are large nerve-ending "onion bulbs" with thick lamellae and a central nerve fiber. These nerve endings respond to deep pressure and vigorous movements; the nerve impulses are conveyed through thick, myelinated nerve fibers to the cortex with high conduction velocity (100 m per second).

The last two types of nerve endings are localized within or near cavernous tissues and signal engorgement of cavernous tissues. Touch may thus be experienced as just touch or as touch with a sexual quality, depending on the degree of engorgement.

A number of factors, such as hormone levels in the tissues—the level of estrogen, in particular—may have a modulating effect. Estrogen deficiency may result in a change in the quality of sensation, so that touch is experienced as disagreeable instead of pleasurable. Nitric oxide is probably of importance for clitoral erection, because neuronal nitric oxide synthetase immunoreactivity has been detected in nerve bundles and nerve fibers within the human glans clitoris and the corpora cavernosa of the clitoris [19].

Most of the sensory inputs from the clitoris are conveyed via the bilateral dorsal clitoral nerves. These nerves have a protected course through the urogenital diaphragm at the base of the clitoris, pass under the urogenital diaphragm, and then join the pudendal nerves. When the pudendal nerve is blocked—for example, as part of anesthesia for childbirth—the clitoris also becomes anesthetic.

Two important reflexes can be evoked by stimulation of the clitoris. The bulbocavernosus reflex is a spinal, somatic, and bilateral phasic reflex. The reflex arc goes through the pudendal nerves and the sacral cord (S2, S3 segments). The reflex can be elicited by pinching the glans, which elicits a response consisting of contraction of the bulbocavernosus and external anal sphincter muscles. A tonic reflex also exists, by which vibratory stimulation of the clitoris causes sustained contraction of pelvic floor muscles [20]; this reflex has been less well studied.

The unstimulated clitoris has a mean total length of 16 mm (±4.3 mm), whereas the glans clitoris measures 3.4 × 5.1 mm (±1.0 mm) [21]. The clitoris is highly androgen sensitive, and administration of exogenous androgens or an increase in androgen level resulting from certain endocrine tumors may cause hypertrophy of the clitoris.

Cavernous Tissue of the Clitoris, Bulbus Urethrae, Labia, and Vagina

The glans clitoris is homologous to the glans penis and the crura clitoridis to the two corpora cavernosa of the penis. Both glans and crura contain cavernous tissue and are surrounded by a firm tunica. Therefore, on sexual stimulation, an effective erection of the clitoris occurs. Questioning of women often reveals that they notice erection of the clitoris in some but not all sexual encounters. The erection of the clitoris may not be simultaneous in time with vaginal lubrication, and it requires more intense sexual stimulation. It occurs during the excitation phase and increases sexual arousal. Drugs such as trazodone hydrochloride, as well as a number of spinal cord disorders, may result in a true priapism of the clitoris.

The ischiocavernous muscles surrounding each of the two crura also make a contribution to erection of the clitoris. During arousal, blood volume in the preputium of the clitoris increases, and this, as well as the tonic contraction of the ischiocavernosus muscles, brings about an elevation of the clitoris, which seems to disappear. The bulbocavernous muscle, which surrounds the introitus vaginae, passes interiorly and inserts at the dorsal surface of the clitoris, forming a sling around the clitoris. Contraction of these muscles increases clitoral erection by compressing the dorsal vein of the clitoris and the cavernous tissue on both sides of the introitus, the bulbus vestibuli. Passive dilation of the vagina results in a reflex contraction of both the bulbocavernosus and ischiocavernosus muscles [22]. In such a way, direct vaginal stimulation—caused, for example, by movements of the penis—may indirectly affect the clitoris and sensory perception from the clitoris. Contractions of female bulbocavernous muscles may assist erection of the male penis.

Vaginal Blood Flow

During the E phase, blood flow increases not only in the vulva but also in the vagina. Great differences are found among women, in part dependent on parity. Thus, Masters and Johnson [1] describe the vulva of parous women as being darker and bluish, possibly indicating a slower circulation due to varicosity of draining veins.

The technique most often used to study sexual arousal in women in the laboratory is to measure the blood flow in the labia and the vagina, directly or indirectly, by measuring temperature gradients, degree of oxygenation, or some similar parameter (see, e.g., Rosen and Beck [23]). When xenon (Xe) 133 washout techniques were used, an average baseline vaginal blood flow of 9.8 ml per minute per 100 g of tissue was calculated [24]. During digital clitoral self-stimulation, blood flow increased up to 28.9 ml per minute per 100 g of tissue.

Electrical stimulation of anterior roots S2 and S3, but not of S4, results in increased vaginal blood flow [25]. Vasoactive intestinal peptide (VIP) is present both in Frankenhäuser's ganglion and in nerve fibers in the vaginal mucosa [26]. It has been shown that systemic infusion of VIP, as well as local injection of VIP in the vaginal wall, results in a dose-dependent increase in vaginal blood flow with subsequent lubrication [27]. Sexual stimulation causes an increase in blood VIP level [26]. VIP has physiologic effects on the uterus, relaxing the isthmus and causing uterine vasodilation.

Two other peptides of the same vasoactive peptide family as VIP—helospectin and pituitary adenylate cyclase activation polypeptide—have also been found in the mucous membranes of the human vagina and in the walls of small vessels [28].

Peptide histidine methionine and peptide histidine valine have also been shown to be present and biologically active in the human vagina and cervix [29,30].

The greater part of the female spongious tissue is localized on both sides of the introitus and around the urethra, especially in the tissues between the vagina and the urethra. These are also the structures that respond to sexual stimulation, especially if the stimulation is directed toward the anterior part of the vagina. Grafenberg's spot, or the G spot, is a particular area localized to the anterior vaginal wall [31]. However, it is not well defined from the anatomic point of view and may not be found in all women [32]. Anatomic studies have shown abundant innervation by thin nerve fibers with a broomlike appearance in the epithelium and other forms of nerve fiber structures in deeper layers of the mucosa in this part of the vaginal wall [33].

Vaginal Lubrication

Vaginal fluids of the nonmenstruating fertile woman are produced by the vagina itself, by Bartholin's glands, by the cervix, and to a lesser extent by upper parts of the uterus, the tubae, and possibly also by ruptured ovarian follicles or even the peritoneal cavity. The lubrication that occurs as part of sexual arousal is due to transudation through the vaginal walls, with a significant contribution from Bartholin's glands. No actively secreting gland cells are found in the vaginal walls, and the formation of lubricating fluid is thought to be the result of a nonsecretory process entirely dependent on increased vaginal blood flow, although lubrication fluid does contain more potassium and less sodium and chloride than plasma [34,35]. Sperm are usually left in the vagina 2–3 days after intercourse, and the vaginal pH increases after the orgasm, which may favor sperm survival. The slippery quality of vaginal lubricant is due to the sialoprotein content [36].

Sexual arousal, either through direct stimulation of the genital region or through cerebral mechanisms, may result in very rapid vaginal lubrication (i.e., within 30 seconds), so that the vaginal walls and the introitus are covered by a lubrication film early in the E phase; this lubrication continues during the P and O phases but to a lesser degree. One further source of lubricating fluid is the paraurethral glands, which empty into the urethra. Because the urethral orifice is situated just above the introitus vaginae, paraurethral secretion may be expressed on the upper side of the penis during intercourse.

Normal lubrication depends both on intact innervation and on normal estrogen levels. Estrogen deficiency—for example, after normal menopause, in pituitary insufficiency or ovarian insufficiency, or during antiestrogen therapy—reduces lubrication capacity; this symptom may be successfully treated by estrogen substitution. Increased genital blood flow and lubrication occur normally in women at night during rapid-eye-movement phases of sleep, similarly to erection in men.

Changes of the Vagina during Sexual Arousal

The unstimulated vagina is a collapsed structure, but during sexual stimulation a cavity is formed. This is partly due to intromission of the penis, but an active process also occurs whereby the muscles in the pelvic area deepen and widen in the upper two-thirds of the vagina. The detailed mechanisms of this are not well known.

Intravaginal pressure and intra-abdominal pressure vary considerably during intercourse. The intravaginal pressure is negative during intromission but positive during female orgasm [37]. However, both interindividual and intraindividual variations are considerable. Some women can dilate their vaginas episodically during the P and O phases, presumably through changes of intra-abdominal pressure and movements of the thoracic diaphragm, and they may be able to contract their vaginas to a smaller volume—the words "the vagina is swallowing" are sometimes used to express what is happening. Some women can expel intravaginal objects with some force.

Physiology of the Uterus during Sexual Arousal and Orgasm

According to Masters and Johnson [1], the cervix elevates during the later part of the E phase, and during the P and O phases the cervical os shows a degree of opening. During orgasm, the uterine muscles contract; the intrauterine pressure first increases and then rapidly decreases after orgasm. These pressure changes may give the uterus suction capacity that facilitates sperm transport. During orgasm, the cervix dips several times down against the posterior vaginal wall where the seminal pool is collected. Studies of women who have undergone subtotal hysterectomy have not revealed any decrease in the capacity to respond sexually or any change in the quality of orgasm [38]. However, for some women and in some types of orgasm, vigorous uterine contractions seem to be of importance.

Oxytocin Secretion

Caressing of erogenous zones of the body, the female breasts in particular, or stimulation of the uterine cervix releases oxytocin from the hypothalamus–posterior pituitary. The oxytocin level is known to rise during sexual arousal [39] and to peak during orgasm [40]. Oxytocin evokes contraction of the smooth muscles in the ducts of the mammary glands, resulting in the ejection of milk from the breast. This is a very old observation—the mythologic name "the Milky Way" comes from the belief that milk was let down from Hera's breasts when she was having intercourse with Zeus.

The involvement of oxytocin in the facilitation of gamete transport is suggested by studies of smooth muscle contractions with oxytocin administration to the myometrium [41]. Release of oxytocin at intercourse may also have an effect on the uterus during delivery but probably not during other parts of pregnancy. There is also a very old belief that childbirth can be initiated by sexual activity.

During lactation, an amenorrheic period that can last for a year or more, women are usually less sexually responsive and find that a lack of vaginal lubrication may diminish coital experience [42]. Sexual desire is usually also diminished. Physiologically, elevated serum prolactin levels may be responsible for this phenomenon.

Muscles of the Pelvic Floor

The anterior part of the pelvic floor through which the urethra and vagina pass is known as the urogenital diaphragm; more posteriorly, the rectum passes through the pelvic diaphragm. The striated muscles of the pelvic floor are innervated by anterior horn cells in Onuf's nucleus [6]. In addition to these muscles, there are others with a purely sphincter function. The sphincter muscles are composed of two types of striated muscle fibers. Fibers of type I are adapted for tonic contraction, and their continuous activity is important in maintaining continence. Type II fibers fire phasically, and their rapid but short contractions are important in guarding against stress incontinence. Spontaneous contractions occur in the resting vagina in the absence of sexual stimulation [36]. These muscles have estrogen receptors, and a minimum level of estrogen in the tissue is necessary to maintain continence. Androgen receptors are also found in the muscles of the pelvic floor; these are important for the development of the pelvic muscles.

The striated pelvic floor muscles are innervated inferiorly from the pudendal nerve (muscles of the urogenital diaphragm) and superiorly from the pudendal plexus sacral segments S3–S5 (pubococcygeus muscle). Childbirth may cause considerable damage both to the connective tissue muscles and to the nerves of the pelvic floor, as shown by measurements of pudendal nerve terminal motor latency [43] as well as by electromyography. However, in most instances a good recovery occurs with time [44]. Good tone and strength of the pelvic floor is thought to be important for orgasmic capacity and pleasure at orgasm.

Orgasm in the Female

Most women describe a sense of warmth in the genital region at orgasm, spreading to lesser or greater parts of the body. During orgasm, a series of synchronous contractions of the sphincter and vaginal muscles also occur [45]; as many as 20 consecutive contractions have been registered, lasting for 10–50 seconds. However, some women report that they do not notice any contractions, so these cannot be used as a definite marker of orgasm. A major effect of pelvic muscle contractions during orgasm is to reduce vasocongestion.

Theoretically, orgasm can be expressed as the sum of what is happening in the body during sexual climax and how the individual experiences this. Much has been written about the female orgasm, but genuine knowledge is sparse.

Some authors talk of three different forms of orgasm [46]:

1. Clitoral, or vulval, orgasm is the type of orgasm women have after clitoral masturbation but also during intercourse. Contractions of the pelvic floor muscles play a prominent part, with activation of bulbocavernosus reflexes. This type of orgasm cannot occur in women with total denervation of the clitoris.
2. Uterine, or vaginal, orgasm is evoked by deep pressure in the vagina or stimulation of the anterior vaginal wall. This type of orgasm occurs only with vaginal penetration and is characterized by a pronounced effect on respiration. Immediately before orgasm the woman gasps, and respiration is suspended until the feeling of orgasm appears, at which point she makes a deep exhalation. With this Valsalva's maneuver, the uterus moves downward. This movement is immediately followed by a sensation of relaxation and sexual satisfaction. The feelings in the genital region are more deeply localized with vaginal orgasm than with clitoral orgasm.
3. "Blended orgasm" is described as a combination of clitoral and vaginal orgasm.

From a physiologic point of view, the reactions and the experience of them might be reasonably expected to be different if sexual stimulation is directed toward the clitoris with or without vaginal penetration. Some have suggested that the two types of orgasm have different "purposes": Vaginal orgasm may increase the possibility of conception, and clitoral orgasm may deepen the sexual experience and thus bind partners together.

Orgasm can be evoked in many different ways—through clitoral stimulation, through vaginal penetration, through anal penetration, or through breast stimulation. Also, stimulation of other parts of the body not primarily thought of as erogenous zones, such as the back of the neck or the hands, may result in orgasm. Orgasm can be reached purely through respiratory movements, and in some women by thought alone. Spontaneous orgasms may occur in patients with lesions in specific parts of the central nervous system. That nongenital means to orgasm exist is of great importance to the neurologically disabled patient and patients with diseases in the genital region.

Most women have the capacity to reach multiple orgasms, and approximately one-third of women regularly report experiencing several orgasms [47], defined as a series of climaxes (O phases) reached during the same P phase. These climaxes may follow each other within 15 seconds, but more often occur at intervals of 1–2 minutes. Women who can achieve multiple orgasms are usually able to climax in a shorter time; the experience is also described as more intense, and a more marked increase in blood pressure is observed. In a laboratory setting, women have been observed reaching orgasm as often as two times per minute for 1 hour.

Female Ejaculation

Female ejaculation is the expulsion of a small amount (less than a teaspoon) of fluid from the urethra (not the vagina) during orgasm [48]. This is a little-studied phenomenon, and controversies exist regarding its mechanism. Intravaginal stimulation, especially of the anterior vaginal wall, increases likelihood of such ejaculation. Spontaneous female ejaculations are rare and are reported by only a small proportion of the female population, although some women claim that female ejaculation can be trained. The fluid expelled is probably urine mixed with secretions from the paraurethral glands, in part homologous with the male prostatic gland. These glands empty partly as a result of contractile elements within them but also due to passive drainage during penile thrusts. Some women have a suburethral diverticulum that empties through the contractions of the pelvic floor muscles at orgasm. Occasionally, ejaculations of considerable volume are reported; in such cases, the fluid expelled is probably only urine, and the woman may complain of incontinence during intercourse. For some women or some couples, female ejaculation and incontinence during intercourse is a cause of great concern, but for others, these phenomena have a positive impact.

EFFECT OF NEUROLOGIC DISEASES ON FEMALE SEXUALITY

Change in Sexual Desire

Most women who experience a change in sexual desire with neurologic disease report it to be diminished. Much less commonly, a temporary increase in libido may occur. In multiple sclerosis, increased libido may be transitory and concurrent with an episode of new symptoms. A kind of "hypersexuality" may also result from a cerebral lesion.

Change in Lubrication

Many women with neurologic disease experience a delay and some decrease in lubrication as a result of their illness. Because lubrication is the counterpart to erection in males and erectile dysfunction is very common in male neurologic patients, a decrease in lubrication could be expected to result from a lesion to those parts of the spinal cord subserving the lubrication mechanism. The erection of the clitoris during sexual arousal also may be lost. Loss of lubrication may be associated with loss of menstruation, which in itself could be the result of a neurologic disorder, especially one involving the limbic cortex–hypothalamus-pituitary circuits. A decrease in lubrication could result from a spinal cord lesion but could also be due to drug treatment. Erectile dysfunction is very common in men taking various medications, including antihypertensives and antidepressant drugs or histamine$_2$ receptor antagonists. Lubrication is a physiologic phenomenon that is almost completely ignored by medical science, and a decrease in lubrication has almost never been reported as an adverse drug reaction. Despite this, the problem must exist.

Change in Orgasmic Capacity and Quality

Other important symptoms of sexual dysfunction in females with neurologic disorders include deterioration in the intensity and quality of orgasms. In most cases, orgasmic sensations are reduced, and orgasms become shorter, less intense, and less agreeable. The changes may be temporary. Antidepressant medication, especially selective serotonin reuptake inhibitors, may lead to anorgasmia.

Orgasmic improvement has also been noted in some neurologic disorders, however. Orgasms may become more easily triggered, enabling multiple orgasms; in some women, the sensation can be intensified—that is, orgasms can become longer lasting, stronger, and more pleasant.

Table 4.1 lists the different types of female sexual dysfunction that can occur in neurologic disorders and compares them to those experienced by males.

SOME SPECIFIC SEXUAL ISSUES IN THE NEUROLOGIC PATIENT

Epilepsy

A review of sexual issues involving patients with epilepsy, along with useful references, is provided by Lundberg [49, 50].

Focal Sexual Epileptic Seizures

Partial epileptic seizures from the sensory cortex may have a sexual sensory aura. Thus, sensations in the genital organs may be part of a focal seizure. Sen-

Table 4.1 Forms of sexual dysfunction in women and men

Women	Men
Problems of desire (D phase according to Kaplan[3])	
1. Total lack of interest in sex	Total lack of interest in sex
2. Loss of desire	Loss of desire
3. Aversion to sex	Aversion to sex
4. Hypersexuality	Hypersexuality
Problems of sexual arousal (E and P phases according to Masters and Johnson,[1] E phase according to Kaplan[3])	
5. Lack of lubrication/insufficient erection of clitoris	Impotence of central type/impotence of reflex type
6. Decreased lubrication	Erection insufficient for intercourse
7. Dryness of the vagina	Inability to sustain erection during intercourse
8. Sustained painful erection of the clitoris	Priapism
Problems with orgasm (O phase according to Masters and Johnson[1] and Kaplan[3])	
9. Total anorgasmia	Total anorgasmia
10. Coital anorgasmia	Coital anorgasmia
11. Retarded orgasm	Retarded ejaculation
12. Anhedonic orgasm	Anhedonic orgasm
13. Spontaneous orgasm	Spontaneous orgasm
14. Coital incontinence	—
15. Female ejaculation	—
16. —	Dribbling ejaculation
17. —	Retrograde ejaculation
18. —	Azoospermia
19. —	Aspermia
Vaginism, dyspareunia, and other genital pain in relation to sexual arousal and activity	
20. Vaginism	Tense pelvic floor
21. Clitoral or labial pain on sexual excitement	Penile or scrotal pain on sexual excitement
22. Superficial dyspareunia	Penile dyspareunia
23. Deep dyspareunia	—
24. Painful orgasm	Painful ejaculation
25. Painful nocturnal erection of the clitoris	Painful nocturnal erection

Source: Adapted with permission from PO Lundberg. Sexologi. Stockholm, Sweden: Liber Utbildning, 1994.

sations described as being like "a hot poker inserted in the vagina," " a pleasant sensation of anal and vaginal constriction and penetration," or a "sensation of clitoral warmth," as well as attacks of genital pain, may occur and may be experienced as sexual or nonsexual. In the very few case reports of such symptoms, almost all of the patients had parasagittal tumors (primary sensory cortex).

Partial complex epileptic seizures may include movements of the pelvis, compulsive masturbation, or undressing. Lubrication ("abundant vaginal discharge") and orgasm may occur as part of an epileptic seizure, but these sexual phenomena are rare and usually occur in patients with complex partial epilepsy, mostly temporal lobe lesions. Sexual automatisms are more frequent with frontal lobe lesions. They are very uncommon in primary generalized epilepsy of the grand mal or petit mal type.

Epileptic Seizures Provoked by Sexual Activity

Epileptic seizures can be provoked by masturbation, orgasm, and specific sexual stimuli, such as a fetish or an enema. Hyperventilation during sexual intercourse may provoke generalized seizures. Sexual fantasies, genital stimulation (masturbation), or orgasm may provoke focal epilepsy, called reflex epilepsy. Only a small number of cases of sexually provoked epileptic seizures have been described, but the problem is probably not often reported by patients, and physicians rarely inquire about it.

Modification of Sexual Behavior in Patients with Epilepsy

Patients with epilepsy can demonstrate changes of sexual behavior or gender dysphoria in the postictal or interictal state. Thus, hypersexuality, pansexuality, erotomania, sexual paranoia, transvestism, exhibitionism, and fetishism, as well as feelings of uneasiness regarding gender identity and sex roles, have been observed in patients with epilepsy. However, the more usual clinical picture in an epileptic patient is a combination of lack of sexual desire and sexual arousal. Epileptic males are also more often single and childless than males in the general population. Studies of patients with different forms of epilepsy show clearly that sexual problems are more common in those with partial complex temporal lobe epilepsy than in patients with primary generalized epilepsy [49,50].

Benign and Malignant Orgasmic Cephalalgia

Severe headache with sudden onset during coitus is an alarming clinical symptom that can be caused by a cerebrovascular catastrophe, such as subarachnoid hemorrhage, ischemic stroke, or intracerebral hemorrhage. However, a benign, but nevertheless very troublesome, recurrent form of headache that begins at or close to orgasm also occurs. This type of headache is called benign orgasmic cephalalgia (BOC) to differentiate it from headache that is a symptom of a cerebrovascular catastrophe, termed malignant orgasmic cephalalgia.

Two types of BOC attacks are seen: short (lasting 1–15 minutes) and long (lasting 2–24 hours). The short attacks, and also some of the longer-lasting ones, belong to the category of headaches usually called benign exertional headaches. Such headaches may occur after maneuvers that raise the intrathoracic pressure, exercises causing a sudden increase in blood pressure, or maneuvers resulting in traction of intracranial structures, such as head rotation and jumping. The pathophysiologic mechanisms behind the short-lasting attacks are largely unknown, although changes in intracranial pressure gradients and traction of intracranial structures are possible explanations. A number of facts point to a vascular cause for the long-lasting headaches. The symptomatology is very similar to that of vascular migraine, and a high frequency of vascular headache of the migraine type is seen in these patients. The beneficial results of beta-blocking agents or calcium channel blockers in the prophylactic treatment of BOC support the view that long-lasting BOC attacks are a form of migraine.

The site of BOC headaches may be occipital; nausea is not infrequent, but vomiting occurs only occasionally. Consciousness is never affected, and a stiff neck does not ever occur. The presence of focal neurologic symptoms or signs precludes the diagnosis of BOC. Most often, an attack of BOC starts at the moment of orgasm, although sometimes it may start earlier, during the stage of sexual excitement. Usually, a patient has had more than one attack. Thus, BOC is a recurrent symptom that can always occur with intercourse or can occur just occasionally. A proper diagnosis and prophylactic treatment usually make it possible for the patient to continue to be sexually active.

For a review of the topic of headache during intercourse, see Lundberg and Osterman [51].

REFERENCES

1. Masters WH, Johnson VE. Human Sexual Response. Boston: Little, Brown, 1966.
2. Levin RJ. The physiology of sexual function in women. Clin Obstet Gynaecol (London) 1980;7:213–252.
3. Kaplan HS. The New Sex Therapy. New York: Brunner/Mazel, 1974.
4. Hulter B, Lundberg PO. Sexual function in women with hypothalamo-pituitary disorders. Arch Sex Behav 1994;23:171–183.
5. Lundberg PO. Sexologi. Stockholm, Sweden: Liber Utbildning, 1994.
6. Schröder HD. Anatomical and pathoanatomical studies on the spinal efferent systems innervating pelvic structures. J Auton Nerv Syst 1985;14:23–48.
7. Mannen T, Iwata M, Toyokura Y, Nagashima K. Preservation of a certain motoneurone group of the sacral cord in amyotrophic lateral sclerosis: its clinical significance. J Neurol Neurosurg Psychiatry 1977;40:464–469.
8. Kojima H, Furuta Y, Fujioka Y, Nagashima K. Onuf's motoneuron is resistant to poliovirus. J Neurol Sci 1989;93:85–92.
9. Donker PJ. A study of the myelinated fibres in the branches of the pelvic plexus. Neurourol Urodyn 1986;5:185–202.
10. Owman C, Rosengren E, Sjöberg N-O. Adrenergic innervation of the human female reproductive organs: a histochemical and chemical investigation. Obstet Gynecol 1967;30:763–773.
11. Yoshida Y, Yoshida K, Kimura T, Toda N. Distribution of NADPH diaphorase-reactive nerves in the human female genital organ. Acta Obstet Gynecol Scand 1995;74:171–176.
12. Whipple B, Komisaruk BR. Elevation of pain thresholds by vaginal stimulation in women. Pain 1985;21:357–367.
13. Whipple B, Josimovich JB, Komisaruk BR. Sensory thresholds during the antepartum, intrapartum and postpartum periods. Int J Nurs Stud 1990;27:213–221.
14. Peters LC, Kristal MB, Komisaruk BR. Sensory innervation of the external and internal genitalia of the female rat. Brain Res 1987;408:199–204.
15. Mould DE. Women's Orgasm and the Muscle Spindle. In B Graber (ed), Circumvaginal Musculature and Sexual Function. Basel, Switzerland: Karger, 1982;93–100.
16. Helström L, Lundberg PO. Vibratory perception thresholds in the female genital region. Acta Neurol Scand 1992;86:635–637.
17. Campbell B. Neurophysiology of the Clitoris. In TP Lowry, T Snyder Lowry (eds), The Clitoris. St Louis: Warren Green, 1976;35–74.
18. Lowry TP. Some Issues in the Histology of the Clitoris. In TP Lowry, T Snyder Lowry (eds), The Clitoris. St Louis: Warren Green, 1976;91–97.
19. Burnett AL, Calvin DC, Silver RI, et al. Immunohistochemical description of nitric oxide synthase isoform in human clitoris. J Urol 1997;158:75–78.
20. Gillian P, Brindley GS. Vaginal and pelvic floor responses to sexual stimulation. Psychophysiology 1979;16:471–481.
21. Verkauf BS, von Thorn J, O'Brien WF. Clitoral size in normal women. Obstet Gynecol 1992;80:41–44.

22. Shafik A. Vaginocavernosus reflex: clinical significance and role in sexual act. Gynecol Obstet Invest 1993;35:114–117.
23. Rosen RC, Beck JG. Patterns of Sexual Arousal. New York: Guilford Press, 1988.
24. Wagner G, Ottesen B. Vaginal blood flow during sexual stimulation. Obstet Gynecol 1980;56:621–624.
25. Levin RJ, Macdonagh RP. Increased vaginal blood flow induced by implant electrical stimulation of sacral anterior roots in the conscious woman: a case study. Arch Sex Behav 1993;22:471–475.
26. Ottesen B. Vasoactive intestinal polypeptide as a neurotransmitter in the female genital tract. Am J Obstet Gynecol 1983;147:208–224.
27. Ottesen B, Pedersen B, Nielsen J, et al. Vasoactive intestinal polypeptide (VIP) provokes vaginal lubrication in normal women. Peptides 1987;8:797–800.
28. Graf A-H, Schiechl A, Hacker GW, et al. Helospectin and pituitary cyclase activating polypeptide in the human vagina. Regul Pept 1995;55:277–286.
29. Palle C, Bredkjor HE, Ottesen B, Fahrenkrug J. Peptide histidine methionine (PHM) increases vaginal blood flow in normal women. Peptides 1990;11:401–404.
30. Palle C, Ottesen B, Fahrenkrug J. Peptide histidine valine (PHV) is present and biologically active in the human female genital tract. Regul Pept 1992;38:101–109.
31. Grüfenberg E. The role of urethra in female orgasm. Int J Sexol 1950;3:145–148.
32. Whipple B, Komisaruk BR. The G Spot, Orgasm and Female Ejaculation: Are They Related? In P Kothari, R Patel (eds), Proceedings: The First International Conference on Orgasm. Bombay, India: VRP Publ, 1991;227–237.
33. Hilliges M, Falconer C, Ekman-Ordeberg G, Johansson O. Innervation of the human vaginal mucosa as revealed by PGP 9.5 immunohistochemistry. Acta Anat (Basel) 1995;153:119–126.
34. Wagner G, Levin R. Vaginal Fluid. In ESE Hafez, TN Evans (eds), The Human Vagina. Amsterdam: Elsevier, 1978;121–137.
35. Wagner G, Levin R. Electrolytes in vaginal fluid during the menstrual cycle of coitally active and inactive women. J Reprod Fertil 1980;60:17–27.
36. Levin RJ. The mechanisms of human female sexual arousal. Ann Rev Sex Res 1992;3:1–48.
37. Fox CA, Wolff HS, Baker JA. Measurement of intra-vaginal and intra-uterine pressures during human coitus by radio-telemetry. J Reprod Fertil 1970;22:243–251.
38. Helström L, Lundberg PO, Sörbom D, Bäckström T. Sexuality after hysterectomy: a factor analysis of women's sexual lives before and after subtotal hysterectomy. Obstet Gynecol 1993;81:357–362.
39. Carmichael MS, Warburton VL, Dixen J, Davidson JM. Relationships among cardiovascular, muscular, and oxytocin responses during human sexual activity. Arch Sex Behav 1994;23:59–79.
40. Murphy MR, Checkley SA, Seckl JR, Lightman SL. Naloxone inhibits oxytocin release at orgasm in man. J Clin Endocrinol Metab 1990;71:1056–1058.
41. Steer PJ. The endocrinology of parturition in the human. Baillieres Clin Endocrinol Metab 1990;4:333–349.
42. Kayner CE, Zagar JA. Breast-feeding and sexual response. J Fam Pract 1983;17:69–73.
43. Tetzschner T, Sørensen M, Jonsson L, et al. Delivery and pudendal nerve function. Acta Obstet Gynecol Scand 1997;76:324–331.
44. Tetzschner T, Sørensen M, Lose G, Christiansen J. Pudendal nerve recovery after a non-instrumental vaginal delivery. Int Urogynecol J Pelvic Floor Dysfunct 1996;7:102–104.
45. Bohlen JG, Held JP, Sanderson MO, Ahlgren A. The female orgasm: pelvic contractions. Arch Sex Behav 1982;11:367386.
46. Singer J, Singer I. Types of Female Orgasm. In J LoPiccolo, L LoPiccolo (eds), Handbook of Sex Therapy. New York: Plenum, 1978;175–186.
47. Kratochvil S. Multiple orgasms in women. Cesk Psychiatr 1993;89:349–354.
48. Whipple B. Research concerning sexual response in women. Health Psychol 1995;17:126–18.
49. Lundberg PO. Sexual dysfunction in patients with neurological disorders. Ann Rev Sex Res 1992;3:121–150.
50. Lundberg PO. Sexual dysfunction in selected neurological and endocrinological disorders. Baillieres Clin Psychiatry 1997;3:113–130.
51. Lundberg PO, Osterman PO. Intercourse and Headache. In AR Genazzani, G Nappi, F Facchinetti, M Martignoni (eds), Pain and Reproduction. Carnforth, UK: The Parthenon Publishing Group, 1988;149–153.

5

Physiology of Male Sexual Function and Dysfunction in Neurologic Disease

Rupert O. Beck

Sexual function in men is divided into three distinct phases: penile erection, orgasm, and detumescence. This chapter focuses on the physiology of penile erection with brief descriptions of orgasm and ejaculation.

Erections are primarily a vascular phenomenon and are dependent on the inter-action between nerves, neurotransmitters, striated and smooth muscle, and tunica albuginea. Cavernous and arterial smooth muscle relaxation results in increased arterial inflow, which, together with decreased venous return, causes an erection. The mechanisms behind this process are explored in detail in this chapter.

PENILE ANATOMY AND VASCULATURE

The erectile tissue of the penis consists of three longitudinal bundles known as the *corpora*. The paired corpora cavernosa function as the main erectile bodies, whereas the corpus spongiosum surrounds the urethra and expands distally to form the glans. Each of the three corpora is surrounded by tunica albuginea—a layer of fibrous tissue that separates the corpora from each other. The cavernous bodies consist of blood-filled spaces called *sinusoids*, the walls of which are made up of bundles of smooth muscle and fibroelastic tissue.

The arterial supply of the penis derives mainly from the paired pudendal arter-ies, which are terminal branches of the internal iliacs. The terminal divisions of the pudendal artery that supply the penis are well recognized, and the following description is a representative summary of what has been written in textbooks [1, 2]. In the perineum, each pudendal artery gives off a perineal branch and then two arteries to the corpus spongiosum—the bulbar artery and the urethral artery. The bulbar artery supplies the proximal corpus spongiosum; the urethral artery pierces the corpus spongiosum and then continues to supply the spongiosum up to and including the glans penis. The pudendal artery continues to the crus of the penis, where it divides into the dorsal penile artery and the deep penile artery. The dorsal

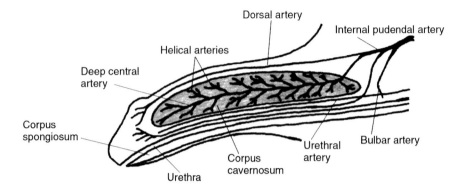

Figure 5.1   Diagrammatic representation of the arterial supply of the human penis.

artery passes distally along the penis between the corpora cavernosa external to the tunica albuginea. Some of its superficial branches supply the skin of the penis. The deep penile artery penetrates the crus of the penis and passes distally as the cavernous artery (Figure 5.1). Numerous anastomotic channels interconnect the arteries of the penis [3, 4]. Studies also demonstrate great variations in the anatomy of the penile vasculature [5]. The venous drainage of the corpora is via small veins within the sinusoids that coalesce to form the emissary veins; these then pass through the tunica albuginea and drain into the deep dorsal vein of the penis.

PHYSIOLOGY OF ERECTION

Two major neurologic pathways of erection are recognized—psychogenic and reflexogenic. Reflexogenic erections are the result of direct stimulation of the genital organs; the afferent impulses are conveyed in the pudendal nerve to S2–S4, and the efferent impulses travel back via the same level sacral roots. Psychogenic erections occur after certain audiovisual or olfactory stimuli or fantasy, and require that long tracts of the central nervous system between cortex, cord, and sympathetic nervous system be intact. Despite the different neurologic input needed to initiate and maintain these two pathways, the final vascular events within the penis are the same. In the flaccid state, the corporeal smooth muscle is tonically contracted, allowing only enough blood to flow through the cavernous tissue to maintain tissue viability (1.4–4.0 ml/minute/100 g tissue) [6]. The blood flows preferentially from the cavernous arteries through the small nutrient vessels of the cavernous tissues to the emissary veins and then out of the corpora. Stimulation of the erectile parasympathetic outflow via psychogenic or reflexogenic pathways releases neurotransmitters that cause cavernous smooth muscle relaxation and vasodilation of the penile arteries. When the cavernous smooth muscle relaxes, blood flow is preferentially shifted from the cavernous arteries and nutrient arterioles into the sinusoidal spaces, and as these fill with blood, they compress the subtunical veins against the tunica albuginea so that venous outflow is impaired. The corpora then fill with blood, resulting in penile tumescence followed by full rigidity. Initially, blood flow increases to approximately 50 ml per minute within the pudendal artery, followed by corporeal pressure rises to 50–80 mm Hg. However, once the penis becomes rigid, blood is actually stored in the sinusoids at a very low flow rate, although the pressure rises to approximately mean systolic blood pressure. This process is described as the veno-occlusive mechanism [7].

NEUROPHYSIOLOGY OF ERECTION

The hemodynamic changes described in the previous section are under neurologic control, although the exact role of the various pathways and neurotransmitters involved remains controversial.

Efferent Pathways

Eckhard [8] was the first to demonstrate that erection in the dog followed stimulation of the pelvic parasympathetic nerves, but that no such response occurred after stimulation of the hypogastric sympathetic nerves. Müller [9], studying the dog, and Root and Bard [10], studying the cat, shed more light on the role of the sympathetic nervous system in erection in these animals. Müller discovered that excision of the entire sacral and most of the lumbar spinal cord abolished reflex penile erections, but erections still occurred if the dog was placed with an excitable female. Root and Bard performed similar experiments in cats, in which they demonstrated that the ability to produce an erection when exposed to an estrous female remained after ablation of sacral parasympathetic pathways. The addition of spinal cord transection anywhere between T11 and L1, or the division of the hypogastric nerves in the cats that had previously undergone parasympathetic ablation, prevented the development of these psychogenic erections. Resection of purely the sympathetic nerves, however, had no effect on psychogenic or reflexogenic erections in cats. Results of hypogastric nerve stimulation vary from species to species; in the rabbit, stimulation causes erection [8]; in the cat, it results in contraction of the penile arteries, causing the erect penis to become flaccid [11]; the latter effect also occurs in dogs and monkeys [12, 13].

Human data relating to the neural pathways involved in the erectile process are limited. Much of the data is retrospective, derived from questionnaires or obtained from patients with isolated neurologic disease. One drawback with human studies is that the completeness of the neurologic lesion produced by any spinal cord injury may be difficult to ascertain. Bors and Comarr [14] published data on a large number of patients with spinal cord injury. All patients with clinically complete lower motor neuron lesions were unable to achieve an erection with genital stimulation; however, 24% reported psychogenic erections. Patients with suprasacral spinal cord injury were able to obtain erections secondary to genital stimulation. The percentage achieving erection secondary to psychic stimulation varied with the level of the injury: For those with cervical injuries, the percentage was 4%; for injuries at T1–T6, 0%; at T7–T12, 8%; and for lumbar injuries, 57%. Patients who have undergone lumbar sympathectomy or retroperitoneal lymph node dissection do not report erectile difficulties [15–18], although they frequently develop retrograde ejaculation from failure of contraction of the bladder neck sphincter.

In humans, the parasympathetic pathways appear to be of prime importance in penile erection, although the sympathetic nervous system also has a role in the development of psychogenic erections and plays an important role in detumescence. This latter conclusion has been drawn from studies with intracavernous injections of α_1-adrenergic agonists in man [19, 20]. These injections result in detumescence, whereas conversely, injections of α_1-adrenergic blockers often result in tumescence and erection [21, 22]. Giulano et al. [23] found that erections can result from inhibition of the sympathetic pathways. They showed that in rats, chemical sympathectomy by administration of the adrenergic neurotoxin 6-hydroxydopamine enhanced the erectile response produced by cavernous electrical stimulation, as did administration of the α_1-blocker phentolamine, which enhanced both the cavernous filling rate and the intracavernous pressure. The β-blocker propanolol decreased the response. Further electrophysiologic studies in rats identified a polysynaptic reflex between the dorsal nerve of the penis and the lumbosacral sympathetic chain. In rats, electrical stimulation of the lumbosacral chain at the L4/L5 level evoked a discharge in the dorsal nerve of the penis, whereas stimulation of the dorsal nerve of the penis evoked a spinally mediated reflex discharge in the lumbosacral chain. The latency of this response was significantly decreased after spinal cord transection at T8, indicating a supraspinal component to this reflex. The hypothesis has been advanced that in rats, afferent inputs during coitus may influence the sympathetic tone of the pelvic organs and in particular induce emission and ejaculation [24].

Further evidence of the role of the sympathetic nervous system has come from studies on a number of patients with dopamine β-hydroxylase deficiency. Dopamine β-hydroxylase is the enzyme that converts dopamine into noradrenaline. In dopamine β-hydroxylase deficiency, noradrenaline and adrenaline are absent from sympathetic nerve endings, with consequent failure of noradrenergic nerve function. However, parasympathetic cholinergic function is preserved. Two men with this condition have been reported, and both have impaired sexual function. One had difficulty in maintaining an erection and had retrograde ejaculation [25], whereas the other was able to maintain an erection, but ejaculation was delayed or absent. In the latter patient, ejaculation was improved by administration of the drug DL-dihydroxyphenylserine, which bypasses the enzymatic defect and results in formation of noradrenaline [26]. This evidence underlines the importance of the sympathetic nervous system in the physiologic closure of the bladder neck and ejaculation.

Afferent Pathways

Stimulation of the penis usually elicits reflexogenic erections. The afferent limb of this reflex is in the pudendal nerve. The glans penis is one of the most sensitive parts of the human body and has a high tactile threshold and low pain threshold. It has a very high receptor density compared to most other parts of the human body [27]; only 10–20% of its nerve endings are encapsulated, the rest being free. Two types of receptors exist: slowly adapting (SA) on the distal side of the glans and rapidly adapting (RA) on the proximal side. The RA receptors respond to movement and are thought important in the maintenance of the erection during vaginal penetration, whereas the SA receptors respond more to pressure and slow movement and may have a role in triggering the ejaculation.

The supraspinal afferent pathways involved in psychogenic erections have not been easy to study. Experiments in monkeys and rats have shown that the hypothalamic and limbic pathways are important in the erectile process and that the medial preoptic anterior hypothalamic area is an important integrating center for sexual function [28]. Lesions at this site inhibit the development of erections in animals. Human studies in these areas are difficult, but bilateral lesions in the ansa lenticularis (produced in the treatment of hyperkinetic syndrome) have been shown to abolish libido and erectile function [28].

EMISSION, EJACULATION, AND ORGASM

Orgasm comprises emission and ejaculation, which, although closely related, are separate phenomena. During emission, which is the first phase of the process, reflex activity in the thoracolumbar sympathetic outflow results in the transfer of semen (formed by the combined secretions of the testes, vasa deferentia, seminal vesicles, prostate gland, and bulbourethral glands) into the urethra, and closure of the bladder neck. After emission, rhythmic contractions of the bulbocavernosus, ischiocavernosus, and periurethral striated muscles result in ejaculation.

Electromyographic [29] and video [30] studies during orgasm have demonstrated the order of events in humans. Emission begins during arousal; the ampulla contracts and ejects its contents (contribution from testes and vasa) into the urethra. Simultaneously, peristaltic-like activity occurs in the seminal vesicles, which also eject their contents into the urethra. The bladder neck closes the moment the first phase of emission begins. Expulsion of the ejaculate is caused by synchronous, rhythmic contractions of the bulbocavernosus, ischiocavernosus, and periurethral striated muscles. Ejaculation is not triggered by the entrance of semen into the urethra as previously thought, because bulbocavernosus and ischiocavernosus ejaculatory contractions still occur when seminal fluid emission has been abolished by administration of phenoxybenzamine.

The central neural control of ejaculatory function remains poorly understood, but it is thought to be a spinal reflex with one afferent limb (sensation from the penis and glans) and several efferent limbs. One efferent limb is probably parasympathetic and controls secretion by the accessory glands during the arousal phase; another is the main sympathetic pathway responsible for closure of the bladder neck and contraction of the smooth muscle within the seminal vesicles, proximal urethra, and prostate, resulting in emission; and the third limb is the somatic motor pathway to the bulbocavernosus and ischiocavernosus muscles, contraction of which causes ejaculation [31].

NEURAL MODULATION OF CAVERNOUS SMOOTH MUSCLE ACTIVITY

The recognition that corporeal smooth muscle tone is critical to erectile function has led to a search for the neurotransmitters involved in both relaxation and contraction of smooth muscle. The most physiologically relevant effector pathways are

(1) parasympathetic nonadrenergic noncholinergic pathways, which decrease smooth muscle tone, probably via nitric oxide and vasoactive intestinal polypeptide (VIP); (2) sympathetic adrenergic pathways, which increase corporeal smooth muscle tone; and (3) a separate parasympathetic cholinergic pathway that indirectly modulates tone by altering sympathetic input.

Many neurotransmitters have been isolated from human and animal cavernous tissue, and in many cases their exact role in the neural modulation of erection and detumescence remains uncertain. The literature concerning this topic is extensive and has been the subject of many reviews [32–33]. A degree of species-to-species variation is likely, and the results of investigations into neurotransmitter effects in one nonhuman species cannot be taken as evidence for that effect in humans. The most rigorously studied neurotransmitters are described in the section that follows; for a more detailed review of the intercellular and intracellular pathways involved, the reader is referred to the article by Christ et al. [33]

NEUROTRANSMITTERS INVOLVED IN CAVERNOUS RELAXATION

Acetylcholine

The primary neurotransmitter for the parasympathetic cholinergic nerves is acetylcholine. For many years, it was considered the sole effector for erections. However, it is clear that this is not the case, as intravenous injections of the anticholinergic atropine fail to block the development of erections [21]. In addition, in vitro experiments on human cavernous tissue taken from men with male erectile dysfunction (MED) showed that atropine could diminish but not block electrically induced relaxation of smooth muscle strips [34]. These experiments pointed to the existence of a noncholinergic parasympathetic pathway.

Nonadrenergic Noncholinergic Neurotransmitters

Many nonadrenergic noncholinergic (NANC) neurotransmitters exist, but the two most important with regard to erectile function are nitric oxide [35, 36] and VIP [37, 38]. That nitric oxide, originally termed *endothelium derived relaxing factor*, has an important role in the relaxation of cavernous smooth muscle is now widely accepted [35, 36]. It is produced by the enzyme nitric oxide synthetase, which is distributed throughout the corpora both in NANC nerves and on the surface endothelium itself. Unlike other neurotransmitters, nitric oxide has a very short half-life, is not stored at nerve endings, and seems to be synthesized on demand. It has its effect via the secondary messenger cyclic guanosine monophosphate [39], which alters calcium and potassium channels within the smooth muscle cell, resulting in smooth muscle relaxation [33]. The oral erectogenic agent sildenafil citrate acts on this metabolic pathway. However, neuronally derived nitric oxide cannot be the only vasorelaxant neurotransmitter involved, because mice lacking neuronal nitric oxide synthetase still achieve full erections [40].

Vasoactive Intestinal Polypeptide

The possible role of VIP as a transmitter mediating relaxation became apparent when it was discovered within the neurons of the hypogastric plexus [41]. Infusion of exogenous VIP onto the vasculature of the penis produces erection in several species, including humans [38, 42], and VIP antibodies have been shown to block the erection produced by electrical stimulation of the pelvic nerve in the dog [43]. A high concentration of VIP is found in the deep arteries of the penis as well as in the nonvascular smooth muscle tissue of the corpus cavernosum. However, intracavernous injection of VIP alone has failed to produce erections in men with MED, indicating again that this is not the sole neurotransmitter involved [44].

Prostaglandins

The widespread use of intracorporeal injections of prostaglandin E_1 (PGE$_1$) for treatment of erectile dysfunction has focused interest on the physiologic function of the prostaglandins in the erectile process. Human cavernous tissue can synthesize various prostanoids that may have a role in smooth muscle contraction (PGF$_2$ and thromboxane A$_2$) or relaxation (PGE$_1$, PGE$_2$) [45–47]. Relaxation may come about through the increase of intracellular concentrations of cyclic adenosine monophosphate, which inhibits various calcium channels and leads to an overall decrease in intracellular calcium, producing relaxation.

NEUROTRANSMITTERS INVOLVED IN SMOOTH MUSCLE CONTRACTION

Detumescence occurs when the cavernous smooth muscle contracts. The vascular sinuses decrease in size, allowing the emissary veins, which are no longer compressed, to drain freely. Studies have shown that the release of noradrenaline from sympathetic nerve terminals with activation of postsynaptic α_1-adrenergic receptors is the primary mediator of this event, although some modulation from the α_2-presynaptic receptors occurs [31, 48]. However, noradrenaline is not the only vasoconstrictor found in penile tissue. Corporeal endothelial cells manufacture endothelin, which has potent vasoconstrictor activity on isolated cavernous smooth muscle strips in vitro [49]. Other vasoconstricting neurotransmitters discovered within the cavernous tissue include thromboxane A$_2$, PGF$_2$, and some leukotrienes [46, 50]. These nonadrenergic mechanisms are thought to help modulate corporeal smooth muscle tone during flaccidity and perhaps detumescence.

PATHOPHYSIOLOGY OF MALE ERECTILE DYSFUNCTION

The pathophysiology of MED is best discussed using a functional classification—psychogenic, neurogenic, arterial, cavernous, venous, or endocrinologic—although frequently several disorders coexist. Neurogenic MED can be the result of many different diseases affecting either the central or peripheral nervous system that can

Table 5.1   Etiologic factors in neurogenic erectile dysfunction

Intracranial lesions
  Temporal lobe
  Hypothalamus
  Ansa lenticularis
Suprasacral spinal cord disease
  Multiple sclerosis
  Spinal cord injury—trauma
  Tumors (benign and malignant, primary and metastatic)
Conus and cauda equina syndromes
  Central disk prolapse
  Tethered cord
  Spina bifida
  Vascular malformations
Pelvic nerve damage
  Major pelvic surgery
Small-fiber or autonomic neuropathies
  Diabetes
  Amyloid
Multiple system atrophy with or without autonomic failure

cause sexual dysfunction (Table 5.1). These are discussed in detail in later parts of this book (Chapters 14, 15, 18, 19, 22, and 23).

REFERENCES

1. Benson GS, Boileau MA. The Penis: Sexual Function and Dysfunction. In JY Gillenwater, JT Grayhack, SS Howards, JW Duckett (eds), Adult and Paediatric Urology. St Louis: Mosby–Year Book, 1991;1599–1642.
2. Lue TF. Physiology of Erection and Pathophysiology of Impotence. In PC Walsh, AB Retik, TA Stamet, E Darracott-Vaughan (eds), Campbell's Urology. Philadelphia: Saunders, 1992;709–728.
3. Reiss HF, Northup HF, Zorgniotti A. Artificial erection by perfusion of penile arteries. Urology 1982;20:284–288.
4. Deysach LJ. The comparative morphology of the erectile tissue of the penis with special emphasis on the possible mechanism of erection. Am J Anat 1939;64;111.
5. Bookstein JJ, Valji K, Parsons L. Pharmacoarteriography in the evaluation of impotence. J Urol 1987;137;333–337.
6. Wagner G. Erection. In G Wagner, R Green (eds), Impotence: Physiological, Psychological and Surgical Diagnosis and Treatment. New York: Plenum, 1981;25–36.
7. Lue TF, Takamura T, Schmidt RA, et al. Haemodynamics of erection in the monkey. J Urol 1983;130:1237–1241.
8. Eckhard C. Untersuchungen Über die Erection des Penis biem Hunde. In C Eckhard (ed), Beitrage zur Anatomie und Physiologie (Vol 3). Geissen, 1863.
9. Müller LR. Klinische und experimentelle studien über die innervation der Blase, des mastdarms und des genitalapparates. Deutsch Z Nervenheilk 1902;21:86.
10. Root WS, Bard P. The mediation of feline erections through sympathetic pathways with some remarks on serial behaviour after deafferentiation of genitalia. Am J Physiol 1947;151:80–90.

11. Bacq ZM. Recherches sur la physiologie et la pharmacologie du système verveux autonome; XII. Nature cholinergique et adrenergique des diverses innervations vasomotrices du penis chez le chren. Arch Int Physiol Biochem 1935;11:311.

12. Carati CJ, Creed KE, Keogh EJ. Autonomic control of penile erection in the dog. J Physiol (Lond) 1987;384:525–538.

13. Diederichs W, Stief CG, Lue TF, et al. Sympathetic inhibition of papaverine induced erection. J Urol 1991;146:195–198.

14. Bors E, Comarr AE. Neurological disturbance of sexual function with special reference to 529 patients with spinal cord injury. Urol Surv 1960;10:191–222.

15. Rose SS. An investigation in sterility after lumbar ganglionectomy. BMJ 1953;1:247.

16. Kedia KR, Markland C, Fraley EE. Sexual function following high retroperitoneal lymphadenectomy. J Urol 1975;114:237–239.

17. Jones DR, Norman AR, Horwich A, Hendry WF. Ejaculatory dysfunction after retroperitoneal lymphadenectomy. Eur Urol 1993;23:169–171.

18. Whitelaw GP, Smithwick RH. Some secondary effects of sympathectomy with particular reference to disturbance of sexual function. N Engl J Med 1951;245:121–130.

19. Brindley GS. New treatment for priapism. Lancet 1984;2:220.

20. De Meyer JM, De Sy WA. Intracavernous injection of noradrenaline to interrupt erections during surgical interventions. Eur Urol 1986;12:169–170.

21. Brindley GS. Pilot experiments on the actions of drugs injected into the human corpus cavernosum penis. Br J Pharmacol 1986;87:495–500.

22. Blum MD, Bahnson RR, Porter TN, Carter MF. Effect of local alpha-adrenergic blockade on human penile erection. J Urol 1985;134:479–481.

23. Guilamo F, Bernabe J, Jardin A, Rousseau JP. Antierectile role of sympathetic nervous system in rats. J Urol 1993;150:519–524.

24. Giulano F, Rampin O, Jardin A, Rousseau JP. Electrophysiological study of relations between dorsal nerve of the penis and the lumbar sympathetic chain in the rat. J Urol 1992;150:1960–1964.

25. Mathias CJ, Bannister R, Cortelli P, et al. Clinical, autonomic, and therapeutic observations in two siblings with postural hypotension and sympathetic failure due to an inability to synthesize noradrenaline from dopamine because of a deficiency of dopamine beta-hydroylase. QJM 1990;75:617–633.

26. Mathias CJ, Bannister R. Dopamine B—Hydroxylase Deficiency and Other Genetically Determined Causes of Autonomic Disorders: Clinical Features and Management. In R Bannister, CJ Mathias (eds), Autonomic Failure: A Textbook of Clinical Disorders of the Autonomic Nervous System (3rd ed). Oxford, UK: Oxford University Press, 1992;721–748.

27. De Groat WC, Booth AM. Neural Control of Penile Erection. In CA Maggi (ed). Nervous Control of the Urogenital System. The Autonomic Nervous System (Vol 3).London: Harwood Academic Publishers, 1993;465–522.

28. De Groat. Neurophysiology of Pelvic Organs. In DN Rushton (ed), Handbook of Neuro-Urology. New York: Marcel Dekker, 1994;55–93.

29. Gerstenberg TC, Levin RJ, Wagner G. Erection and ejaculation in man: assessment of the electromyographic activity of the bulbocavernosus and ischiocavernosus muscles. Br J Urol 1990;65:395–402.

30. Mitsuya H, Asai J, Suyama K, et al. Application of x-ray cinematography in urology. 1. Mechanisms of ejaculation. J Urol 1960;83:86–95.

31. Hoyle CHV, Lincoln J, Burnstock G. Neural Control of Pelvic Organs. In DN Rushton (ed), Handbook of Neuro-Urology. New York: Marcel Dekker, 1994;1–54.

32. Lerner SE, Melman A, Chist GJ. A review of erectile dysfunction: new insights and more questions. J Urol 1993;149:1246–1255.

33. Christ GJ, Richards S, Winkler A. Integrative erectile biology: the role of signal transduction and cell to cell communication in coordinating corporal smooth muscle tone and penile erection. Int J Impot Res 1997;9:69–84.

34. Saenz de Tajada I, Blanco R, Goldstein I, et al. Cholinergic neurotransmission in human corpus cavernosum. I. Responses of isolated tissue. Am J Physiol 1988;254:H459–H467.

35. Azadzoi KM, Kim N, Brown ML, et al. Endothelium-derived nitric oxide and cyclooxygenase products modulate corpus cavernosum smooth muscle tone. J Urol 1992;147:220–225.

36. Rajfer J, Aronson WJ, Bush PA, et al. Nitric oxide as a mediator of relaxation of the corpus cavernosum in response to non-adrenergic, noncholinergic neurotransmission. N Engl J Med 1992;326:90–94.

37. Polak JM, Gu J, Mina S, Bloom SR. Vipergic nerves in the penis. Lancet 1981;2:217.

38. Steers W, McConell J, Benson GS. Anatomical localisation and some pharmacological effects on vasointestinal peptide in human and money corpus cavernosum. J Urol 1984;132:1048–1053.
39. Furchgott RF, Jothianadan D. Endothelium dependant and independent vasodilation involving cyclic GMP: relaxation induced by nitric oxide, carbon monoxide and light. Blood Vessels 1991;28: 52–61.
40. Burnett AL, Nelson RJ, Calvin DC, et al. Nitric oxide–dependent penile erection in mice lacking neuronal nitric oxide synthase. Mol Med 1996;2:288–296.
41. Dail WA, Moll MA, Weber K. Localisation of vasoactive intestinal polypeptide in penile erectile tissue and in the major pelvic ganglion of the cat. Neuroscience 1983;10:1379–1386.
42. Takahashi Y, Aboseif SR, Bernard F, et al. Effects of intracavernosal simultaneous injections of acetylcholine and vasoactive intestinal polypeptide on canine penile erection. J Urol 1992;148:446–448.
43. Aoki M, Matsuzaka J, Yeh K-H et al. Involvement of vasoactive intestinal polypeptide VIP as a humoral mediator of penile erection in the dog. J Androl 1994:15:174–182.
44. Kiely EA, Bloom SR, Williams G. Penile responses to intracavernosal vasoactive intestinal peptide alone and in combination with other agents. Br J Urol 1989;64:191–194.
45. Christ GJ, Maayani S, Valcic M, Melman A. Pharmacological studies of human erectile tissue: characteristics of spontaneous contractions and alterations in alpha-adrenoceptor responsiveness with age and disease in isolated tissues. Br J Pharmacol 1990;101:375–381.
46. Melman A, Maayani S, Schwartzman M. Prostaglandin synthesis as a putative biochemical correlate of spontaneous myotonic oscillations in the isolated human penile erectile tissue [abstract 1028]. J Urol 1986;135(pt 2):361A.
47. Andersson K-E, Wagner G. Physiology of penile erection. Physiol Rev 1995;75:191–236.
48. Hedlund J, Andersson KE, Mattiasson A. Pre- and postjunctional adreno- and muscarinic receptor functions in the isolated human corpus spongiosum urethrae. J Auton Pharmacol 1984;4:241–249.
49. Saenz De Tejada I, Carson MP, De Las Morenas A, et al. Endothelin: localisation, synthesis, activity and receptor types in human penile corpus cavernosum. Am J Physiol 1991;261(4 pt 2): H1078–H1085.
50. Hedlund J, Anderson KE, Fovaeus M, et al. Characterisation of contraction-mediating prostanoid receptors in human penile erectile tissues. J Urol 1989;141:182–186.

6
Consequences of the Neuropathic Bladder and Bowel for Patients

Scott Glickman and Julia Segal

The central urogenital neural pathways extend from the frontal lobes to the conus medullaris, connecting peripherally via the second, third, and fourth sacral roots. The central neurology of the anorectum is not well described, but the tracts might be expected to be very closely aligned, because both the bladder and the anorectum develop from the urorectal septum.

Disease of the conus medullaris may produce damage isolated to genitourinary and coloanal functions. Much more commonly, however, central neural damage affecting these organs is associated with other neural, and therefore other peripheral, dysfunctions. Therefore, consideration of the effects on patients of central neural damage to the urinary or proctocolonic tracts often includes issues not only of associated sensory loss but also of limb paralysis; spasticity; cognitive and behavioral problems; movement disorders, such as tremor; and communication.

The enduring impacts of damage result from persistent neuropathology. These impacts can be classified broadly as symptoms, impairments, disabilities, handicaps, secondary pathologies (both physical and psychological), and emotional and behavioral consequences. The impairments, disabilities, and handicaps categories are taken from the World Health Organization's international classification of impairments, disabilities, and handicaps [1] and can be defined as follows:

Impairment—the reduction or loss of a basic function in the central nervous system. This impairment might be slowing of neural conduction or loss of communication across a spinal cord transection. An example of impairment in the peripheral nervous system would be the loss of receptive relaxation in the filling bladder.

Disability—the dysfunctional impact resulting from an impairment (e.g., failure to store or void urine or feces). Some disabilities are multifactorial, with additional contributions from the environment or equipment. For example, a paraplegic person's ability to transfer from a wheelchair to a toilet depends as much on the accessibility of the toilet as on the power-to-weight ratio of the upper limbs.

Handicap—the way in which an individual is personally disadvantaged. It represents the ways in which a person is impeded from fulfilling an expected or intended role that would be achievable under normal circumstances. Being forced to live in isolation or having to endure ridicule because of a disability are handicaps.

Secondary pathologies are pathologic complications. Typical examples are urinary tract calculi produced because of poor voiding or reflux nephropathy resulting from a hyperreflexic bladder. Bowel-associated complications include hemorrhoids, rectal prolapses, and anal fissures. These may develop because of constipation or straining to overcome rectal hypocontractility. Incontinence of both urine and feces macerates skin. Incontinence lowers the resistance of such affected skin to pressure sores, for which neurodisabled people are at high risk. Ineffective urinary voiding predisposes to bladder infections. Psychological problems also may present as secondary complications. This aspect is discussed later.

Except for renal failure resulting from reflux nephropathy, septicemia from pressure sores, and suicidal depression, life-threatening risks from the primary neuropathology are rare. Instead, it is the quality of living that is affected. For each individual, these effects are uniquely personal.

Although clinicians should be aware that the consequences of pathology may fit into any one of the categories cited above, patients generally perceive problems as being due to the primary pathology, disabilities, or handicaps.

For conditions in which the primary pathology is incurable, restorative rehabilitation is not possible (Figure 6.1). Furthermore, partial restoration of function commonly serves no useful purpose. For example, if someone is incontinent of urine at a liter or more per day, reduction of volume by 50% may be of no

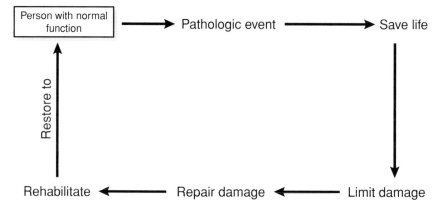

Figure 6.1   Restorative rehabilitation paradigm. Rehabilitation in this paradigm encapsulates the processes that follow after the pathology is no longer the focus of attention. (Reprinted with permission from S Glickman, J McKimm. Disability and Rehabilitation: A Medical Tutor's Handbook. London: British Brain and Spine Foundation, 1996.)

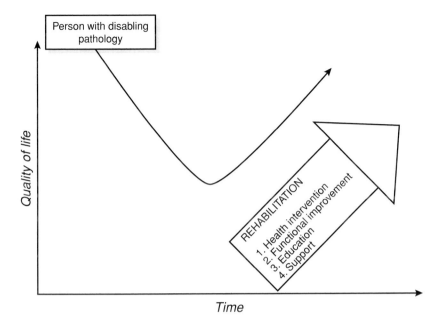

Figure 6.2   Glickman's rehabilitation paradigm. (Reprinted with permission from S Glickman, J McKimm. Disability and Rehabilitation: A Medical Tutor's Handbook. London: British Brain and Spine Foundation, 1996.)

value in terms of quality of living, because the fear of embarrassment or the social isolation may remain unchanged. A much better management approach uses a paradigm for rehabilitation of people with persistent disabling pathology (Figure 6.2) [2]. This paradigm is defined as a goals-directed process for facilitating improvements in quality of living for people with disabling pathology by preventing or limiting processes that are physically, psychologically, or socially detrimental and by appropriately addressing health, abilities, education, and support.

The various ways in which bowel and bladder dysfunctions can affect people obviously are more numerous than can be presented in any chapter. The reason is that the influences on each person depend on the physical, psychological, and social contexts in which the individual experiences the problems. Therefore, what follows is intended merely to illustrate some examples within the various categories.

IMPAIRMENTS

Impairments present as symptoms and signs. The nature and type of impairments that present are considered in Chapter 3.

Symptoms

Symptoms are subjective evidence of disease that are perceived by the patient and that result from impairments. Urgency, dysuria, and pain are symptoms.

Signs

Signs are objective clinical indications of the presence of pathology, impairments, and disabilities. Frequency, hesitancy, constipation, and incontinence are signs. The distinction between symptoms and signs in the context of rehabilitation is crucial. Patients may complain of abnormalities, such as frequency of seven times per day, because they do not appreciate that this is normal for the population. Even when neuropathology obviously is present, patient complaints, such as frequency or constipation, should not necessarily be taken at face value, because they may not stand up to objective assessment. In cases in which people complain of problems that are not abnormal, education would be the treatment of choice. In some cases, complaints may be due to comorbid pathology. For example, polydipsia can occur typically with diabetes mellitus, diabetes insipidus, or even a belief that excessive drinking is necessary to "cleanse the system."

DISABILITIES—PRACTICAL ISSUES

The functions of the bladder and rectum are to store and void their waste contents effectively. Impairments can undermine these functions. For example, loss of sensitivity to rectal fullness may predispose someone to bowel incontinence, because the patient would not have been made aware of the need to use the toilet. The impairments of hypocontractility of the bladder and bowel produce voiding disabilities. The central nervous system impairment of inhibitory neuronal function may produce detrusor hyperreflexia, which leads to a storage disability because of reflux of urine. If detrusor contraction force exceeds outlet sphincter resistance, then incontinence occurs. Some refer to this incontinence as "firing off."

The neural conditions that produce bladder and bowel disabilities rarely do so in isolation. Stroke, multiple sclerosis, Parkinson's disease, traumatic brain and spinal cord injuries, and hereditary spastic parapareses are notable examples. Other neural tract impairments and disabilities associated with these pathologies may contribute substantially to the symptoms and signs. For example, aphasia may prevent someone from asking for a catheter, suppository, or commode. Lower limb paralysis or ataxia may prevent someone from getting to the lavatory in time, with incontinence being the result.

The environment can also contribute to disability. The social model of disability implies that the environment or society generates the disability. For example, wheelchair users may not have access to toilets because of failures in the design of facilities. Conversely, consideration of impaired people in the design of buildings, transport services, and so forth can enable them. In a similar way, equipment can contribute to disability. For example, urine or stoma bags that leak produce incontinence.

HANDICAPS—PRINCIPLES AND PRACTICAL ISSUES

Clinical practices directed at survival and recovery focus on interfering with the destructive natural history of pathologic processes. Humans are both physical and social beings. Often, physical, psychological, and social issues are inextricably linked. Rehabilitation medicine is holistic and is directed at the physical, psychological, and social impacts of the disabling pathology. People who live with such pathology require holistic approaches because these impacts, which are interconnected, affect health, function, and quality of life.

Handicaps are imposed by people. This can occur in a variety of ways. Avoiding, disempowering, and treating people maliciously because of their abnormalities are all very common behaviors. A variety of legislation has emerged in countries around the world to counter this behavior and enforce equity. Examples include the Americans with Disabilities Act of 1990 and Great Britain's Disabilities Discrimination Act of 1995. Contemporary Western societies formally reject invalidation of people with disabilities.

Ignorance also encourages handicaps. If people are not given appropriate or complete information for effective self-management, their failure to cope is not surprising. Physiologically normal people typically take health and normality for granted. People who acquire disabling pathologies develop problems to which they may never have been exposed or with which they have had no experience. When information is lacking, superstitions, old wives' tales, or other nonsense tends to fill the void. For example,

- A 60-year-old woman with multiple sclerosis presented with constipation and urinary frequency. The urinary frequency followed the patient's self-treatment of her constipation, because she believed that increasing her fluid intake to exceed 8 liters per day would cure her bowel disorder.
- A 50-year-old patient with multiple sclerosis suffered with urgency and urge incontinence because she believed her anticholinergic therapy could produce urinary retention that would cause her whole body to become edematous.

Education is very important in the rehabilitation of disabled people. Therefore, teaching is an integral part of neurorehabilitation services.

There is a powerful mechanism for handicap that cannot be changed through legislation. It is the prejudice disabled people have about their own conditions [3]. This prejudice can arise from cultural or deep-rooted beliefs. For example, a 50-year-old female patient with multiple sclerosis presented reporting that she isolated herself in her home because she felt *ashamed* to have others know she had to rush to the lavatory because of urgency.

Another example is that of a 21-year-old woman with multiple sclerosis who presented for a full rehabilitation medical assessment denying that she had any bowel-associated problems. Further direct questioning revealed that she was incontinent of feces at least once each week. On being challenged, she stated that she thought such a subject was improper to discuss with a doctor.

The latter example highlights what may be a general phenomenon. In 1982, Leigh and Turnberg [4] found that, even among patients who presented to a gastroenterology service with diarrhea and fecal incontinence, fewer than 50% of them were prepared to reveal information spontaneously about their incontinence.

It is worth noting that some handicaps are produced through legislation. Excluding women from voting handicapped them because they were unable to directly contribute to the democratic process. This exclusion did not stand the test of time. Preventing blind people from driving cars may well endure. Not all handicapping legislation is bad; however, with advances in technology, future legislation may overturn what is vital for safety in today's societies. With advances in medicine and technology, many handicaps for disabled people eventually may be eliminated.

One must appreciate that other people, too, can experience handicaps as a result of a person's disabling pathology. Although for many basic functions, independent capabilities are expected and desired, interdependence rather than independence is the norm. Handicaps obtained by association may be referred to as indirect handicaps. In rehabilitation medical services, relief of distress for others and prevention of unnecessary burdens on social and other services are associated aims.

Handicaps may be reflected in any personal, social, or societal context. These include areas as wide-ranging as nutrition, sexual activity, housework, parenting, social relations, residential placement, employment, traveling, and dependence on health services. This list inevitably is incomplete. The following sections discuss representative issues in these areas as they concern individuals with bladder and bowel problems.

NUTRITION

Ideas about nutrition and its relationship to bowel and bladder functions may lead people to follow diets that are beneficial. However, all too often these ideas are foolish or detrimental. A young woman with multiple sclerosis was convinced that her bladder and bowel symptoms were caused by allergies. Consequently, she gave up eating virtually everything except rice. She persisted with this diet until she became seriously malnourished.

Another young woman with multiple sclerosis spent so much money on vitamins and minerals that she believed would cure her upset bladder that her financial situation became dire.

SEXUAL ACTIVITY

People often fear that bladder or bowel problems will adversely affect their sex lives. Where sexuality is concerned, practical, emotional, and symbolic issues typically are interconnected and are sometimes difficult to disentangle. This topic is discussed in more detail in Chapter 7.

HOUSEWORK

Bladder and bowel problems may not have a direct effect on a person's ability to do housework but may contribute to pressures on family members or social services in this area. Time taken to assist a partner with toileting may interfere with housework and add to it considerably. The additional work, and the impossibility of asking someone else to do it, may force a partner to give up employment.

PARENTING

Bladder and bowel problems can have practical effects on parenting. Visits to the park can be curtailed if no toilet is nearby. For an otherwise mobile parent, running may not be acceptable if it induces "leakage." Even quite small children may become involved in helping parents to or from a toilet.

Some children find themselves helping their parents in even more intimate ways. Children may believe they are parenting their parent, which effectively means they have lost a parent and must grow up too fast. This can have deleterious effects on their relationships and on the psychological welfare of both parties. Children should be protected from having to assume such a reversed role until they are adults themselves.

A person's ability to command respect as a parent may be undermined by his or her own reduced self-respect. Being incontinent often diminishes self-respect. As a result, people try to hide their disabilities from their children. When this fails, parents may believe they are failing in their primary parenting tasks. In such situations, social service agencies may need to become involved.

SOCIAL RELATIONS

Being unable to sit through a conversation, film, or child's school performance because of toileting needs may disrupt family life. Sometimes, the individual's partner finds the preoccupation with bladder and bowel care more of a problem than does the person with the disability. The partner may be the one who presents the problem to the doctor.

If a parent or the home smells because of incontinence, the child may be embarrassed. This embarrassment may discourage the child from bringing friends home or encourage the child to leave the family home at the first available opportunity. Conversely, the child may feel the weight of responsibility to care for the disabled parent, which constrains the child from establishing an independent social life.

When bowel management requires considerable time, a decision may need to be made as to whether this time should be taken from family and social time or from work time. Often, such decisions are made by default. Partners commonly avoid discussing issues involving intimate functions. Furthermore, men commonly value their work over their contributions toward other aspects of family welfare. This may have adverse effects on the family.

Sometimes disabilities may provoke violence due to frustration. For example,

- A woman was furious with her disabled husband because he always had "bowel accidents" on the rare occasions when she went out. She believed he did it deliberately as an expression of his anger at her having an independent life and to prevent her from going out any more. In a counseling session, she reported that she "exploded" and dragged him across the carpet, inducing carpet burns.

RESIDENTIAL PLACEMENT

In 1965, Miller et al. [5] stated that "control of excretory functions is the most likely single factor that determines a patient's admission to hospital." This is likely to be as true today of nursing home placements. With the increasing employment of women outside the home, the migration of working people and students away from their parents, and the increasing dependence of society on statutory services for care of incontinent people, resources are more and more likely to be strained.

The success of bowel or bladder management may be the factor that determines whether some disabled people can continue to live in their own homes. Incontinence management adds considerably to the costs of care because of needs for consumables, such as incontinence pads, catheters, laundry, and labor. Therefore, extra charges may be levied by care institutions, limiting choices for residence.

Personal assistants may interpret patients' demands for toileting as exploitative or an attempt to exert power over or exact revenge against them or against the forces that made the patient disabled. Such interpretations may be entirely wrong. Interpersonal skills may be compromised by associated cognitive deficits or communication impairments. Education of assistants (professional and informal) about the consequences of neurologic diseases on communication may be beneficial to everyone concerned.

EMPLOYMENT

People commonly are identified by their work. Loss of work has wide-ranging implications, from loss of income to loss of respect. Employment may be undermined by bladder or bowel disabilities in a variety of ways. For example,

- A 47-year-old man who developed tetraparesis from cervical spine osteomyelitis had to give up full-time work as a lawyer, because his daily bowel management unpredictably could take up so much time that he was uncertain he could keep morning appointments.
- A 30-year-old receptionist with multiple sclerosis lost her job because she constantly smelled of urine.
- A 32-year-old teacher with multiple sclerosis gave up work because urgency and running to the toilet so frequently prevented her from properly supervising the children in her charge.

Employment may be affected if a person feels worthless or dirty. Although society no longer invalidates people because of disability, patients may invalidate themselves. In practical terms, this attitude may discourage disabled people from continuing with employment. However, a different reason may be declared for giving up employment:

• A woman reported quitting work in a bank; she could not manage any more, because she could not predict when she would need to go to the toilet. On further inquiry, she said she had experienced a "near accident" in the toilets, which so upset her that she lost the will to battle against the management's unjust attempts to terminate her contract.

TRAVEL

Both short-distance and long-distance travel may be affected by bowel or bladder disabilities. Some people need to plan journeys from toilet to toilet. Other people do not venture out for fear of accidents. Shopping trips and visits to distant relatives may be affected equally.

One accident may be sufficient to prevent an individual from going out for years. On the other hand, the disabilities may be useful pegs on which to hang a reluctance to travel, which has other roots. Obtaining information about aids, such as urine bags or car toilets, may be sufficient to enable some people to find a new ability to travel; for others, providing such information may draw attention to the fact that deeper reasons exist for not wishing to leave the house or locality.

Many people with neurogenic bowel or bladder problems have associated disabilities, such as visual disturbances. Often, these people do not have the capability of independent car travel. Reliance on public transport limits the ability to address toileting needs.

DEPENDENCE ON HEALTH SERVICES

Glickman et al. [6] surveyed general practitioners caring for postrehabilitation spinal cord injury patients; the survey revealed that, in the previous 12 months, 71% of the patients presented with urologic problems and 50% with colonic problems. Annual rates of consultation with primary care services among these patients greatly exceeded the national norms. Bowel and bladder issues featured strongly among the reasons for the contacts.

PSYCHOLOGICAL ISSUES

Acquired incontinence may encourage people to feel as though they have returned to childhood and may call up all the associated issues of dependence and powerlessness. However, the "authorities" are different, in some cases being partners, children, associates, and even statutory services personnel. Also, incontinence may provoke changes in body image, sometimes even producing beliefs about bodily disintegration.

Inevitably, the quality of any person's life depends on how that person interprets and evaluates the symptoms, disabilities, and handicaps. This is determined not only by the physical and social circumstances, but also by the character and psychological makeup of the individual. The spectra for interpretation can be very wide.

In the immediate aftermath of a significant loss, people generally feel that their worlds have collapsed. People need time to grieve for losses; a 2-year adjustment period is considered common before individuals feel that life is worth living even with the losses. Losing normal bowel and bladder functions is such a loss. Moreover, individuals still have to contend with the anxieties, frustrations, and depression caused by the need to live with disabilities and handicaps.

A survey of bowel dysfunction in 115 spinal cord injury patients conducted by Glickman and Kamm [7] revealed that bowel dysfunctions were considered by these patients to be among their most distressing disabilities. These disabilities produced major psychological problems. Patients with the greatest bowel disabilities also scored highest on the Hospital Anxiety and Depression Scale [8].

BEHAVIORAL REACTIONS

Behavioral responses to the problems may be anything from stoic or phlegmatic to hysterical. Some individuals may choose to exploit their disabilities for secondary gains. Sometimes, communication difficulties prevent patients from seeking help appropriately.

Some people feel inhibited from discussing issues of such an intimate nature as bladder or bowel problems, because they do not know respectable words to convey their stories. Some people resent having to resort to euphemisms with childish overtones to avoid using "offensive" language. Clinical terms may not have shared meanings. To facilitate the consultation, doctors may need to take the initiative by providing words and clarifying their meanings.

CONCLUSION

The breadth of the consequences of neurogenic bowel and bladder dysfunctions on patients appears to be matched only by their depth for given individuals and their families. Approaches to minimizing the impacts at any level can contribute greatly to patients' health and welfare.

REFERENCES

1. World Health Organization. International classification of impairments, disabilities and handicaps: a manual of classification relating to the consequences of disease. Geneva: World Health Organization, 1980.
2. Glickman S, McKimm J. Disability and Rehabilitation: A Medical Tutor's Handbook. London: British Brain and Spine Foundation, 1996.
3. Segal JC. Counselling People with Multiple Sclerosis and Their Families. In H Davis, L Fallowfield (eds), Counselling and Communication in Health Care. Chichester, UK: Wiley, 1991.
4. Leigh RJ, Turnberg LA. Faecal incontinence: the unvoiced symptom. Lancet 1982;1(8285): 1349–1351.
5. Miller H, Simpson CA, Yeates WK. Bladder dysfunction in multiple sclerosis. BMJ 1965;1:1265–1269.

6. Glickman S, Dalrymple-Hay M, Phillips GF. Spinal cord injury after rehabilitation: the general practice experience. Br J Ther Rehab 1996;3:168–171.
7. Glickman S, Kamm MA. Bowel dysfunction in spinal-cord-injury patients. Lancet 1996;347:
1651–1653.
8. Zigmond AS, Snaith RP. The hospital anxiety and depression scale. Acta Psychiatr Scand
1983;67:361–370.

7
Impact of Neurologic Disability on Sex and Relationships

Barbara J. Chandler

Sexuality is one of the most complex aspects of human life. Sexual expression is dependent on functioning anatomic and physiologic systems that are influenced by cognitive and emotional processes. Annon [1] has described sex as a truly psychosomatic process. Sexual development starts in utero, in keeping with the genetic constitution of the fetus. As the hormonal environment develops, the anatomic characteristics denoting maleness or femaleness emerge. Sexual development at this stage may be compromised by rare disorders of genetic makeup, by endocrine abnormalities, or by exogenous toxins. At birth, a gender is assigned and, in the vast majority of people, will be the gender they assume throughout their lives. From this point, sexual development is described by Bancroft [2] as continuing along three main strands:

1. Sexual differentiation, which started in utero
2. Sexual responsiveness
3. The capacity for intimate dyadic relationships

Dyadic refers to the unique relationship between two individuals and encompasses both sexual and nonsexual interactions.

These strands become integrated during adolescence to form mature adults who should feel confident and at ease with their gender and sexual identity and should be able to form intimate relationships that allow full expression of their sexuality. Abuse, disease, disability, and psychological or social stress may compromise this developmental process or produce morbidity in sexual and relationship functioning in the mature adult.

Given the complex interplay of physical, cognitive, emotional, and social factors in sexual expression, the high prevalence of sexual difficulties is not surprising. Using standardized measures of sexual and relationship functioning amongst a population attending their general practitioners in Britain, Rust et al. identified a prevalence of 20% for sexual dysfunction and 30% for relationship dysfunction [3]. Because of the intensely personal and private nature of sex, patients are reticent in presenting sexual problems, and health care professionals are reticent in screening for such problems [4–7].

69

SEXUAL EXPRESSION IN ADULT LIFE

Sexual Response

The pioneering work of Masters and Johnson [8] in the 1960s allowed an understanding of the physiology of human sexual response. They divided sexual response into four phases: excitement, plateau, orgasm, and resolution. Any such division is somewhat arbitrary, but their working definition has proved valuable in understanding some aspects of sexual dysfunction. Difficulties in the excitement phase manifest as vaginismus, dyspareunia, and erectile dysfunction, whereas difficulties in the orgasmic phase include premature ejaculation, delayed ejaculation and orgasm, and anorgasmia. Completion of the sexual response cycle is not essential for a satisfying and "complete" sex life. Stanley [9] proposed that sexual response be viewed as a ladder that each individual ascends and descends, going only as far as desired in a sexual encounter (Figure 7.1). Except at the stage of imminent orgasm, individuals may comfortably move up and down the rungs of the ladder and enjoy the sensations and emotions at each level. On different occasions, they may move to different points on the ladder and move at different rates. No obligation exists to achieve a particular rung. This conceptualization can be a useful tool in treating individuals and couples with sexual difficulties related to "performance."

One of the myths of sexual behavior is the concept of "the norm." The norm of sexual responsiveness within a dyadic relationship is probably unique to each couple, but their perception of the norm may enhance or detract from their sex life, depending on whether the reality of their experience is in accordance with their expectations.

Sexual Arousal

Bancroft [2] described a state of central arousability that determines the individual's capacity for reacting to an appropriate stimulus with a sexual response. Sexual desire depends on the level of arousability and is influenced by other factors, such as mood, cognitive processes (including internal imagery), level of fatigue, and the social context or environment. A complex interplay is found between neurotransmitters and the endocrine system, which affects both sexual desire and sexual response. Changes in sexual desire occur in association with damage to cognitive processes, as in traumatic brain injury or degenerative neurologic conditions and with the use of drugs—for example, dopaminergic agents used in the treatment of Parkinson's disease. Dopamine is undoubtedly important in sexual functioning, both as a direct neurotransmitter and through its effect on prolactin levels. However, the effect of dopaminergic agents on the sexual drive of patients with Parkinson's disease is not consistent, and other factors, including the individual's previous sexual experiences and current state of well-being, as well as the functioning of the dyadic relationship, are also important in determining their sexual interest [10–12]. Changes in sexual desire or arousal present a problem if the individual or couple is concerned about the change. Low sexual desire is a common dysfunction, particularly among women, and is frequently associated with lack of sexual arousal and orgasm [13–15]. Low sexual desire may be unmasked by the restoration of function in

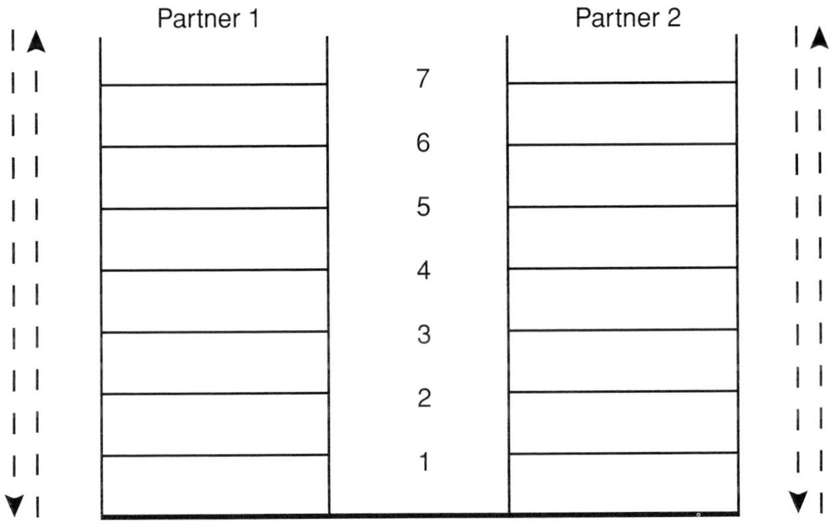

Place on ladder	Cognitions/emotions	Physical change
7	Relaxation, somnolence	Reversal of changes
6	Orgasm	Orgasmic changes
5	Intense arousal, imminent orgasm	Full erection/lubrication
4	Increasing arousal	Full erection/lubrication
3	Moderate sexual arousal	Partial erection/start of lubrication
2	Increasing pleasure	Minimal genital sensation
1	Pleasure in physical contact	None
Ground	No sexual thoughts or feelings	None

Figure 7.1   Sexual response ladders in a dyadic relationship. (Adapted with permission from E Stanley. Dealing with fear of failure. BMJ 1981;282:1281–1283.)

one partner. For example, a man with erectile dysfunction may report how supportive and understanding his partner has been for the duration of this problem. Restoration of his potency may force the couple to recognize that his partner has low sexual interest and does not wish to resume penetrative sex. Successful treatment of a partner may so disturb the dynamics of the relationship that significant difficulties arise within the relationship (Figure 7.2).

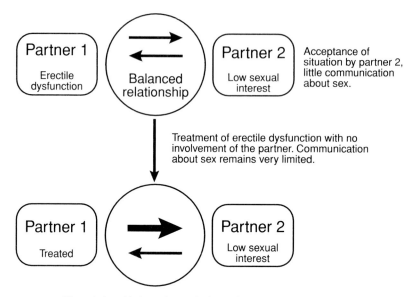

Figure 7.2   Interplay of sexual functioning and the dyadic relationship.

Dyadic Relationship

One of the goals of sexual development within adolescence and early adult life is the acquisition of skills to allow the formation of intimate dyadic relationships. These relationships change and mature throughout life, and sexual expression generally occurs within this setting. Other than in masturbation and fantasy, sex is experienced within a relationship [16]. Indeed, the couple has been described as the true unit of sexual expression [17].

To understand the dynamics of sexual expression within a relationship, three distinct but interactive components must be considered:

1. Partner 1
2. Partner 2
3. The relationship

This triad of sexual expression is illustrated in Figure 7.3.

In addressing the sexual problems with which one or both partners may present, these three parameters can be examined and treatment planned according to the degree to which each is contributing to the dysfunction. The interaction of these variables is influenced by external factors, such as social environment and finances, and by internal factors, such as illness. The addition of neurologic disease or injury may cause a major disruption to the dynamics of the system, resulting in dysfunction of one, two, or all three components. Sex is only one form of communication

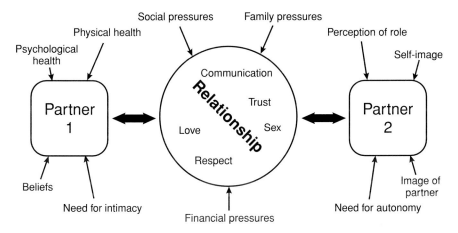

Figure 7.3 Triad of sexual expression. Each partner experiences the physical and psychological factors illustrated, and these contribute to the dynamic equilibrium. The equilibrium can be altered. For example, ill health in partner 1 may result in financial pressures, role changes, and alteration in the autonomy and desire for intimacy of both partners. On the other hand, ill health might increase the bond of love and respect, resulting in increased communication and intimacy. If change results in a dysfunctional situation, intervention may be required to restore the equilibrium. See also Figure 7.5.

within a relationship. Relying on sex as the only means of intimate communication places too great a demand on it, and a sexual dysfunction can then result in a serious relationship problem. Spence commented that, in the management of sexual problems, "Failure to consider the interactional aspects of sexual behavior, the couple's general relationship and the influence of the family and sociocultural environment is likely to result in failure to tackle some important sources of influence over sexual functioning and hence less effective therapy" [18].

Frank et al. [17] illustrated the complex interplay of sexual experience and the functioning of the dyadic relationship in a study of American couples. One hundred volunteers from various predominantly middle-class groups whose marriages were "working" were studied. Forty percent of the men reported some sexual dysfunction (e.g., erectile or ejaculatory problems), and 50% reported some sexual difficulty (e.g., difficulty relaxing, being attracted to someone other than their partner). Among the female partners, 63% described some dysfunction (e.g., arousal or orgasmic problems) and 77% reported some difficulties. In 5–10% of cases, it became apparent that one partner thought the marriage was working and was not aware of the marital distress experienced by the spouse. As the authors suggested, caution is needed in interpreting the results, because the numbers are small and the study is based on a self-selected group. Nevertheless, this study highlights the following points:

1. Sexual dysfunction can exist within a functioning dyadic relationship.
2. When a sexual problem is being examined, the individual's partner and the functioning of the relationship should be considered.
3. Sexual or relationship difficulties may be perceived by only one partner.

In a study of patients seen in general practice in London, Golombok et al. [19] also found a high incidence of sexual dysfunction in the context of sexual relationships that the partners described as satisfying. The actual incidence of sexual dysfunction is therefore a poor indicator of the number of people who are likely to request help with the problem. A similar phenomenon is evident among people with neurologic disability. For example, although at least 50% of people with multiple sclerosis experience a change in their sex lives, not all are concerned about this; therefore, not all require help. Szasz et al. [20] estimated that a minimum of one in four people with multiple sclerosis is concerned about his or her sexual dysfunction and may require help. A similar figure was found in a study among people with neurologic disability due to various different causes [21].

Sexual Expression

Sexual expression is one of the most complex human functions. It involves the recognition of erotic stimuli, whether external or a product of internal imagery; the peripheral response of the body, with the visible changes of sexual excitement; monitoring of this response; and the emotional consequences of sexual arousal. Within the context of the dyadic relationship, the individual must also monitor the response of his or her partner in physical and emotional terms. Emotions, cognitions, and behaviors are influenced by past experience, prevailing conditions, attitudes, expectations, and fears. Bancroft [2] simplified the approach to this complex system by examining it in terms of a linked circle of events—the psychosomatic circle of sex. The circle may be entered at any point, and it may also be broken at any point, resulting in various manifestations of dysfunction. An adapted version of his original description is shown in Figure 7.4. The physical elements of the circle are described elsewhere in this book (see Chapters 4 and 5).

Cognition, Behavior, and Emotions

Thoughts about sex are open to many influences, such as upbringing, religious beliefs, education, perceived social norms, attitudes, expectations, fears, and past experience. Disorders of cognition that may accompany progressive conditions (e.g., multiple sclerosis) or trauma (e.g., head injury) may therefore have a major impact on sexual expression.

Anxiety

Anxiety alone may not inevitably impair sexual response, and some studies have suggested an enhancement of arousal in response to certain anxiety-provoking situations [2]. However, anxiety has been well recognized as contributing to the development of some sexual dysfunctions, such as sexual aversion disorders, vaginismus, erectile dysfunction, or dyspareunia [18]. In treating such disorders, reduction of anxiety plays a major role in the therapy [8, 22].

Barlow [23] proposed that the various components of anxiety may affect sexual responsiveness and performance in different ways. The physiologic compo-

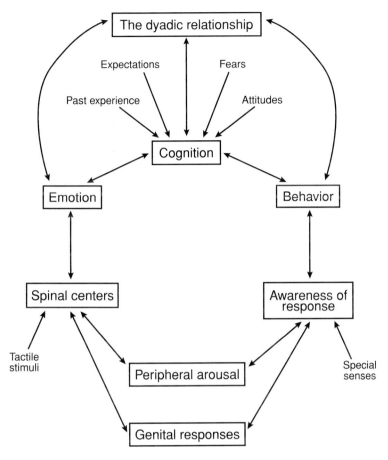

Figure 7.4 Psychosomatic circle of sex in neurologic disability. (Adapted with permission from J Bancroft. Human Sexuality and Its Problems. Edinburgh, UK: Churchill Livingstone, 1989.)

nents, such as increased heart rate and blood pressure, also occur during sexual arousal. Anxiety may therefore facilitate this part of the sexual response cycle. However, the cognitive and emotional components of anxiety may inhibit sexual responsiveness through the cognitive pathways of sexual arousal.

Anxiety may be instrumental in maintaining and initiating a sexual problem. For example, one episode of failure may generate a fear of failure on the next occasion that the couple make love. This fear of failing to perform adequately may result in further failure. The ensuing anxiety may become so severe as to result in avoidance of the stressful situation. This behavior may then be interpreted in a variety of ways by the partner, leading to possible accusations of lack of love, infidelity, and so on, that have a direct impact on the functioning of the relationship.

In the context of chronic disease or disability, the individual may have fears about specific issues, such as incontinence, pain, spasticity, or precipitation of a catastrophic event.

Pain

Disorders of the sexual response cycle due to either physical or psychological factors may result in pain on intercourse. During the excitement phase, the uterus increases in size and rises in the pelvis, pulling the cervix out of the way of the thrusting penis. The upper two-thirds of the vagina balloon, and the vagina becomes lubricated by a transudate. If vaginal entry is attempted when these changes of the excitement phase have not occurred, discomfort or pain may be experienced. This discomfort may generate anxiety about sexual intercourse and result in the establishment of a dysfunctional cycle. Pain may also be caused by a specific disease process; for example, superficial dyspareunia may be due to perineal dysesthesia in multiple sclerosis, or pain may be caused by moving inflamed joints in arthritis [24].

Fear of Precipitating Major Illness

Fear that sexual activity will cause further deterioration or precipitate a specific event, such as myocardial infarction, is common during the recovery and rehabilitation period [25]. In their original laboratory work, Masters and Johnson [8] recorded marked changes in heart rate and blood pressure during sexual activity. On average, the heart rate increased to 100–175 beats per minute during the plateau phase of the sexual response cycle and to 110–180 beats per minute during the orgasmic phase. In males, systolic blood pressure rose by 40–100 mm Hg and diastolic pressure by 20–50 mm Hg; the increase was slightly less marked in females. However, these rather alarming figures may not reflect the changes outside the laboratory; Bancroft [2] suggested that the added stress or excitement of the laboratory situation may have contributed to an artificial elevation of values. More recent research suggests that cardiac changes during sex with an established partner are of modest severity and are similar to the changes that occur on climbing two flights of stairs [26] or completing stage 1 of the Bruce Exercise Test [27]. Such information can be incorporated into a cardiac rehabilitation program, and the reassurance it provides may prevent the development of anxiety-triggered sexual dysfunctions. However, sexual activity with a new partner in unfamiliar surroundings such as a hotel room, perhaps associated with a heavy meal or excessive alcohol intake, may result in greater and possibly damaging cardiovascular changes [2, 27].

Expectations

Unrealistic expectations may lead to sexual and relationship dysfunction. These expectations may be generated by myths the individual or couple have received from childhood, their peer group, and the media. Some commonly held beliefs that can lead to perceptions of failure and dysfunction are shown in Table 7.1.

All of these myths can lead to unrealistic expectations and a cycle of failure [9, 28–30]. Spence [18] listed some additional erroneous ideas that can interfere with sexual functioning and apply particularly to the dyadic relationship and to women (Table 7.2).

Table 7.1   Examples of myths in sexual expression

1. The size of the penis and the tightness of the vagina determine the amount of pleasure a couple experiences when making love.
2. Physical contact must always lead to sexual expression.
3. Sexual activity should always involve sexual intercourse.
4. Sexual activity involves a fixed path that should always end in simultaneous orgasm.
5. A man cannot be in love and fail to get an erection with his partner.
6. Men should know instinctively how to be sexually competent.
7. Sex must be natural and spontaneous.
8. "Handicapped people have no sexual needs or desires . . . or have perverted or excessive sexual desires" [45].

Sources: Adapted from B Zilbergeld. Men and Sex. London: Fontana, 1978; W Guirgius. Sex Therapy with Couples. In D Hooper, W Dryden (eds), Couple Therapy: A Handbook. Buckingham, UK: Open University Press, 1991; and C DeLoach, BG Greer. Adjustment to Severe Physical Disability: A Metamorphosis. New York: McGraw-Hill, 1981.

Table 7.2   Myths concerning relationships and women

1. All couples have sexual intercourse several times per week.
2. If sex is not good, something must be wrong with the relationship.
3. A woman should always take part in sex if her partner makes approaches.
4. A woman should always be capable of intercourse, even as a passive recipient.
5. Respectable women should not masturbate or use fantasy.
6. Respectable women do not communicate their sexual needs and preferences to their partners.

Source: Adapted with permission from S Spence. Psychosexual Therapy: A Cognitive Behavioural Approach. London: Chapman & Hall, 1991.

As Spence [18] commented, the women's movement has caused a shift away from some of these attitudes, but the new liberation has brought along some new myths that may have equally negative effects (Table 7.3).

Many of these myths can be particularly damaging for couples with disabilities. Changes in functional ability may necessitate a change in emphasis away from penetrative sex or orgasm. The need to catheterize or perform an intracavernosal injection may take away the spontaneity of sexual expression. If one partner usually initiated sex, it may now be necessary for the other partner to initiate. Depending on how tightly held these beliefs are, the individual or couple may have varying degrees of difficulty adjusting.

Failure can only be defined in terms of the perception of success. Unrealistic ideas of what constitutes a successful sex life can result in a cycle of failure. Stanley [31] described the concept of successful and "normal" sex that many couples present to her as their goal: "An erect penis entering a lubricated vagina giving orgasm in both partners, preferably simultaneously, is a typical picture. Anything short of this achievement is perceived as failure." This goal clearly represents an amalgamation of some of the myths outlined in Table 7.1. As the author explains,

Table 7.3   New myths held by women

1. The woman must be able to achieve orgasm.
2. The woman must initiate sex with her partner.
3. The woman must give her partner plenty of feedback about her sexual likes and dislikes.

"if this is the expectation of success in a long term relationship, there will be many experiences of failure." Enabling individuals to explore their perceptions of sexuality and what they understand as "normal" or "successful" sex is an important aspect of treating sexual dysfunction. This is particularly the case when acquired disability requires the individual or couple to adapt to a different pattern of sexual expression.

Past Experience

In treating people with sex and relationship problems after neurologic disease or trauma, ascertaining how they functioned before the onset of disability is important. For example, erectile dysfunction secondary to multiple sclerosis used to be treated with intracavernosal injections, and more recently with an oral erectogenic agent, but neither of these treatments will restore the patient's sex life if a breakdown of communication and trust has occurred in the partnership. Indeed, studies have shown that one of the factors predicting resumption of a satisfactory sex life after a major insult (acquired disease or injury) is good quality of sex life and good functioning of the dyadic relationship before the event [32–34]. Paradoxically, those relationships formed before the onset of disease or trauma may be more adversely affected than those formed subsequently because of the number of adjustments that must be made [35–37]. Mona et al. [38] found that sexual self-esteem was lower in individuals who acquired their disability in later life than in individuals who acquired their disability at a younger age. This finding supports the hypothesis proposed by Cole [28] that "notions of sexual self" may be interrupted by acquired disability and result in adjustment problems.

Other, hitherto undisclosed traumas may have occurred in the past that surface when another stress is added in the form of acquired disability. Sexual abuse, rape, or a traumatic childhood may affect the ability of the individual to form an intimate relationship and respond sexually [39, 40]. These influences on the cognitive pathways of sexual responsiveness may need to be addressed before the issues surrounding the disability can be approached.

Attitude

In his book *Stigma: The Management of Spoiled Identity*, Goffman [41] states, "we believe the person with a stigma is not quite human. On this assumption we exercise varieties of discrimination, through which we effectively, if often unthinkingly, reduce his life chances." A clear example is seen in regard to attitudes toward the sexual expression of people with disabilities. The idea that people with disabilities do not have sexual feelings and should not attempt a sexual relationship still exists [38, 42–45]. The attitude of the health care professional may influence the individual's willingness to present a sexual difficulty or seek information. An inquiry by a health care professional and implicit permission to discuss sexual issues may in itself be therapeutic [1, 20]. On the other hand, a dismissive approach or a misinterpretation of the needs of the patient may damage an already compromised self-esteem and fail to address the problem [5].

INFLUENCE OF NEUROLOGIC DISABILITY ON SEX AND RELATIONSHIPS

Neurologic disease has an obvious impact on sexual functioning. In adolescence and early adult life, it affects how individuals form intimate relationships and how they start to explore their sexuality. This impact stems from basic difficulties, such as how to meet friends when major mobility problems exist, to having the confidence to make friends when self-image may be challenged by apparent and hidden impairments.

At a slightly later stage, the onset of disease or disability affects the functioning of the individual, his or her partner, and their relationship; for those not in a relationship, it affects the ability to meet potential partners and establish a liaison. The marital dyad has been described as the most important social context within which the psychological aspects of chronic illness are managed [46]. The outcome of the disability with regard to sexual functioning should therefore be viewed from the perspective of each partner and the relationship.

Adolescents

One of the prerequisites for developing a close relationship is the opportunity to meet with other people and, in particular, with a peer group. In this way the adolescent gains skills and confidence in social interaction. Studies of physically disabled adolescents have shown these young people to be limited in terms of social contact. In a study of young people with myelomeningocele and cerebral palsy, 70% of those with disabilities stated that they were lonely and had limited social lives. More than 60% of this group did not see their friends outside school, and 50% had never visited their friends at home [47]. Limited mobility may make the individual dependent on parents for transport to and from friends and places of socialization. Social isolation has been described as a phenomenon among severely disabled young people. Hallum [48] commented, "Because of the triad of prejudice, stereotype and discrimination, social attitudes toward people with physical impairments create barriers beyond those caused by the physical limitations alone." In another study of adolescents with myelomeningocele, Borjeson and Lagergren [49] found that 46% of the young people studied felt that their social contacts were very poor or that they had no affinity with their peers at school.

Hallum noted that the attitude that young people with disabilities do not wish to form intimate relationships is still prevalent. Despite this, the young people themselves continue to develop sexually and to have hopes and aspirations with regard to future relationships. In a study of teenagers with spina bifida, Dorner [50] found that 65% hoped to marry, and approximately one-half thought they would be able to have children; similar figures have been found in other studies [51].

If young people with disabilities are to meet the developmental milestones of sexuality, they need appropriate education and a person to whom they can turn for advice. Sex education programs must be adapted to meet the individual needs of someone with a disability [52]. In designing a sex education video for young adults with spina bifida, Blackburn et al. [53] ascertained that individuals wished to know about urinary and bowel management in sexual relationships, genetic risks, contraception, penile appliances, comfortable positions for lovemaking, and methods of sexual fulfillment other than penetrative sex. Clearly, some of these issues are not covered in the usual school sex education program. Many queries and difficulties become apparent only after the individual has left school; the individual may then wish to seek help from their doctors or other health care professionals. How the request for information and help is handled may vary considerably depending on the interests of the person from whom the information was requested. In the future, services may be more uniform if the recommendations of Lewin and King [54], that sexual medicine should be an integral part of many medical and surgical specialties, are accepted. At present, services are fragmented. In a survey of British rehabilitation physicians, 50% expressed dissatisfaction with the services they were able to offer for sex and relationship problems, and 39% indicated dissatisfaction with the services they could access. Despite this, 90% stated that they felt this area of health care should be addressed within rehabilitation medicine [55]. In a discussion of the sexual health of adolescents with cystic fibrosis, Sawyer [7] commented, "Care of the disease is absolutely necessary but of itself it is not sufficient if we wish to achieve success in terms of quality as well as length of life."

Partner with an Acquired Disability

Sexuality is a fundamental aspect of all people, whatever their level of physical or cognitive functioning. To illustrate the way in which acquired disability can affect sexual functioning and the continuance of intimate relationships, three specific examples have been chosen:

1. A traumatic physical condition—spinal injury
2. A traumatic condition with marked effects on cognition—head injury
3. A degenerative condition with physical and cognitive sequelae—Parkinson's disease

Spinal Injury

Spinal injury results in an immediate disruption of the psychosomatic circle, breaking the link between cognitive processes and physiologic response (see Figure 7.4). Spinal cord injury is more common among men, and more studies of sexual function have been carried out in this group. Erectile and ejaculatory capability after injury are determined by the level and completeness of the lesion.

Among patients with complete lesions, reflex erectile capability is more likely to be preserved with high upper motor neuron lesions. The incidence ranges from 100% erectile capability in patients with lesions at the cervical level to no erectile capability in some patients with lower lesions, particularly if the lesions were of the lower motor neuron type. Psychogenic erections are more likely to be preserved in cases of incomplete lesion. In a small proportion of patients, psychogenic erections may be preserved in the absence of reflex erections; this finding suggests the possibility of a different mechanism of erection, a concept supported by animal work (see Chapter 5) [2, 56, 57]. The consequence of spinal cord injury in women is analogous, with the effect on vaginal lubrication and orgasm being determined by the type of lesion [58]. Evidence suggests that the outcome for restoration of the individual's sex life is better if sex is approached early rather than late in the process of rehabilitation [34]. This involves acknowledging to patients that problems do occur as a consequence of spinal cord injury and presenting the opportunity for patients and their partners, if patients are currently in a relationship, to raise their concerns [59–61].

One consequence of spinal cord injury is that the patient may spend a lengthy time in a hospital or rehabilitation unit. During this period, many procedures are carried out on parts of the body that under normal circumstances would be considered private or personal. In particular, the genitalia, instead of being part of sexual arousal, become part of a bladder or hygiene regime. The concept of a person with disabilities as asexual may begin in the process of rehabilitation [44, 45]. A publication about sexuality produced by the Spinal Cord Injury Association encourages individuals to set about the task of reclaiming their bodies—that is, to take control over when and how intimate procedures are carried out [62]. This is an important goal for the re-establishment of self-esteem and the perception of the sexual self. A further part of sexual rehabilitation is for the individual and his or her partner to explore which parts of the body now respond to erotic stimuli. Individuals with spinal injury report that different areas of their body become responsive, depending on the level of the lesion. Some people describe orgasmic experiences in the absence of any sensation from the genitalia [62]. Some couples automatically begin this process of exploration and discovery; others may require "permission" from a health care professional to move away from their concept of "normal" sexual activity. They may also need time to grieve for the loss of their previous sex life in addition to the other losses that result from spinal injury. Despite the major disruption to normal physiologic functioning caused by spinal cord injury, individuals can establish fulfilling sex lives with their partners [63].

Traumatic Brain Injury

Traumatic brain injury is well recognized as causing profound and often destructive effects on the family and social network. Increased depression and anxiety on the part of the spouse is common and may persist [64–66]. Sexual problems after injury are also common, although no consistent pattern of sexual dysfunction exists [67, 68]. Dysfunction may result from factors within the individual, within the partner, or within the relationship. The most damaging deficits for sexual expression within a dyadic relationship appear to be those affecting cognitive functioning. Factors affecting the brain-injured individual include depression, anxiety, low motivation, lack of a partner, and, in a small number, reduced testosterone level [68, 69]. As a result, sexual desire and frequency of intercourse may be reduced. O'Carroll et al. [70], in a study of people who had been admitted to the hospital for a minimum of 24 hours after a closed head injury over a 15-year period, found that 50% of the males had scores in the dysfunctional range on a standardized assessment tool of sexual functioning (the Golombok Rust Inventory of Sexual Satisfaction, GRISS [71]). The study also suggested that sexual dysfunctions did not resolve with time.

Increased sexual expression may be seen in some patients after traumatic brain injury. Patients who present as more sexually demanding post-injury are more likely to have frontal lobe damage [68, 72]. The mechanism is therefore different from that involved in the hypersexuality associated with dopaminergic therapy, discussed earlier. The end result may be similar, however, with increased demands placed on the partners, who may be unsure as to whether they should always acquiesce or whether they can say "no" to some sexual contact. Inappropriate comments by the patient may alienate friends and family members, and this reaction may contribute to the increasing isolation experienced by couples in whom one partner has a brain injury [66]. Inappropriate comments to health care professionals may result in a label of "behavioral problem," which, paradoxically, may detract from the efforts that should be made to help the individual relearn socially acceptable behavior [73].

Neurologic trauma often results in the patient's spending long periods within an institution, whether a hospital or a rehabilitation center. Many of these patients are young and are at a stage of having high interest in sex. Older patients may have been in long-term relationships and may never have experienced an extended period of separation before. How these patients deal with their sexual feelings at this time depends on their level of cognitive and physical functioning, their emotional state, their relationship with their partner (if they have one), and their environment. Masturbation and sexual fantasy may have played an important part in their sexual expression in the past, or these activities may develop as new strategies for dealing with the current circumstances. Little privacy exists within a hospital or rehabilitation unit. Masturbation may quickly be labeled as a behavioral problem, when in fact the individual simply needs to be given some privacy. If, by implicit or explicit behavior, professionals convey the message that this activity is dirty or perverted, the patient may begin to feel that it is true, and self-esteem, already damaged by disease or disability, may fall even further. Alternatively, such disapproval may offer fuel to a behavior that can be used to manipulate staff by gaining attention. Increased sexual behavior may make patients, particularly women, very vulnerable. Safety issues, such as preventing sexually transmitted disease and pregnancy and protecting the individual from sexual abuse, must be considered.

Parkinson's Disease

Sexual expression is affected by Parkinson's disease, and, as is often the case, the cause of the sexual dysfunctions is multifactorial. With the onset of a chronic disease, changes take place within the individual and the dyadic relationship that may enhance or detract from the ability to respond sexually. The alteration in mobility, self-image, and role within the family; social changes; and the influence of

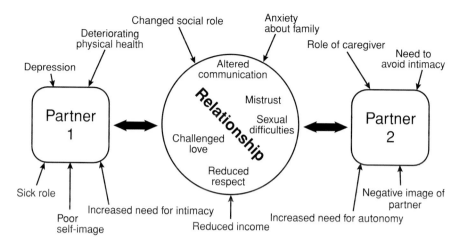

Figure 7.5 Triad of sexual expression in the context of acquired disability. The partners experience physical and psychological changes to their lives that may hinder their ability to respond sexually. One set of changes in response to acquired disability in partner 1 is illustrated. Many different responses may occur.

drugs and associated conditions, such as depression, may all contribute to changes in the dynamics of the dyadic relationship and in sexual functioning. Figure 7.5 illustrates how sexual and relationship dysfunction may arise in response to the onset of acquired disease or disability.

Brown et al. [74] studied couples attending a Parkinson's Disease Society residential weekend. Forty-four couples were eligible to take part in the study. Those who agreed to participate were 23 male patients, 11 female patients, 11 male spouses, and 27 female spouses. They found that more than one-half the male patients and their spouses indicated likely sexual dysfunction as measured by the GRISS [71]. More than one-third of the female patients indicated a possible problem, although none of their male spouses scored in the problem area. When relationship satisfaction was examined (using the Golombok Rust Inventory of Marital State [75]), slightly fewer than one-half the male patients and slightly more than one-half the female spouses indicated likely marital dissatisfaction, whereas few of the female patients and their spouses scored in the dissatisfaction range. Hypersexuality was not specifically assessed, but five female spouses reported excessive demands from their male partners. Whether this finding reflected hypersexuality in the male or reduced desire in the woman could not be assessed in this study.

In another study of 25 young people with Parkinson's disease (age range, 36–56 years), Wermuth and Stenager [76] found a particularly high incidence of altered sex life among women. Seventy percent of the women described reduced libido compared with 20% of men. The main conclusion of this study was that health care professionals should be more aware of the potential for altered sex lives in patients with Parkinson's disease and should be able to discuss this subject with patients [76].

A number of studies have reported increased sex drive in patients with Parkinson's disease who are being treated with dopaminergic agents [10, 11]. A dose-related effect has been shown in some reports [77]. Evidence exists that, in some patients, this change represents a true increase in sexual drive rather than simply a manifestation of frontal disinhibition or a psychotic state [78]. In other instances, the effect is more complex, because the improvement in general well-being and ability that accompanies the initiation of L-dopa therapy may be sufficient to effect a restoration of sexual interest [10]. A study of 19 Parkinson's disease patients taking L-dopa found three patterns of altered sexual functioning after treatment. One group experienced a general improvement, which included a slight improvement in sex life depending on age, previous sex life, and availability of a partner. The second pattern was a specific stimulation of sex drive. This pattern occurred in three men and was transient, despite continuation of the drug. The third pattern was the occurrence of sexual disinhibition in patients who developed an "acute brain syndrome" on treatment [79]. Whatever the cause of the alteration in sexual drive, it may be the source of considerable distress to the partner and may challenge the stability of the dyadic relationship, which may already be weakened by the impact of chronic disease and the associated change in lifestyle and roles.

Nondisabled Partner

Masters and Johnson [8] observed that there is no such thing as an uninvolved partner. In response to an individual's acquisition of disability, his or her able-bodied partner may experience a turmoil of emotions, including fear, anxiety, pity, shame, anger, helplessness, hopelessness, loneliness, depression, worry, and sadness [80]. To these may be added resentment, guilt, confusion, and despair. The social context and expectations of the community may dictate that the partner should nurture, understand, and care for the disabled individual. This mass of emotions and associated thoughts may have a detrimental effect on both the physiologic and psychological processes of sexual expression. In the effort to achieve a good rehabilitation result, the partner may be drawn into the role of caregiver and assistant therapist. The dual roles of sexual partner and caregiver are incompatible for many people. The difficulty of responding sexually to a person toward whom the individual feels "motherly" may place an enormous strain on the relationship and may trigger negative emotions in both partners. Alternatively, the partner may be excluded from the rehabilitation process and be left feeling alone and forgotten [16]. Professionals in rehabilitation must guard against making assumptions about the degree and nature of involvement that relatives would like in the rehabilitation and caregiving process.

A common complaint from the spouse of a person with altered cognitive functioning is that "he [or she] is not the person I knew before." This person is not the person the spouse chose as a sexual partner, the person with whom he or she wished to spend the rest of life and with whom he or she could lower defenses and become vulnerable in the act of making love. Thoughts such as these may progress to feelings of aversion, which may in turn trigger feelings of guilt and contribute to the anxiety and depression that are very frequent among spouses of individuals with altered cognitive function. Changes in the behavioral aspects of functioning are the most damaging to interpersonal relationships [64–66, 70, 81]. In a study of the wives of soldiers injured during military service, a marked reduction in sexual activity was found among those couples in whom the husband had sustained a spinal or brain injury compared to nondisabled couples. In the case of those with spinal injury, the reason was the altered physiology; however, when the husband had a brain injury, wives reported a feeling of dislike toward physical contact with their husbands [66].

In treating sexual dysfunctions, consideration of the partner is important. Restoring a male patient's erectile function may be relatively easy, but if his partner is experiencing the doubt and confusion outlined earlier, this treatment may be insufficient to effect a restoration of the couple's sex life together. Indeed, as Vermote and Peuskins [82] described, such a scenario could challenge the "brittle equilibrium" based on nursing that is holding the relationship together. The only way to move forward in this setting is to focus on the issues for each partner and the relationship, if the partners are willing to do this. In a study of couples attending a clinic for diabetes patients, the researcher observed that men could progress through the clinic to implant surgery with no reference to the partner. The author described how some of the female partners feared a successful treatment outcome, as this would be "an unwelcome disturbance of [their] post–sexual adjustment" [83]. As Hartman et al. [80] stated, "a physical disability is never experienced exclusively by the individual."

Relationship

Sexual expression within an intimate relationship represents a declaration of commitment and trust that allows the partners to lower their defenses and experience a vulnerability that they would not generally choose in any other setting. With the onset of acquired illness or disability and its attendant feelings of fear, loss, role change, and the potential for further loss, previous assumptions about the relationship may be challenged. Factors associated with but not part of the illness or disability may play a very strong role in creating a crisis in the relationship. Indeed, disability may be a confounding factor in attempts to elicit the cause of the dysfunction. Rodgers and Calder [46], in a study of couples in whom one partner had multiple sclerosis, found that among those participants who felt their relationship had deteriorated over the years, all attributed the change to the disease; those whose relationships had fluctuated, however, attributed this fluctuation to general stressful events rather than to the multiple sclerosis. Abrams [37], in reviewing the literature on the impact of spinal injury on marital stability, found that low income and unemployment may be the most significant predictors of marital termination among paraplegic patients. These are conditions commonly associated with disability [20, 37, 84, 85]. The aim of a therapeutic intervention is to restore the functioning of the relationship; however, this attribute is very difficult to measure and, as Abrams points out, nondivorce does not necessarily represent a successful outcome—that is, a healthy, functioning relationship.

Evidence indicates that progressive disability can be more damaging to relationships than static conditions; a gradually increasing dependence on a spouse places a huge stress on the relationship [86]. Marriages that begin before the onset of disease or disability are recognized as high-risk relationships because of the number of unexpected adjustments that have to be made [35, 86].

Disability may have a positive impact on a couple's sex life. Kreuter et al. [63], in a study of 49 partners (39 women and 10 men) of patients with spinal cord injuries, found that nearly one-half of the partners considered their current sex life to be as good as (3 men, 8 women) or better than (1 man, 10 women) their previous sex life. Positive changes to the sex life that were cited included increased playfulness, prolonged foreplay, and feelings of sexual equality. The authors speculate that focusing on sensuality rather than achievement in sexual expression may have contributed to the feelings of sexual equality. Moving away from performance goals has already been discussed as one of the aims of therapy for sexual dysfunctions [31].

Individuals without a Sexual Partner

People may have concerns about their sexuality when they are not in a current relationship. In many ways, such individuals may have more difficulty in seeking help, because no partner is present to legitimize their concern about sex. They may have questions about masturbation, about the likelihood of difficulties should they establish a relationship, about the difficulties of meeting people, or about sexual orientation. Anger, sadness, or resentment about the breakup of a relationship may be present. The perceived role of the disability in the failed relationship may need exploration. Low self-esteem is a frequently expressed feeling when a relationship has failed, and the presence of disability may exacerbate this condition. Patients may be uncertain as to how to start exploring their sexuality [87] and may easily be discouraged from pursuing their concerns. As Cole et al. [59] described, "In some cases the physician's personal anxieties regarding sexuality make him virtually inaccessible to the patient who wishes to seek advice on this subject. The subtly rebuffed patient cannot distinguish between the physician's discomfort and the appropriateness of his sexually oriented questions or needs." Therapy exploring an individual's concept of sexual expression and sexuality may be helpful, and such therapy has been carried out successfully both on a one-to-one basis and in a group setting [88].

Different Perceptions of Men and Women

The importance of viewing sexual problems within the partner-partner-relationship triad (see Figure 7.3) is illustrated by studies that have examined male and female perceptions of sex and relationships. A study of 28 couples attending a sexual and marital clinic found a closer association between sexual and marital problems for men than for women [89]. Indeed, when male sexual dysfunction was present, it had a significant positive correlation with poor marital state as perceived both by the men and the women. This was not the case when female sexual dysfunction was present. The authors concluded that "male sexual performance may be more susceptible to marital problems and consequently aggravate the situation, whereas female sexual dysfunction may be less intrusive as far as the relationship is concerned."

Frank et al. [17], in their study of couples in "working relationships," found that the husbands tended to underestimate the occurrence of sexual dysfunction in their wives. For example, 33% of women had difficulty maintaining excitement, but only 15% of their partners thought their wives had this problem ($P <.01$). A similar discrepancy was seen in a study of patients with Parkinson's disease [74].

Apparently, women do not always take part in sexual activity because they wish to. A further example is provided by Hulter and Lundberg [90] in a study of women with advanced multiple sclerosis. When asked how frequently they would like to have intercourse, 13 of the 47 women said they would prefer not to have intercourse at all.

MANAGEMENT OF SEX AND RELATIONSHIP PROBLEMS AMONG PEOPLE WITH NEUROLOGIC DISABILITY

Many authors have expressed the opinion that health care professionals should be proactive in offering information and help with regard to sexual functioning [34, 59, 91]. However, professionals may have their own fears and embarrassment about sexuality. This situation is compounded by a lack of training in sexual medicine and methods of dealing with relationship issues [4, 6, 7, 54].

Understanding sexual expression within the dyadic relationship (see Figure 7.3) has important therapeutic implications. Halvorsen and Metz [36] commented, "Because sexual intimacy and marital intimacy are inextricably united, brief marital therapy is also an essential component of competent sex therapy." Zimmer found that the negative emotions identified in couples experiencing sexual dysfunction were similar to those in couples experiencing marital dysfunction and were significantly different than those of couples who were not experiencing sexual or relationship difficulties [92]. Marital and sex therapy are now recognized as being clinically interrelated, with the emphasis of a particular treatment session being determined by the problems the couple present [93, 94].

P-LI-SS-IT Model

One of the most useful models for approaching sexual and relationship problems, and one particularly applicable to the nonspecialist, is the P-LI-SS-IT model proposed by Annon [1]. It has been described as a hierarchical model, with the depth of interaction depending on the skill and experience of the professional concerned [1, 93, 95]. The key to approaching problems of sexual functioning and relationship conflict is for the professional to develop a trusting and permission-giving rapport with the patient.

P—Permission

Patients who have experienced a major illness or operation or have acquired a disability are often hoping to be asked whether they have concerns about sex but are too reticent to initiate the discussion [5, 6]. Giving patients permission to discuss sexual problems may involve simply creating a trusting and confidential relationship in which patients can express their concerns. This alone may be therapeutic, and no further action may be required. Alternatively, the individual or couple may need to talk about these issues on a number of occasions and sometimes may need more specific help.

LI—Limited Information

Giving information to patients and their partners can address concerns or provide reassurance that may restore confidence in their sex life. The information may concern the disease or disability in relation to sexual functioning, facilitate coping strategies, or dispel firmly held myths about sexual expression (see Table 7.1). Zilbergeld proposed a number of commonly held beliefs about male sexuality that he termed myths—for example, "in sex, as elsewhere, it's performance that counts," or "all physical contact must lead to sex" [28]. A study at a psychosexual clinic in London found that a group of men with sexual dysfunction showed a significantly greater belief in Zilbergeld's myths of sexual functioning than did a nondysfunctional control group [96].

SS—Specific Suggestions

After a full history is established, supported by an examination and sometimes by laboratory tests, suggestions can be offered about treatment. In sexual medicine, the examination can be a therapeutic tool, just as is the permission to discuss sexual issues. Treatment may include alteration of current drug regimes, psychosexual therapy, counseling, relationship therapy, or medical treatment for specific conditions, such as intracavernosal injection of alprostadil for erectile dysfunction or use of carbamazepine for perineal dysesthesia. Referral to another service agency or specialty, such as specialist relationship counseling, clinical psychology, psychosexual medicine, or urology, may be indicated at this stage.

IT—Intensive Therapy

At this stage, skilled treatment with a trained sex therapist is indicated. The number of patients requiring intervention at this level is small.

Rarely does sexual disorder have a single cause, and failure to appreciate the wider context may lead to a therapeutic failure. Halvorsen and Metz [35] stated this succinctly: "Even when an organic factor is present, it is essential to treat the principle psychological factors that can complicate the organic problem or that could have resulted from it."

Fertility

No discussion of sexuality is complete without consideration of the possible outcome of sexual activity. It is easy to forget that once sex is resumed, pregnancy may occur. If the couple are planning pregnancy, they may require genetic counseling, information about fertility, and methods of assisted conception. For example, after spinal cord injury, fertility is reduced in the male, and optimum bladder management is important to maintain sperm quality [97]. Spinal injury is not a contraindication to pregnancy, and fertility is largely unaffected in women. Antenatal care is best provided through a department with experience in the provision of obstetric care to women with spinal cord injuries or through close liaison

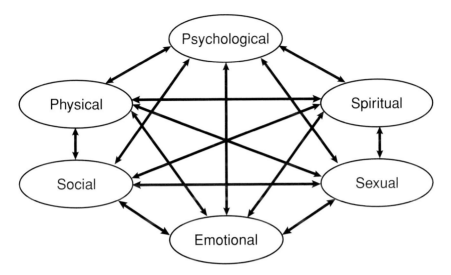

Figure 7.6 Aspects of personhood and their interactions.

between the spinal injury unit and obstetric team. The risk of pressure sores and urinary tract infection is somewhat increased during pregnancy, and autonomic dysreflexia is a risk in those with lesions above T6 [98–100]. However, with appropriate care, pregnancy can be managed successfully.

Contraception

Unless a couple wants to achieve a pregnancy, contraception should be discussed. Some methods, such as the intrauterine device, may be contraindicated in individuals with paraplegia because of the lack of abdominal sensation should a problem arise. Some oral contraceptives are contraindicated when a risk of thromboembolism exists. Impairment of manual dexterity may preclude the use of barrier methods, such as diaphragms or condoms. Patients should be encouraged to discuss contraceptive issues with their general practitioner or family planning clinic; where appropriate, liaison between these services and the neurologist or neurorehabilitation personnel can take place. An excellent review of contraception has been written by John Guilleband [101].

SUMMARY

Sex is a fundamental part of each individual's life that interacts with all other aspects of human functioning (Figure 7.6). It achieves its most intense and most meaningful expression within the dyadic relationship. Stresses affecting the physical, psychological, and social life of an individual will also impact his or her partner in an intimate relationship. The acquisition of neurologic disease or trauma resulting in disability may challenge assumptions about sexual functioning, roles within a relationship, and concepts of "normal" sexual behavior for disabled persons and their partners. Patients need reassurance that addressing issues of sexual health is relevant within many health care disciplines, and voicing concerns is permissible. Disease and disability by no means dictate an end to sexual expression. The clinician may need to guide those concerned into examining their perceptions of sexuality and perhaps dispel myths, provide information, and give permission to explore new means of sexual expression.

REFERENCES

1. Annon JS. The Behavioural Treatment of Sexual Problems: Brief Therapy. New York: Harper & Row, 1976.
2. Bancroft J. Human Sexuality and Its Problems. Edinburgh, UK: Churchill Livingstone, 1989.
3. Rust J, Golombok S, Pickard C. Marital problems in general practice. Sex Marital Ther 1987;2(2):127–130.
4. Finger WW, Hall ES, Peterson FL. Education in sexuality for nurses. Sex Disabil 1992;10:81–89.
5. Young EW. Patients' plea: tell us about our sexuality. J Sex Educ Ther 1984;10:53–56.
6. Weston A. Challenging assumptions. Nurs Times 1993;89:26–31.
7. Sawyer SM. Reproductive and sexual health in adolescents with cystic fibrosis. BMJ 1996;313: 1095–1096.
8. Masters WH, Johnson VE. Human Sexual Response. London: Churchill, 1966.
9. Stanley E. Dealing with fear of failure. BMJ 1981;282:1281–1283.
10. Goodwin FK. Behavioural effects of L-dopa in man. Semin Psychiatry 1971;3(4):477–491.
11. Weinman E, Ruskin PE. Levodopa dependence and hypersexuality in an older Parkinson's disease patient. Am J Geriatr Psychiatry 1994;3:81–83.
12. Vogel HP, Schiffter R. Hypersexuality—a complication of dopaminergic therapy in Parkinson's disease. Pharmacopsychiatry 1983;16:107–110.
13. Warner P, Bancroft J. Members of Edinburgh Human Sexuality Group. A regional clinical service for sexual problems: a 3 year study. Sex Marital Ther 1987;2:115–126.
14. Bancroft J and Coles. Three years' experience in a sexual problem clinic. BMJ 1976;1:1575–1577.
15. LoPiccolo J, Stock WE. Treatment of sexual dysfunction. J Consult Clin Psychol 1986;54:158–167.
16. Neumann RJ. The forgotten other: women partners of spinal cord injured men, a preliminary report. Sex Disabil 1979;2:287–292.
17. Frank E, Anderson C, Rubenstein D. Frequency of sexual dysfunction in "normal" couples. N Engl J Med 1978;299:111–115.
18. Spence S. Psychosexual Therapy: A Cognitive Behavioural Approach. London: Chapman & Hall, 1991.
19. Golombok S, Rust J, Pickard C. Sexual problems encountered in general practice. Br J Sex Med 1984;11:171–175.
20. Szasz G, Paty D, Maurice WL. Sexual dysfunctions in multiple sclerosis. Ann N Y Acad Sci 1984;436:443–452.
21. Chandler BJ, Brown S. Sex and relationship dysfunction in neurological disability. J Neurol Neurosurg Psychiatry 1998;65:877–880.
22. Kaplan HS. The New Sex Therapy. London: Bailliere Tindall, 1974.
23. Barlow DH. Causes of sexual dysfunction: the role of anxiety and cognitive interference. J Consult Clin Psychol 1986;54:104–148.
24. Blake DJ, Maisiak R, Alarcon GS, et al. Sexual quality of life of patients with arthritis compared to arthritis free controls. J Rheumatol 1987;14:570–575.
25. Seidl A, Bullough B, Haughey B, et al. Understanding the effects of a myocardial infarction on sexual functioning: a basis for sexual counselling. Rehabil Nurs 1991;16:255–263.
26. Larson JL, McNaughton MW, Ward Kennedy W, Mansfield LW. Heart rate and blood pressure responses to sexual activity and a stair climbing test. Heart Lung 1980;9:1025–1030.

27. Nemec ED, Mansfield L, Ward Kennedy J. Heart rate and blood pressure responses during sexual activity in normal males. Am Heart J 1976;92:274–277.
28. Zilbergeld B. Men and Sex. London: Fontana, 1978.
29. Cole SS. Women, sexuality and disabilities. Women Ther 1988;7:277–294.
30. Guirgius W. Sex Therapy with Couples. In D Hooper, W Dryden (eds), Couple Therapy: A Handbook. Buckingham, UK: Open University Press, 1991.
31. Stanley E. Nonorganic causes of sexual problems. BMJ 1981;282:1042–1044.
32. Bancroft J. Impact of environment, stress, occupational, and other hazards on sexuality and sexual behavior. Environ Health Perspect 1993;101(suppl 2):101–107.
33. Bowers MB, Woert MV, Davis L. Sexual behaviour during L-dopa treatment for parkinsonism. Am J Psychiatry 1971;127:1691–1693.
34. Miller S, Szasz G, Anderson L. Sexual health care clinician in an acute spinal cord injury unit. Arch Phys Med Rehabil 1981;62:315–320.
35. Halvorsen JG, Metz ME. Sexual dysfunction, part 1: classification, aetiology and pathogenesis. J Appl Board Fam Pract 1991;5:51–61.
36. Halvorsen JG, Metz ME. Sexual dysfunction, part 2: diagnosis, management and prognosis. J Appl Board Fam Pract 1992;5:177–192.
37. Abrams KS. The impact on marriages of adult onset paraplegia. Paraplegia 1981;19:253–259.
38. Mona LR, Gardos PS, Brown RC. Sexual self views of women with disabilities: the relationship among age of onset, nature of disability and sexual self esteem. Sex Disabil 1994;12:261–277.
39. Cotgrove AJ, Kolvin I. Child sexual abuse. Hosp Update 1996;22:401–406.
40. Jehu D. Sexual dysfunctions among women clients who were sexually abused in childhood. Behav Psychother 1989;17:53–70.
41. Goffman E. Stigma: The Management of Spoiled Identity. London: Penguin, 1963.
42. Litvinoff S. The Relate Guide to Sex in Loving Relationships. London: Vermillion, 1992.
43. Becker JB, Abel GG. Sex and disability: treatment issues. Behav Med Update 1983;4(4):15–20.
44. Greengross W. Entitled to Love. National Fund for Research into Crippling Disease. London: Mallaby Press, 1976.
45. DeLoach C, Greer BG. Adjustment to Severe Physical Disability: A Metamorphosis. New York: McGraw-Hill, 1981.
46. Rodgers J, Calder P. Marital adjustment: a valuable resource for the emotional health of individuals with multiple sclerosis. Rehabil Couns Bull 1990;34:24–32.
47. Anderson EM, Clark L, Spain B. Disability in Adolescence. New York: Methuen, 1982.
48. Hallum A. Disability and the transition to adulthood: issues for the disabled child, the family and the paediatrician. Curr Probl Pediatr 1995;25:12–50.
49. Borjeson MC, Lagergren J. Life conditions of adolescents with myelomeningocele. Devel Med Child Neurol 1990;32:698–706.
50. Dorner S. Adolescents with spina bifida: how they see their situation. Arch Dis Childhood 1976;51:439–444.
51. Castree BJ, Walker JH. The young adult with spina bifida. BMJ 1981;283:1040–1042.
52. Blackburn M. Sexuality, disability and abuse: advice for life . . . not just for kids. Child Care Devel 1995;21:351–361.
53. Blackburn MC, Carlton I, Bax MCO, Grant D. You, your partner and continence: an introduction to sexuality, disability and continence. Eur J Pediatr Surg 1993;3(suppl I):24–25.
54. Lewin J, King M. Sexual medicine. BMJ 1997;314:1432.
55. Chandler BJ, Brown S. How Are Sex and Relationship Problems Dealt with by Rehabilitation Physicians? Clin Rehabil 1998;12:181–182.
56. Bors E, Comarr AE. Neurological disturbances of sexual function with special reference to 529 patients with spinal cord injury. Urol Surv 1960;10:191–222.
57. Higgins GE. Sexual response in spinal cord injured adults: a review. Arch Sex Behav 1979;8: 173–196.
58. Berard EJJ. The sexuality of spinal cord injured women: physiology and pathophysiology: a review. Paraplegia 1989;27:99–112.
59. Cole TM, Chilgren R, Rosenberg P. A new programme of sex education and counselling for spinal cord injured adults and health care professionals. Paraplegia 1973;11:111–124.
60. Courtois FJ, Charvier KF, Leriche A, et al. Clinical approach to erectile dysfunction in spinal cord injured men: a review of clinical and experimental data. Paraplegia 1995;33:628–635.
61. Ide M, Ogata H. Sexual activities and concerns in persons with spinal cord injuries. Paraplegia 1995;33:334–337.

62. Hooper M. Spinal Cord Injured Men and Sexuality. London: Spinal Injuries Association, 1992.
63. Kreuter M, Sullivan M, Siosteen A. Sexual adjustment after spinal cord injury (SCI) focusing on partner experiences. Paraplegia 1994;32:225–235.
64. McKinlay WW, Brooks DN, Bond MR, et al. The short term outcome of severe blunt head injury as reported by relatives of the injured persons. J Neurol Neurosurg Psychiatry 1981;44:527–533.
65. Oddy M, Humphrey M, Uttley D. Stresses upon the relatives of head injured patients. Br J Psychiatry 1978;133:507–513.
66. Rosenbaum M, Najenson T. Changes in life patterns and symptoms of low mood as reported by wives of severely brain injured soldiers. J Consult Clin Psychol 1976;44:881–888.
67. Garden FH. Incidence of sexual dysfunction in neurologic disability. Sex Disabil 1991;9:39–47.
68. Elliott ML, Biever LS. Head injury and sexual dysfunction. Brain Inj 1996;10:703–717.
69. Clark JDA, Raggatt PR, Edwards OM. Hypothalamic hypogonadism following major head injury. Clin Endocrinol 1988;29:153–165.
70. O'Carroll RE, Woodrow J, Marouns F. Psychosexual and psychosocial sequelae of closed head injury. Brain Inj 1991;5:303–313.
71. Rust J, Golombok S. The Golombok Rust Inventory of Sexual Satisfaction. Windsor, UK: NFER-Nelson, 1986.
72. Sandel ME, Williams KS, Dellapietra L, Derogatis LR. Sexual functioning following traumatic brain injury. Brain Inj 1996;10:719–728.
73. Strauss D. Biopsychosocial issues in sexuality with the neurologically impaired patient. Sex Disabil 1991;9:49–67.
74. Brown RG, Jahanshahi M, Quinn N, Marsden CD Sexual function in patients with Parkinson's disease and their partners. J Neurol Neurosurg Psychiatry 1990;53:480–486.
75. Rust J, Bennun I, Crowe M, Golombok S. The Golombok Rust Inventory of Marital State. Windsor, UK: NFER-Nelson, 1988.
76. Wermuth L, Stenager E. Sexual problems in young patients with Parkinson's disease. Acta Neurol Scand 1995;91:453–455.
77. Quinn NP, Toone AE, Marsden CD, Parkes JD. Dopa dose dependent sexual deviation. Br J Psychiatry 1983;142:296–298.
78. Harvey NS. Serial cognitive profiles in levodopa induced hypersexuality. Br J Psychiatry 1988;153:833–836.
79. Bowers JR, Woert MV, Davis L. Sexual behavior during L-dopa treatment for parkinsonism. Am J Psychiatry 1971;127:127–129.
80. Hartman C, MacIntosh B, Englehardt B. The neglected and forgotten sexual partner of the physically disabled. Soc Work 1983;28:370–374.
81. Liss M, Willer B. Traumatic brain injury and marital relationships: a literature review. Int J Rehabil Res 1990;13:309–320.
82. Vermote R, Peuskins J. Sexual and micturition problems in multiple sclerosis patients: psychological issues. Sex Disabil 1996;14:73–82.
83. Webster L. Working with couples in a diabetic clinic: the role of the therapist in a medical setting. Sex Marital Ther 1992;7:189–196.
84. Townsend P, Phillimore P, Beattie A. Health and Deprivation: Inequality and the North. Beckenham, Kent, UK: Croom Helm, 1988.
85. Martin J, White A. The Financial Circumstances of Disabled Adults Living in Private Households. OPCS Surveys of Disability in Great Britain. Report. London: Her Majesty's Stationery Office, 1988.
86. Woollett SL, Edelmann RJ. Marital satisfaction in individuals with multiple sclerosis and their partners; its interactive effect with life satisfaction, social networks and disability. Sex Marital Ther 1988;3:191–196.
87. Becker JV, Abel GG. Sex and disability: treatment issues. Behav Med Update 1983;4:15–20.
88. Zilbergeld B. Group treatment of sexual dysfunction in men without partners. J Sex Marital Ther 1975;1:204–214.
89. Rust J, Golombok S, Collier J. Marital problems and sexual dysfunction: how are they related? Br J Psychiatry 1988;152:629–631.
90. Hulter BM, Lundberg PO. Sexual function in women with advanced MS. J Neurol Neurosurg Psychiatry 1995;83:83–86.
91. Szasz G. Sex and disability are not mutually exclusive: evaluation and management. West J Med 1991;154:560–563.
92. Zimmer D. Interaction patterns and communication skills in sexually distressed and normal couples: two experimental studies. J Sex Marital Ther 1983;9:251–265.
93. Sager CJ. The role of sex therapy in marital therapy. Am J Psychiatry 1976;133:555–558.

94. Zimmer D. Does marital therapy enhance the effectiveness of treatment for sexual dysfunction? J Sex Marital Ther 1987;13:193–209.
95. Dupont S. Multiple sclerosis and sexual functioning—a review. Clin Rehabil 1995;9:135–141.
96. Baker CD, De Silva P. The relationship between male sexual dysfunction and belief in Zilbergeld's myths: an empirical investigation. Sex Marital Ther 1988;3:229–238.
97. Rutkowski SB, Middleton JW, Truman G, et al. The influence of bladder management on fertility in spinal cord injured males. Paraplegia 1995;33:263–266.
98. Robertson DNS, Guttmann L. The paraplegic patient in pregnancy and labour. Proc R Soc Med 1963;56:381–387.
99. Young BK, Kutz M, Klein SA. Pregnancy after spinal cord injury: altered maternal and fetal responses to labour. Obstet Gynaecol 1983;62:59–63.
100. McCunniff DE, Dewan D. Pregnancy after spinal cord injury. Obstet Gynaecol 1984;63:757.
101. Guilleband J. Contraception: Your Questions Answered. Edinburgh, UK: Churchill Livingstone, 1993.

II
INVESTIGATIONS

8
Urodynamics

Michael J. Swinn

The term *urodynamics* was introduced in the 1950s and refers in its broadest sense to any test of urinary tract function. In practice, investigative techniques are mostly restricted to the lower urinary tract, enabling the two functions of the bladder, urine storage and voiding, to be studied.

In the past, the lower urinary tract was assessed using static investigations, such as intravenous pyelography and cystourethroscopy, but the techniques currently employed reflect dynamic activity. Indeed, a wide range of urodynamic tests are available, from simple, noninvasive tests, such as uroflowmetry, to more sophisticated techniques, such as videocystometrography, which requires catheterization and radiographic screening of the patient.

The clinician must be alert to the potential for upper urinary tract damage to occur in neurogenic bladder disorders, with transmission of high pressures to the ureters and kidneys. Once the limits of mural distensibility have been reached, ureteral and renal damage can result. Therefore, renal function is commonly assessed in patients at risk, with estimation of serum creatine levels and upper urinary tract ultrasonography.

UROFLOWMETRY

Uroflowmetry is the simplest urodynamic investigation. Originally, a kymograph was used to record the weight of urine passed over time. Other methods have used weight transducers or the principle of air displacement. The most commonly used modern method involves a rotating disc at the base of a urine receptacle; the amount of energy required to keep the disc spinning at a constant velocity is calculated, and this energy is proportional to the force of urine flow. Whichever method is used, the result is the generation of a uroflow curve, which is a graphic representation of the rate at which urine is voided (Figure 8.1).

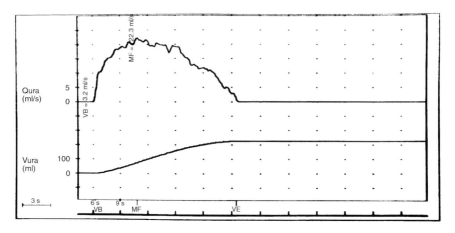

Figure 8.1   Normal uroflow curve. In the top trace, the flow curve follows a parabola. The maximum flow rate was recorded at 22.3 ml per second. The lower trace represents the volume of urine voided. The total voided volume can be read as approximately 220 ml. (MF = maximum flow [ml/sec]; Qura = flow of urine; VB = void begin; VE = void end; Vura = volume of urine [ml].)

Flowmeters may, in addition, derive and calculate a range of parameters for each void, including the maximum rate of urine flow, the mean rate of urine flow, the voided volume, and the flow time. Because of the uncritical placement of measurement markers in any machine-read system, the clinician must be vigilant. Spurious spikes often result when the subject directs the flow to different parts of the urine receptacle, and whereas the objective observer might wish to disregard such phenomena, an electronic uroflowmeter duly records them and produces a corresponding set of results.

For a flow curve to be meaningful, the voided volume should be at least 150–200 ml. Patients should void in privacy, in a position they are used to and when a normal desire to void is felt. Poulsen and Kirkeby showed that, although voided volume is largest in the morning, maximum flow rate is highest in the afternoon [1]. Consequently, if multiple voidings are performed for comparison or to monitor disease progression, the investigator should ensure that they are performed at the same time of day.

Significant information may be learned by examining the shape of the flow curves. The normal flow curve is unbroken and bell-shaped, with little or no asymmetry of the bell. Obstruction (for example, due to prostatic enlargement) usually gives rise to an unbroken curve with pronounced asymmetry: After the maximal flow rate has been reached, the curve follows an elongated, flattened course until voiding is completed (Figure 8.2). Constriction, such as that due to a urethral stricture, usually results in a long, unbroken, flat plateau curve (Figure 8.3). A fractionated or discontinuous flow curve, characterized by one or more episodes in which flow is zero (Figure 8.4), is seen in detrusor-sphincter dyssynergia. However, none of these features is sufficiently specific to be diagnostic.

More information regarding lower urinary tract function can be gained by combining uroflowmetry with ultrasonography of the bladder. An assessment of the residual urine volume has been shown to be an important factor when form-

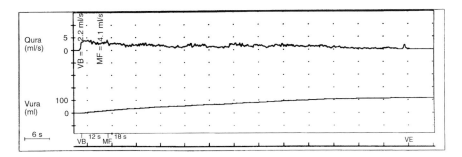

Figure 8.2   Uroflow curve compatible with prostatic obstruction. (MF = maximum flow [ml/sec]; Qura = flow of urine; VB = void begin; VE = void end; Vura = volume of urine [ml].)

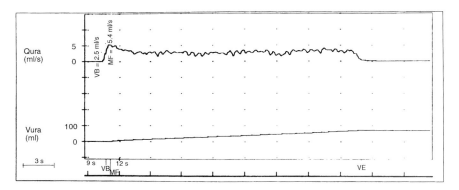

Figure 8.3   Uroflow curve compatible with urethral stricture. (MF = maximum flow [ml/sec]; Qura = flow of urine; VB = void begin; VE = void end; Vura = volume of urine [ml].)

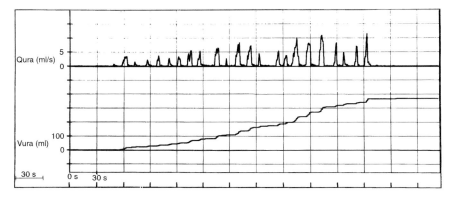

Figure 8.4   Uroflow curve demonstrating the intermittent flow seen in detrusor-sphincter dyssynergia. (Qura = flow of urine; Vura = volume of urine [ml].)

ing a management plan for the patient with a neurogenic bladder [2]. Because incomplete bladder emptying can act as a stimulus to further unwanted detrusor contractions, a patient with a large residual is likely to gain symptomatic benefit from self-catheterizing on a regular and frequent basis.

The flow of urine generated in any single void is a product of the detrusor pressure (together with abdominal pressure) and the outflow resistance. Although a simple flow test with residual measurement can provide the examiner with some information regarding lower urinary tract function, it reveals little about the storage phase. Information about the relative contributions made by the detrusor and the outflow resistance is inevitably absent. A poor flow could be the result either of poor detrusor function or of high outflow resistance (or both), and a normal flow can be obtained by abdominal straining to overcome bladder outflow obstruction.

Cystometry, on the other hand, allows the investigator to make a more complete assessment of bladder function, because the behavior of the bladder on filling can be studied, and the relationship between detrusor pressure and flow is recorded throughout the voiding phase.

CYSTOMETRY

The term *cystometry* is usually taken to mean the measurement of detrusor pressure during controlled bladder filling and subsequent voiding. Cystometry can be used to assess detrusor activity, sensation, capacity, and compliance.

Detrusor pressure cannot be measured directly, but because the total intravesical pressure is the sum of the abdominal pressure and the pressure exerted by the detrusor muscle, detrusor pressure can be calculated by subtracting the abdominal pressure from the measured intravesical pressure. For the purposes of cystometry, rectal pressure is usually recorded and taken as a measure of abdominal pressure.

To perform cystometry, the investigator catheterizes the patient with a small-diameter (8 French) filling catheter. A 1-mm-diameter plastic pressure line is used to measure intravesical pressure and is "railroaded" into the bladder by inserting its end into the side hole close to the tip of the catheter. When the pressure line is in the bladder, it is disengaged from the filling catheter, and any residual urine is drained. A free-flow test is performed before cystometry, so that the residual urine obtained represents a natural postmicturition residual. The uroflow curve is thus obtained in the absence of the urethral catheter, which can distort the flow.

Once the urethral catheter and intravesical pressure line have been carefully fixed with tape, the patient turns to the left lateral position, and a similar, but covered, pressure line is inserted into the rectum. Care must be taken to avoid undue bending of the terminal part, as such bending can lead to suboptimal transmission of pressure and error in recording. Both pressure lines are then flushed with saline, the filling solution (saline) is connected to the catheter, and both transducers are set to zero by using the balancing function of the urodynamic machine.

The International Continence Society has established the convention that "zero pressure" is set to atmospheric pressure. The transducer is therefore never set when exposed to intravesical pressure. A three-way tap exists at the junction of each pressure line and its transducer, so that a reading of zero can be set when the transducer is closed to the pressure line and open to air. An alternative method is to set the transducers to zero before the pressure lines are inserted into the patient. So the investigator can check that both pressure lines are recording satisfactorily and that subtraction of the abdominal pressure from the intravesical pressure is adequate, the patient is asked to cough, which increases abdominal and intravesical pressures.

The bladder is filled at a rate controlled by an infusion pump. A filling rate of less than 10 ml per minute is termed *slow-fill cystometry*; this fill rate approaches physiologic rates, which are generally less than 2 ml per minute. A filling rate of between 10 and 100 ml per minute is termed *medium-fill cystometry,* and a rate greater than 100 ml per minute is termed *rapid-fill cystometry*. The rate of filling can have a considerable influence on the resulting measurements. The faster the fill, the lower the compliance (as defined on the next page); detrusor instability can be provoked by filling the bladder rapidly. Slow-fill cystometry should be used in the investigation of patients with neurologic abnormalities, particularly patients with spinal cord trauma, to minimize the risk of artifactual detrusor activity [3].

Throughout the study, continuous and simultaneous recordings of rectal (abdominal) and intravesical pressure are made, and from these the detrusor pressure is calculated. The investigator should watch the trace carefully so that any potentially misleading rises in pressure, for example, due to patient movement, can be appropriately annotated. During bladder filling, the patient is asked to suppress any sensed bladder contraction, and the temporary suspension of active filling can help at this stage. The bladder volume at which the subject first experiences a sensation of filling is noted. Similarly, the bladder volumes at which the patient reports a normal desire and a strong desire to void are marked by the investigator on the urodynamic trace (Figure 8.5). The former is defined as the level of filling at which the subject would normally pass urine but at which voiding could be

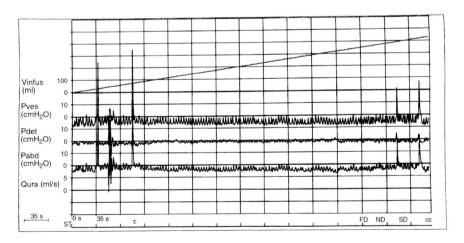

Figure 8.5 Normal filling cystometry. The sawtooth appearance in the intravesical and rectal pressure traces is caused by the pressure changes brought about by the subject's respiration. The detrusor pressure is calculated by subtracting one from the other. (c = cough; cc = cystic capacity; FD = first desire to void; ND = normal desire to void; Pabd = abdominal [rectal] pressure; Pdet = detrusor pressure; Pves = intravesical pressure; Qura = flow of urine; SD = strong desire to void; ST = start; Vinfus = volume infused.)

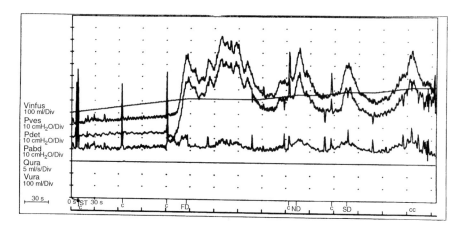

Figure 8.6   Filling cystometry demonstrating detrusor hyperreflexia. The rises in intravesical pressure are independent of any increases in abdominal pressure but rather are due to rises in detrusor pressure. (c = cough; cc = cystic capacity; FD = first desire to void; ND = normal desire to void; Pabd = abdominal [rectal] pressure; Pdet = detrusor pressure; Pves = intravesical pressure; Qura = flow of urine; SD = strong desire to void; ST = start; Vinfus = volume infused; Vura = volume of urine.)

delayed if necessary, and the latter is defined as the level at which there is a persistent desire to void without the fear of leakage.

Bladder filling is usually terminated when maximal capacity has been reached but the filling has not become painful for the patient. At this point, the filling catheter is removed and the patient is encouraged to void. The flow rate is recorded, and the detrusor pressure during the voiding phase is calculated as before. Postvoid residual can be determined either by ultrasonography or by insertion of a different catheter.

Conventional cystometry is carried out under highly unphysiologic conditions. In addition to the artifacts that can be caused during the filling phase, the presence of the intravesical pressure line can distort the flow. These problems have been recognized, and methods have become available for recording bladder pressures over longer periods. *Ambulatory urodynamics* allows the bladder to fill naturally and without attachment of the patient to a urodynamics machine.

Two types of abnormal pressure rise are seen on bladder filling in patients with neurologic disease affecting the bladder: hyperreflexic contractions and poor compliance. Hyperreflexic contractions are sudden, involuntary, phasic contractions of the detrusor muscle. Any rise in detrusor pressure on bladder filling may be considered abnormal, although commonly a sudden rise of 15 cm H_2O is taken as the threshold above which hyperreflexia is said to occur (Figure 8.6). If the urethral closure pressure is exceeded during such a pressure rise, then incontinence results (Figure 8.7). When similar contractions occur in the absence of neurologic disease, the bladder is described as "unstable."

Compliance is the term applied to the innate ability of the bladder to expand without a significant rise in intravesical pressure. This important property is part of the mechanism protecting the upper urinary tracts from vesicoureteric reflux of urine and is often affected by neurologic disease. The expansion of bladder

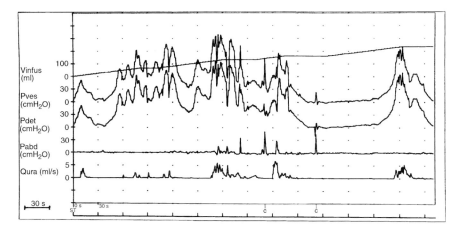

Figure 8.7   Filling cystometry showing detrusor hyperreflexia associated with incontinence. (c = cough; Pabd = abdominal [rectal] pressure; Pdet = detrusor pressure; Pves = intravesical pressure; Qura = flow of urine; ST = start; Vinfus = volume infused.)

urothelium, the viscoelastic properties of bladder muscle, and possibly the active relaxation of the detrusor on bladder filling are thought to be important factors contributing to compliance. A rise in pressure on bladder filling of more than 3.3 cm H_2O at a bladder volume of 100 ml has been considered by some to be abnormal, whereas others have defined a pressure rise of 6 cm H_2O, regardless of bladder volume, as the upper limit of normal (Figure 8.8) [4].

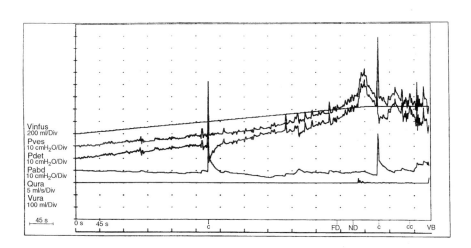

Figure 8.8   Filling cystometry demonstrating loss of compliance. Intravesical and detrusor pressure increase gradually as filling progresses. (c = cough; cc = cystic capacity; FD = first desire to void; ND = normal desire to void; Pabd = abdominal [rectal] pressure; Pdet = detrusor pressure; Pves = intravesical pressure; Qura = flow of urine; VB = void begin; Vinfus = volume infused; Vura = volume of urine [ml].)

A reduction in compliance sometimes occurs as the bladder approaches its maximal capacity; it may occur at lower volumes if rapid filling is used. In the latter instance, the temporary suspension of filling allows the detrusor pressure to fall. Knowledge of the rate of filling and of the total infused volume are therefore required for accurate interpretation of compliance as measured by a urodynamics machine. In cases in which pressure rises are suspected of being artifactual, stepwise filling of the bladder should be used [5]. In this procedure, the bladder is filled with the infusant intermittently.

The precise mechanisms involved in the reduction of compliance in pathologic states remain unclear, although it seems likely that some change occurs in the viscoelastic properties of the bladder wall. A loss of compliance is seen in various neurologic disorders, such as spinal cord injury, suggesting that a neurologic component may be deficient. Other conditions that reduce compliance include infection, bladder carcinoma, and fibrosis (e.g., postradiotherapy or due to long-term catheterization).

During voiding cystometry, the detrusor pressure and flow rate are continuously and simultaneously recorded. In addition to the separate graphic recordings of each of these parameters over time, a computer-generated plot can be made showing their relationship to each other, termed the *pressure/flow plot*. This plot can provide useful information regarding urethral resistance. In the theoretical case in which the detrusor contracts against no resistance, the detrusor pressure is reflected precisely in the flow rate produced. In practice, and particularly in pathologic conditions, the urethra does not remain completely passive, and its influence on flow can be significant.

VIDEOCYSTOMETROGRAPHY

If the fluid used to fill the bladder is radio-opaque and radiographic screening is used during cystometry, structural and functional information can be obtained. This type of study is termed *videocystometrography* (VCMG). The bladder can be visualized, and measures including the presence of ureteric reflux or detrusor-sphincter dyssynergia, the level of any outflow obstruction, and the degree of support to the bladder base during coughing can all be assessed using this technique. Because of the expense of the equipment, the extra time and expertise required, and the exposure to radiation involved in VCMG, it is not routinely undertaken. However, it is particularly useful in diagnosing stress incontinence and in determining the exact site of bladder outlet obstruction in individuals with a high pressure/low flow voiding pattern.

LEAK-POINT PRESSURE

Two types of leak-point pressure are evaluated, abdominal or Valsalva leak-point pressure and detrusor leak-point pressure. The first refers to the minimum vesical pressure produced by the subject's straining that is sufficient to cause leakage of urine. A measure of sphincter strength, it is used in the investigation of stress incontinence. The detrusor leak-point pressure is the detrusor pressure at which leakage occurs in the absence of stress maneuvers; it is also measured during filling cystometry. An elevated detrusor leak-point pressure of more than 40 cm H_2O is reported to be a reliable prognostic indicator for the development of upper urinary tract disease (see Chapter 24) [6]. Bloom et al. [7] treated a group of children who had high detrusor leak-point pressures with urethral dilatation and noted an improvement in bladder compliance and a corresponding fall in leak-point pressure. The suggestion is that high outlet resistance causes a reduction in compliance, and this in turn causes a deterioration in ureteric and then renal function. The measurement of leak-point pressure can be affected if the filling catheter used is larger than size 10 French.

Most patients with a significant residual demonstrated by ultrasonography can be managed satisfactorily with intermittent self-catheterization and anticholinergic medication, as in most cases the regular and frequent complete emptying of the bladder protects the upper renal tracts. However, in patients with neurogenic bladders for whom intermittent self-catheterization is not possible, complete patient management should include cystometry and detrusor leak-point pressure estimation, so that those who are at high risk of upper urinary tract damage can be identified at an early stage.

URETHRAL PRESSURE PROFILOMETRY

The urethral pressure profile indicates the intraluminal pressure along the length of the urethra with the bladder at rest. Ideally, the intraurethral pressure would be measured by a urethral catheter with multiple pressure sensors along its length and with simultaneous recording of the intravesical pressure. The pressure gradient along the urethra and the change in this gradient over time could then be recorded. Such a catheter is not available, however, and most urethral pressure profiles are measured using a single pressure recording on a catheter withdrawn at a constant rate. By following this procedure, the investigator can obtain a plot of urethral pressure against distance, the urethral pressure profile (Figure 8.9).

The most common method used, the perfusion catheter technique, was first described by Brown and Wickham in 1969 [8]. A small-bore catheter bearing symmetrical side holes 5 cm from its end is continuously perfused at a fixed rate of between 2 and 10 ml per minute and is slowly withdrawn down the urethra by an automatic puller at a constant rate of less than 7 mm per second. The catheter is connected to a pressure transducer, and the pressure required to perfuse the catheter at a constant rate is recorded. This pressure is the pressure needed to just lift the urethral wall off the catheter. This technique requires that there be a degree of distensibility in the urethral wall and also that a tight seal be present, so that not just the resistance to flow but also the pressure exerted by the walls of the urethra is recorded. This measurement forms the basis for a static or "resting" urethral pressure profile. If a strain is applied, for example, by the patient's coughing, then a "stress" urethral pressure profile is obtained. The latter is used in the investigation of stress incontinence [9].

Urethral pressure can also be recorded using a balloon catheter or a microtransducer. In the balloon catheter technique, a cylindrical balloon covering the side holes on the tip of a catheter is filled with saline and connected to an external pressure transducer. The balloon is usually 5 or 10 mm long, and therefore the urethral pressure is averaged over this length. Expelling the system of small air

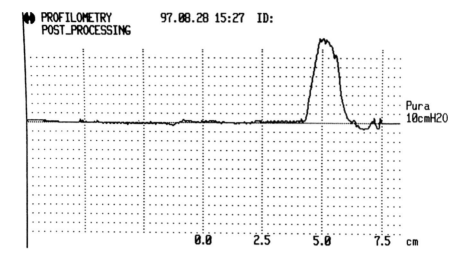

Figure 8.9   A urethral pressure profile showing a maximum urethral closure pressure of approximately 90 cm H$_2$O. (Pura = urethral pressure.)

bubbles is very difficult. In the microtransducer method, one or more pressure transducers are mounted on the side of a urethral catheter [10]. In this technique, care must be taken to ensure consistent positioning of the microtransducer within the urethra, because the results vary slightly according to the direction it is facing. Conventionally, it is placed laterally.

No well-defined range of normal values exists, and an overlap has been found in the values measured in groups of normal subjects and in subjects with stress incontinence [11]. However, provided suitable attention is paid to technique, the results are reproducible, and urethral pressure profilometry can be a useful investigative tool in some clinical and research settings.

CONCLUSIONS

The main function of urodynamic investigations is to provide information so that appropriate management can be instituted. A patient with urgency and frequency shown to have a large postmicturition residual almost invariably gains symptomatic benefit from intermittent self-catheterization. A patient with detrusor hyperreflexia and a small residual is likely to improve by taking anticholinergic medication. In addition, urodynamics has a role in the investigation of urinary symptoms in those patients for whom the nature of the underlying neurologic disorder is unclear.

The clinician should bear in mind at all times that abnormalities seen on urodynamic testing are generally not specific for a particular disorder. For example, the phasic rises in intravesical pressure on filling cystometry caused by detrusor hyperreflexia are indistinguishable from those caused by detrusor instability. Thus, urodynamics should be regarded as offering descriptive rather than diagnostic information.

REFERENCES

1. Poulsen EU, Kirkeby HJ. Home monitoring of uro-flow in normal male adolescents: relation between flow-curve, voided volume and time of day. Scand J Urol Nephrol 1988;114:58–62.
2. Fowler CJ. Investigation of the neurogenic bladder. J Neurol Neurosurg Psychiatry 1996;60:6–13.
3. Thomas DG, O'Flynn KJ. Spinal Cord Injury. In AR Mundy, TP Stephenson, AJ Wein (eds), Urodynamics (2nd ed). Edinburgh, UK: Churchill Livingstone, 1994;348–349.
4. McGuire EJ. Neuromuscular Dysfunction of the Lower Urinary Tract. In PC Walsh, RF Gittes, AD Perlmutter, TA Stamey (eds), Campbell's Urology. Philadelphia: Saunders, 1986;616.
5. Coolsaet BL, Van Duyl WA, Van Mastright R, van der Zwart A. Stepwise cystometry of urinary bladder. Urology 1973;2:255–257.
6. Wang SC, McGuire EJ, Bloom DA. A bladder pressure management system for myelodysplasia—clinical outcome. J Urol 1988;140:1499–1502.
7. Bloom DA, Knechtel JM, McGuire EJ. Urethral dilation improves bladder compliance in children with myelomeningocele and high leak point pressures. J Urol 1990;144:430–433.
8. Brown M, Wickham JEA. The urethral pressure profile. Br J Urol 1969;41:211–217.
9. Asmussen M, Lindstrom K, Ulmsten U. Simultaneous urethrocystometry and urethral pressure profile measurement with a new technique. Acta Obstet Gynecol Scand 1975;54:385–386.
10. Millar HD, Baker LE. Stable ultraminiature catheter tip pressure transducer. Med Biol Eng Comput 1973;11:86–89.
11. Hilton P, Stanton SL. Urethral pressure measurement by microtransducer: the results in symptom-free women and those with genuine stress incontinence. Br J Obstet Gynaecol 1983;90:919–933.

9
Clinical Neurophysiology

David B. Vodušek and Clare J. Fowler

Clinical neurophysiologic techniques have been used to examine the motor innervation of the sphincters and pelvic floor, sensory innervation of pelvic structures, and, most recently, autonomic sudomotor activity. Such tests are sometimes referred to as *uroneurophysiologic* and have been used mostly in urogynecology, neurourology, and proctology research, although some have found their way into routine diagnostic investigations.

The equipment used for uroneurophysiology is standard clinical neurophysiology equipment, except for some specially constructed electrodes and stimulating devices that have been adapted to urogenitoanal anatomy.

ELECTROMYOGRAPHY

Electromyography (EMG) of the pelvic floor is performed for two quite distinct, although related, purposes. Kinesiologic EMG is used to examine the pattern of activity of a particular muscle, whereas conventional EMG is used to demonstrate whether a muscle is normally or abnormally innervated.

Kinesiologic Electromyography

The choice of muscle for EMG depends on the aims of the investigation. Routine EMG performed as part of urodynamic studies usually uses a single channel for recording from the urethral or anal sphincter muscle. Because the sphincters are small, circular muscles, the two sides are assumed to react in a similar fashion; however, as was shown for the levator ani muscle, this may not always be the case [1].

For noninvasive EMG recordings, various surface electrodes have been devised (Figure 9.1). Small skin-surface electrodes can be applied to the perineal skin. For

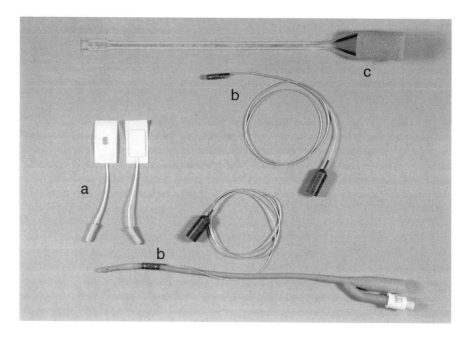

Figure 9.1   Various types of surface electrodes used for recording electromyographic activity from the pelvic floor. (a = stick-on surface electrodes; b = catheter-mounted ring electrodes for urethral sphincter recording; c = vaginal sponge-mounted electrode.)

intravaginal placement, a disposable electrode mounted on a foam pad is available [2], and other custom-built intravaginal recording devices have been described [3]. Anal plugs have been used to record from the anal sphincter, and catheter-mounted ring electrodes have been used to record from the urethral sphincter [4]. Recordings with surface electrodes are prone to artifacts that may be difficult to identify, and the amplitude of muscle activity recorded in this way is usually low. These problems can be overcome by using intramuscular needle electrodes, the most common of which is the concentric needle electrode.

Concentric needle electrodes for recording EMG signals are widely available and robust devices. Although they are needles and are therefore painful for the subject, they are easily introduced and their position can be readily adjusted; however, they also may be dislodged by movement. Lacking some of those drawbacks is the double-wire hooked electrode, which can be introduced into the muscle via a needle cannula. The cannula is then withdrawn and the wires remain in place. The advantages of this type of recording are good stability and painlessness once in place; the disadvantage is that position cannot be adjusted once the wires are placed.

Normal sphincter activity consists of continuous activity at rest that may be increased voluntarily or reflexively. Such activity has been recorded for up to 2 hours [5] and even after subjects have fallen asleep [6, 7]. This physiologic spontaneous activity depends on prolonged activation of tonic motor units, not on rapidly changing activation and inactivation of various motor units [7]. The amount of recorded tonic activity is influenced by physiologic and technical factors. It depends on the uptake area of the electrode; with a concentric needle electrode, activity from one to five motor units is usually recorded per detection site. Although tonic activity is found in both sphincters, it is not found in all recording sites of the levator ani muscle [8] and is practically never seen in the bulbocavernosus muscle [7].

Typically, the tonic motor unit potentials (MUPs) occur regularly at low frequencies. In a study of 39 such motor units from the anal sphincter in 17 subjects, the range of discharge rates was found to be 2.5–9.4 Hz (mean of 5.3 ± 1.8 Hz) [7]. Any reflex or voluntary activation procedure is reflected by an initial increase in the firing frequency of these motor units, and, with any stronger activation, new phasic motor units are recruited. The signals of these phasic units are of higher amplitude, and their discharge rates are faster and more irregular. A small percentage of motor units with an intermediate activation pattern may also be encountered [7]. The different types of MUPs may differ not only in amplitude but also in duration, as evidenced by EMG frequency analysis [9]. Both the urethral and anal sphincters show short-lasting voluntary activation times (typically less than 1 minute [10]), which is also the case for the pubococcygeal muscle [8]. In continent females, the pubococcygeal muscle reveals patterns of activity similar to those of the urethral and anal sphincters at most detection sites [8], whereas in women with stress incontinence, the patterns of activation and coordination between the two sides may be lost (Figure 9.2) [1].

On voiding, all EMG activity in the urethral sphincter ceases before detrusor contraction. Coordinated detrusor-sphincter activity is lost when lesions are found between the lower sacral segments and the pons, so that no sphincter inhibition is seen preceding detrusor contractions—a pattern of activity called *detrusor-sphincter dyssynergia* [11]. The pelvic floor muscle contractions of non-neuropathic voiding dyssynergia may be a learned abnormal behavior [12] and may be encountered in women with dysfunctional voiding [13].

The striated anal sphincter relaxes with defecation [14]. Paradoxic sphincter activation during defecation has been described in Parkinson's disease and termed *anismus* [15].

Electromyography to Examine Motor Unit Details

Needle EMG may help to differentiate between normal, denervated, and reinnervated muscle and possibly myopathic muscle. Concentric needle or single fiber EMG electrodes can be used.

The needle electrode must be appropriately placed in the target muscle. The bulbocavernosus muscle in the male and the subcutaneous part of the anal sphincter in both sexes are easily accessible. The levator ani muscle can be located by transrectal or transvaginal palpation and reached transcutaneously. In men, the urethral sphincter is approached through a single transperineal insertion approximately 4 cm in front of the anus with the needle directed toward the apex of the prostate; the finger of the free hand is used to palpate

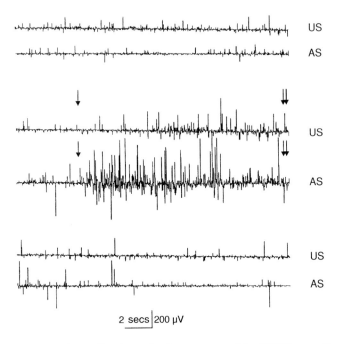

Figure 9.2   Concentric needle electrode electromyographic (EMG) recording from the urethral sphincter (US) and the anal sphincter (AS) of a 47-year-old parous woman with mild genuine stress incontinence, with comfortably full bladder. This type of recording is called *kinesiologic* because it demonstrates only the overall pattern of muscle activity. The three pairs of channels constitute continuous recordings. The woman was instructed to be as relaxed as possible. During the time period between the single and double arrows, she was asked (and continually verbally admonished) to contract the pelvic floor muscles ("as if she would hold urine"). In the first and third pair of recordings, continuous firing of motor unit potentials is seen; on voluntary contraction, a well-demarcated increase in EMG activity can be observed in the anal sphincter, whereas in the urethral sphincter this increase is delayed and less pronounced.

the apex of the prostate, and the electrode is directed toward the finger in the rectum. Because the urethral sphincter is the only striated muscle located in the midline at the apex of the prostate, the muscle can be located with some certainty. In women, the urethral sphincter is anatomically separate from the pelvic floor musculature [16]; it can be approached perineally with a needle insertion 0.5 cm lateral to the urethral orifice (the authors suggest one skin insertion per side), or it can be reached transvaginally using a Sims' speculum to retract the posterior vaginal wall. The latter approach is less uncomfortable [17], although a paraurethral injection of local anesthetic lessens discomfort and does not appear to alter the EMG signal. The position of the needle should be adjusted to several sites in a systematic way so that the same motor unit is not analyzed repeatedly.

Needle recording electrode	Needle tip and recording surface	Pickup	Needle diameter	Filter settings	Activity recorded
Concentric needle electrode Central insulated platinum wire inside a steel cannula.	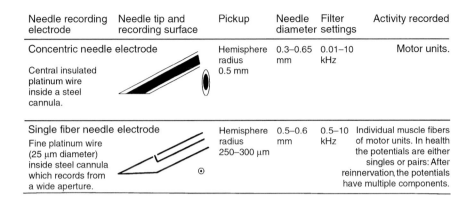	Hemisphere radius 0.5 mm	0.3–0.65 mm	0.01–10 kHz	Motor units.
Single fiber needle electrode Fine platinum wire (25 µm diameter) inside steel cannula which records from a wide aperture.		Hemisphere radius 250–300 µm	0.5–0.6 mm	0.5–10 kHz	Individual muscle fibers of motor units. In health the potentials are either singles or pairs: After reinnervation, the potentials have multiple components.

Figure 9.3 Structure and recording characteristics of concentric needle and single fiber needle electrodes. (Modified and reprinted with permission from CJ Fowler. Pelvic Floor Neurophysiology. In JW Osselton, CD Binnie, R Cooper, et al. [eds], Clinical Neurophysiology: EMG, Nerve Conduction and Evoked Potentials. Oxford, UK: Butterworth–Heinemann, 1995;233–252.)

Concentric Needle Electrode Electromyography: Normal Findings

The electrode most commonly used in EMG is the concentric needle electrode. It consists of a central insulated platinum wire that is encased within a steel cannula, the tip of which is ground to give an elliptical area of 580×150 µm (Figure 9.3). This type of electrode has the recording characteristics necessary to record spike or near activity from approximately 20 muscle fibers. The number of motor units recorded therefore depends on both the local arrangement of muscle fibers within the motor unit and the level of contraction of the muscle.

The long-established method of concentric needle electrode EMG [18, 19] can provide information on insertion activity, abnormal spontaneous activity, MUPs, and interference pattern.

In a normal skeletal muscle, initial placement of the needle elicits a short burst of insertion activity that is due to mechanical stimulation of excitable membranes. This phenomenon may also be seen in the sphincters, although it may be difficult to discern because of the reflex, pain-induced burst of motor unit activity. Insertion activity is recorded at a sensitivity setting of 50 µV per division, which is also the gain used to record spontaneous activity. Tonic MUPs are the only normal activities at rest, but phasic MUPs can be activated reflexively or voluntarily.

MUPs are analyzed at sensitivity settings that allow their full display. The commonly used time scale is 5 or 10 milliseconds per division, with an amplification of 50–500 µV per division. The commonly used amplifier filter settings for concentric needle electrode EMG are 5–10,000 Hz.

The amplitude of an MUP is largely determined by the activity of those muscle fibers closest to the recording electrode. Other fibers within a 0.5-mm radius of the recording electrode contribute little to the amplitude, but in a nor-

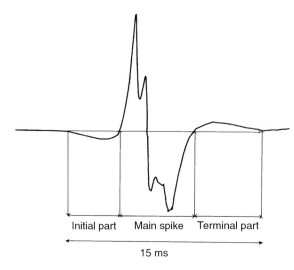

Initial part   Main spike   Terminal part

15 ms

Figure 9.4   Motor unit potential recorded with a concentric needle electrode. The spike of the motor unit is produced by the muscle fibers closest to the electrode, whereas the late phases result from activity in more distant fibers. (Reprinted with permission from CJ Fowler. Pelvic Floor Neurophysiology. In JW Osselton, CD Binnie, R Cooper, et al. [eds], Clinical Neurophysiology: EMG, Nerve Conduction and Evoked Potentials. Oxford, UK: Butterworth–Heinemann, 1995;233–252.)

mal motor unit the existence of more than two or three fibers belonging to the same motor unit is unlikely. Amplitude is highly sensitive to needle position, and very minor adjustments of the electrode result in major changes; for example, a change in position of 0.5 mm alters the amplitude from tenfold to a hundredfold.

The duration of a motor unit signal is the time between the first deflection and the point at which the waveform finally returns to the baseline (Figure 9.4). The duration depends on the number of muscle fibers within the motor unit and is little affected by the proximity of the recording electrode to the nearest fiber. The difficulty in making this measurement is defining the exact point of return to the baseline (Figure 9.5). The phases of a motor unit potential are defined by the number of times the potential crosses the baseline. A unit that has four phases or more is said to be *polyphasic*. A related parameter is a turn, which is defined as a shift in direction of a potential of greater than a specified amplitude.

Using the standard recording facilities available on all modern EMG machines, individual MUPs can be captured and their amplitude and duration measured. To allow identification of MUPs and ensure that the late components of complex potentials are not due to superimposition of several MUPs, the same potential must be captured repeatedly using a trigger and delay line. The trigger device starts the oscilloscope sweep when an incoming signal achieves a particular preset value; the delay line causes the triggering signal to be displayed not from the moment of triggering, but after an interval of some 1–5 milliseconds. The result is that the triggering potential appears repeatedly in the center of the oscilloscope screen. MUPs can also be identified if they appear repeatedly in a prolonged recording of EMG activity. Both approaches favor identification of relatively larger MUPs and become less reliable on stronger activation of

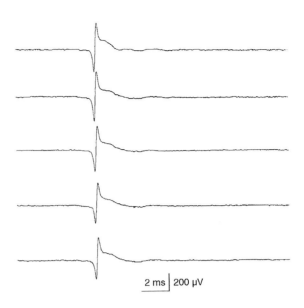

Figure 9.5 Concentric needle electrode electromyographic (EMG) recording from the urethral sphincter of a 37-year-old man with an atypical perineal pain syndrome without neurologic deficit. The trigger and delay facility of the EMG apparatus is used. The figure illustrates the occasional difficulty in measuring the duration of a motor unit potential: The onset of the potential is well demarcated, but the offset is not.

2 ms | 200 μV

muscle. Some computer-averaging programs for MUPs do not have these drawbacks. Instead of MUP analysis, an automatic quantitative analysis of the interference pattern using the turns/amplitude plot has been suggested [20], but such analysis has yet to be demonstrated as more valuable than individual motor unit analysis in assessing reinnervation.

MUPs are mostly below 1 mV and are certainly below 2 mV in the normal urethral and anal sphincters. Most are shorter than 7 milliseconds in duration (Figure 9.6), and few (less than 15%) are longer than 10 milliseconds. Most are biphasic and triphasic, but 15–33% may be polyphasic. Normal MUPs are stable—their shape on repetitive recording does not change [10, 21–26].

In addition to tonic firing of motor units (in sphincters), new MUPs are recruited voluntarily and reflexively. By such maneuvers the amount of recruitable motor units is estimated. Normally, MUPs should intermingle to produce a full interference pattern on the oscilloscope—that is, loss of the baseline when the muscle is contracted powerfully or during a strong cough.

Single Fiber Electrode Electromyography: Method and Normal Findings

A single fiber electrode has similar external proportions to a concentric needle electrode. It is made of a steel cannula 0.5–0.6 mm in diameter with a bevelled tip. It does not have the recording surface at the end, however; instead, a fine insulated platinum or silver wire embedded in epoxy resin is exposed through an aperture on the side 1–5 mm behind the tip. The platinum wire that forms the recording surface has a diameter of 25 μm and picks up activity from within a

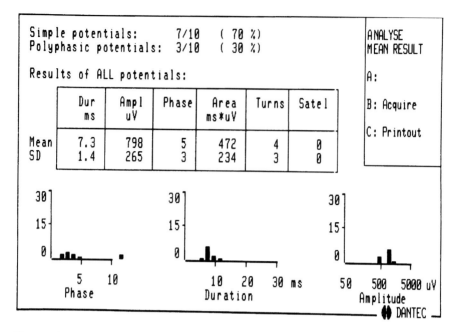

Figure 9.6   Summary of analysis of 10 individual motor units recorded from the anal sphincter with a concentric needle electrode. The mean duration is 7.3 milliseconds. (Ampl = amplitude; Dur = duration; Satel = satellites; SD = standard deviation.)

hemispheric volume 300 µm in diameter. This is quite a bit smaller than the volume of muscle tissue from which a concentric needle electrode records—the latter has an uptake area 1 mm in diameter. Because of the arrangement of muscle fibers in a normal motor unit, a single fiber electrode records only one to three single muscle fibers from the same motor unit. When a single fiber electrode is used for recording, the amplifier filters are set so that low-frequency activity (0.5–10.0 kHz) is eliminated. Thus, the contribution of each muscle fiber appears as a biphasic positive-negative action potential.

The single fiber electrode EMG parameter that reflects motor unit morphology is the fiber density. The fiber density is the mean number of muscle fibers belonging to an individual motor unit per detection site. To measure fiber density, recordings must be made from 20 different detection sites and the number of component potentials to each motor unit recorded and averaged. The normal fiber density for the anal sphincter is less than 2 (Figure 9.7) [27, 28]. Small changes with age have been reported; women have significantly greater fiber density than men (1.52 ± 0.50 versus 1.43 ± 0.14) [29].

The single fiber electrode is also suitable for recording instability of motor unit potentials or "jitter" [30]. Due to its technical characteristics, a single fiber electrode is able to record even small changes that occur in motor units due to reinnervation, but it is less suitable for detecting changes due to denervation itself—that is, abnormal insertion and spontaneous activity.

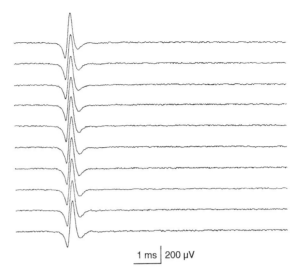

Figure 9.7 Single fiber electrode electromyographic recording from the anal sphincter of a 66-year-old man with idiopathic Parkinson's disease. The fiber density measured was 2 fibers per detection site.

1 ms | 200 µV

Electromyographic Findings Due to Denervation and Reinnervation

After complete denervation, all motor unit activity ceases, and electrical silence may be seen for several days. Ten to twenty days after the denervating injury, insertion activity becomes more prolonged, and abnormal spontaneous activity in the form of short biphasic spikes (fibrillation potentials) and biphasic potentials with prominent positive deflections (positive sharp waves) can be recorded (Figure 9.8). With axonal reinnervation, MUPs appear again—at first short and biphasic or triphasic, but soon becoming polyphasic, serrated, and prolonged [31, 32].

In perineal muscles, complete denervation can be observed after traumatic lesions to lumbosacral spine and damage to the cauda equina. Most lesions, however, cause partial denervation. In partially denervated muscle, some MUPs remain and mingle eventually with abnormal spontaneous activity. Because the MUPs in sphincter muscles are also short and mostly biphasic or triphasic, considerable EMG experience is required to recognize abnormal spontaneous activity in the presence of signals from a few surviving motor units (Figure 9.9).

In muscle with longstanding partial denervation, a peculiar abnormal insertion activity—repetitive discharges—appears. These discharges are comprised of repetitively firing groups of potentials with so little jitter between the potentials that the activity is thought to be due to ephaptic or direct transmission of impulses between muscle fibers [33]. However, this activity may be found in the striated muscle of the urethral sphincter without any other evidence of neuromuscular disease, and it has been hypothesized that it causes impaired relaxation of the muscle when it is spontaneous and profuse [34].

Partially denervated muscle, by definition, shows a loss of the number of motor units. The loss is difficult to estimate, however, because the amount of motor unit activity recorded depends on needle position and voluntary activation.

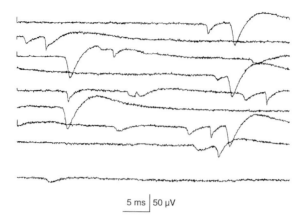

5 ms | 50 µV

Figure 9.8   Concentric needle electrode electromyographic recording from the left half of the anal sphincter of an 18-year-old man 3 weeks after a severe cauda equina injury due to a burst fracture of L3 vertebra (with asymmetric flaccid paraparesis pronounced on the left, and urinary retention, obstipation, flaccid sphincters, and asymmetric sensory loss pronounced on the left in the saddle area). The left side of the anal sphincter was completely denervated. The only activity detected was increased insertion-activity showers of positive sharp waves (shown) and single positive sharp waves or fibrillation potentials at several detection sites without needle movement. No motor unit potentials could be obtained on voluntary contraction or reflex excitation. No M wave was detectable on pudendal nerve stimulation in the perineum. No stimulation over the back was performed due to the presence of a postoperative wound. (Needle was moved just before recording.)

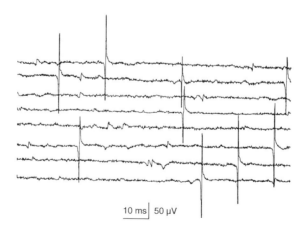

10 ms | 50 µV

Figure 9.9   Concentric needle electrode electromyographic recording from the urethral sphincter of a 34-year-old man 4 months after a lumbar paravertebral shot wound without direct trauma to nervous system structures. The fibrillation potentials shown discharged at a relatively regular and long interdischarge interval. (Needle was at rest.)

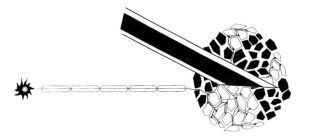

Figure 9.10   Reinnervated motor unit recorded with a concentric needle electrode. (Reprinted with permission from CJ Fowler. Pelvic Floor Neurophysiology. In JW Osselton, CD Binnie, R Cooper, et al. [eds], Clinical Neurophysiology: EMG, Nerve Conduction and Evoked Potentials. Oxford, UK: Butterworth–Heinemann, 1995;233-252.)

In partially denervated muscle, collateral reinnervation takes place. Provided some intact motor units still exist within the muscle, surviving motor nerves sprout and grow out to reinnervate those muscle fibers that have lost their nerve supply; the result is a change in the arrangement of muscle fibers within the unit. Whereas in healthy muscle it is unusual for two adjacent muscle fibers to be part of the same motor unit, after reinnervation several muscle fibers, all belonging to the same motor unit, come to be adjacent to one another (Figure 9.10). Early in the process of reinnervation, the newly outgrown motor sprouts are thin and therefore conduct slowly, so that the time taken for excitatory impulses to spread through the axonal tree is abnormally prolonged. This is reflected by prolongation of the waveform of the muscle action potential, which may have small, late components. Neuromuscular transmission in these newly grown sprouts may also be insecure, so that the motor unit may show instability. In skeletal muscle, with time, and provided no further deterioration occurs in innervation, the reinnervating axonal sprouts increase in diameter and thus increase their conduction velocity; as a result, activation of all parts of the reinnervated motor unit becomes more synchronous, which has the effect of increasing the amplitude and reducing toward normal the duration of the MUPs measured with a concentric needle electrode. This phenomenon may be different in the sphincter muscles, in which long-duration motor units (Figure 9.11) seem to remain a prominent feature of reinnervated motor units [35].

Several conditions occur in which gross changes of reinnervation may be detected in motor units of the pelvic floor. After a cauda equina lesion, the MUPs are likely to be prolonged and polyphasic [23]. Similar marked changes are seen in patients with lumbosacral myelomeningoceles.

Neuropathic changes can be recorded in sphincter muscles of patients with multiple system atrophy [35]. Multiple system atrophy is a progressive neurodegenerative disease that, particularly in its early stages, is often mistaken for Parkinson's disease but is poorly responsive to antiparkinsonian treatment. Autonomic failure causing postural hypotension and cerebellar ataxia causing unsteadiness and clumsiness may be additional features. In both women and men with this condition, uri-

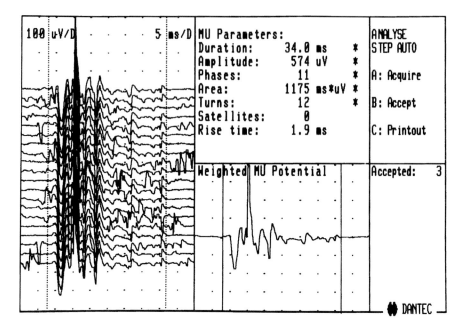

Figure 9.11   Example of motor unit recorded with a concentric needle electrode showing changes of chronic reinnervation. Recordings of the potential are shown in a falling leaf display in the left panel; the "weighted potential" or effective average is shown as a single trace in the lower panel. (D = division; MU = motor unit.)

nary incontinence occurs early, often some years before the onset of obvious neurologic features [36]. As part of the neurodegenerative process, motor units are lost in Onuf's nucleus, so that partial but progressive denervation of the sphincter occurs; recorded motor units show changes of reinnervation, with signals becoming markedly prolonged (Figure 9.12). Such changes can also be demonstrated in the bulbocavernosus muscle [37]. Sphincter EMG has been demonstrated to be of value in distinguishing between idiopathic Parkinson's disease and multiple system atrophy [35, 38], but the changes may not be obvious in the early phase of disease [37]. Similar changes of chronic reinnervation may be found in some patients with other parkinsonian syndromes, such as progressive supranuclear palsy [39]. These changes can also be demonstrated as an increase in fiber density on single fiber electrode EMG (Figure 9.13) [26].

Electromyographic Changes in Genuine Stress Incontinence

Because of the suspected role of denervation in the genesis of genuine stress incontinence, EMG techniques have been used to examine the extent of nerve damage after childbirth and to assess women with genuine stress incontinence. Single fiber electrode EMG was used to measure fiber density in the external anal

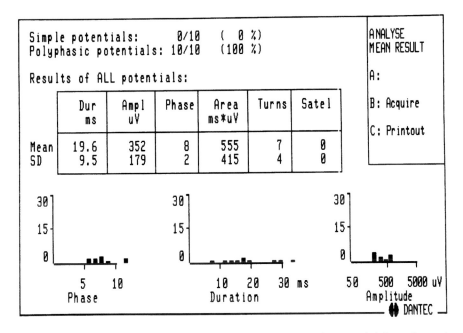

Figure 9.12 Summary of analysis of 10 individual motor units recorded from the anal sphincter with a concentric needle electrode as in Figure 9.6. The mean duration is 19.6 milliseconds— a finding that, in the absence of a history of local disease, is highly suggestive of a diagnosis of multiple system atrophy. (Ampl = amplitude; Dur = duration; Satel = satellites; SD = standard deviation.)

sphincter, and an increase was demonstrated in women with urinary stress incontinence [40]. A meticulous study in Manchester, United Kingdom, looked at the relationship between stress incontinence, genitourinary prolapse, and partial denervation of the pelvic floor [41]. Women with normal urinary control who were parous had an increase in fiber density in the pubococcygeal muscle with age that was slightly higher than that of age-matched nulliparous women. Women with stress incontinence without prolapse had much higher fiber densities than comparable age-matched control subjects. Fiber densities were similar in those with stress incontinence with prolapse and in those with prolapse alone, and were significantly higher than in asymptomatic women. Thus, it was concluded that the pubococcygeal muscle is partially denervated and then reinnervated in women with stress incontinence, genital prolapse, or both. Using a concentric needle electrode to examine the pubococcygeal muscle after childbirth, the Manchester group found a significant increase in the duration of signals from individual motor units after labor and vaginal delivery [42]. The changes were most marked in women who had urinary incontinence 8 weeks after delivery and who had had a prolonged second stage and had given birth to heavier babies.

The concentric needle electrode EMG changes found in these studies were subtle compared to those that occur after a cauda equina lesion or in multiple sys-

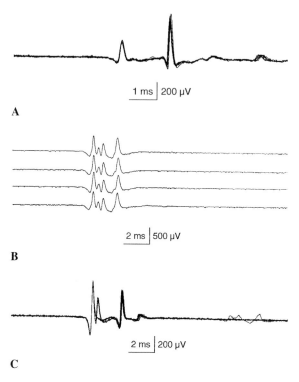

Figure 9.13 (**A**) Single fiber electrode electromyographic (EMG) recording from the urethral sphincter of a 53-year-old nulliparous woman diagnosed with possible multiple system atrophy (parkinsonism poorly responsive to L-dopa therapy and recent onset of mixed urinary incontinence). Recording shows a complex potential with two well-demarcated spikes and two small late components. Ten consecutive discharges are superimposed to show jitter, which is relatively small. For fiber density measurement, only the two large spikes can be counted. (**B**) Single fiber electrode EMG recording (same point as in **A**) shows a complex potential of four spikes. (**C**) Single fiber electrode EMG recording (same point as in **A**) shows a complex potential of four spikes (only three can be counted for fiber density measurement, being 200 V). The second spike has a large percentage of blocks (10 consecutive discharges are superimposed).

tem atrophy. Great care must be taken in any study of genuine stress incontinence that uses an EMG technique to define the control group and obtain an adequate sample of relevant EMG parameters from each subject.

Electromyographic Changes in Women with Urinary Retention and Obstructed Voiding

For many years, isolated urinary retention in young women was said either to be due to psychogenic factors or to be the first symptom of onset of multiple sclerosis [43]. However, concentric needle electrode EMG in this group has demon-

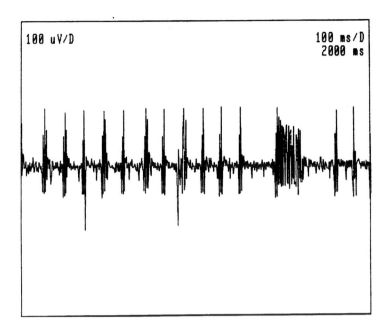

Figure 9.14 Series of 11 complex repetitive discharges followed by a brief decelerating discharge.

strated that many such patients have profuse complex repetitive discharges and decelerating burst activity in the urethral sphincter muscle (Figure 9.14) [44]. This pathologic spontaneous activity was proposed to lead to sphincter contraction, which endures during micturition and causes obstruction to flow. Positive proof of this has only recently been demonstrated by combined concentric needle electrode EMG and kinesiologic EMG analysis of a group of females with dysfunctional voiding [13].

The complex repetitive discharges have a very characteristic auditory quality over the loudspeaker on the EMG machine and sound like a helicopter or motorcycle engine. The decelerating bursts produce the myotonic-like sound that has been likened to underwater recordings of whales. Complex repetitive discharges may be difficult to distinguish from chronically reinnervated motor units, except that the potentials show much less jitter [34].

Why this activity occurs is not known, but in the syndrome described by one of the authors, it was associated with polycystic ovaries [44]. The explanation probably lies in some as yet unidentified hormonal abnormality to which the striated muscle is peculiarly sensitive. Loss of stability of membranes within the striated muscle allows ephaptic transmission to manifest as the complex repetitive discharges. Typically, patients with this syndrome are premenopausal, and the condition shows greatest incidence among women younger than 30 years of age. The clinical presentation of what is primarily a disorder of sphincter relaxation depends on the secondary effect it has on the detrusor—either instability or failure of contractility can occur (see Chapter 25).

Detrusor instability with this disorder of sphincter relaxation presents as urgency, frequency, and possibly incomplete emptying. Detrusor failure presents as urinary retention with a bladder capacity in excess of 1 liter without sensation of urgency. The condition may fluctuate, and although it may have a spontaneous onset in some individuals, it can also follow an event such as administration of a general anesthetic. The hypothesis is that the precipitating event may have an adverse effect on a precariously compromised detrusor muscle and, by tipping the balance, cause retention.

Because concentric needle electrode EMG detects both changes of denervation and reinnervation such as occur with a cauda equina lesion, as well as abnormal spontaneous activity, some have argued that this test is mandatory in women with urinary retention [45]. The test should certainly be carried out before stigmatizing a woman as having "psychogenic urinary retention."

Electromyographic Changes in Primary Muscle Disease

As is evident from the foregoing sections, EMG changes reflect pathologic changes in the structure of the motor unit. Changes in EMG due to disease of the muscle fibers are much more subtle. Although in skeletal muscle the typical features of myopathy are said to be showers of small, low-amplitude polyphasic discharges from units recruited at mild effort, such changes have not been reported in the pelvic floor, even in patients known to have generalized myopathy [46]. Pelvic floor muscle involvement in limb-girdle muscular dystrophy in a nulliparous female has been reported, but concentric needle electrode EMG of her urethral sphincter was reported to be normal [47].

Little is yet known about what might be expected of an EMG recording from muscle that has been subject to a severe stretch injury, such as occurs during childbirth, but changes may well occur that reflect the rupture of individual muscle fibers and injury to small intramuscular nerves.

Conclusion on Electromyography as a Diagnostic Tool

In the authors' view, concentric needle electrode EMG is the most important investigation for diagnostic uroneurology, as it allows the whole spectrum of changes in the course of denervation and reinnervation to be observed. Concentric needle electrode EMG allows recording of pathologic spontaneous activity and quantification of MUP parameters and permits a measure of reinnervation from motor unit duration that is quite as robust as estimates of fiber density using single fiber electrode EMG. Furthermore, the concentric needle electrode can be used at the same diagnostic session for recording motor evoked responses or reflex responses.

A caveat should be mentioned, however. A common misconception is that the amount of denervation that has occurred can be accurately measured by performing EMG. As explained in the preceding sections, denervation causes fibrillation activity and a reduction in the total number of motor units; however, fibrillations are difficult to identify with certainty in the pelvic floor, and no good method currently exists for estimating the number of motor units. Information

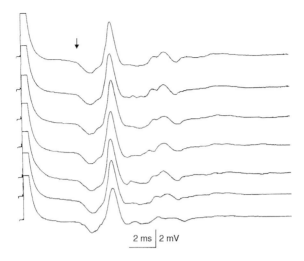

Figure 9.15 Concentric needle electrode electromyographic (EMG) recording from the bulbocavernosus muscle. Recording is from a 41-year-old male patient 1 year after a fall on the back, after which the patient claimed to have problems with defecation; no proctologic or neurologic deficits were seen on examination (on concentric needle electrode EMG examination, the responses to stimulation of the pudendal nerve and bulbocavernosus reflex were all found to be normal as well). The M wave was elicited by electrical stimulation with a conventional bipolar surface electrode "pushed" into the perineum anterior to the anus (using the electrical stimulator of the Mystro EMG machine [Medelec, Old Woking, UK]).

about denervation is therefore hard to obtain, but analysis of MUPs allows changes due to reinnervation to be identified.

NERVE CONDUCTION

Motor Conduction Studies

Measurement of motor conduction velocity is the routine method of functional evaluation of limb motor nerves. However, the technique requires access to the nerve at two well-separated points and measurement of the distance between them—a requirement that cannot be met in the pelvis. Another electrophysiologic parameter, the terminal motor latency of a muscle response, can be measured with a shorter length of motor nerve accessible [48]. The muscle response is the compound muscle action potential or M wave [48]. Terminal motor latency of the pudendal nerve can be measured by recording with a concentric needle electrode from the bulbocavernosus muscle (Figure 9.15) or from the anal or urethral sphincter muscles in response to bipolar stimulation at the perianal or perineal surface. The latencies of motor-evoked potentials (MEPs) from the perineal muscles

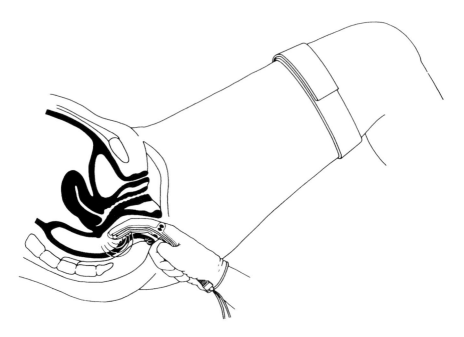

Figure 9.16   St. Mark's stimulator.

obtained by this means are between 4.7 and 5.1 milliseconds [49]. Similar latencies have been obtained from the anal sphincter using the same method of stimulation and recording [21, 50].

The more widely used technique of obtaining the pudendal terminal motor latency
relies on stimulation with a special surface electrode assembly fixed on a gloved
index finger. This technique was developed at St. Mark's Hospital in London [51],
and so is often referred to as the *St. Mark's stimulator* (Figure 9.16). It consists of
a bipolar stimulating electrode fixed to the tip of a gloved finger with the recording
electrode pair placed 3 cm proximally on the base of the finger. The finger is inserted
into the rectum and stimulation is performed close to the ischial spine. When this
stimulator is used for measurement, the terminal motor latency for the anal sphincter MEP is typically around 2 milliseconds. If a catheter-mounted electrode is used,
responses from the urethral sphincter can also be obtained. Amplitudes of the MEP
have unfortunately not proved contributory. The difference in latencies obtained by
the perineal and transrectal methods have not yet been explained.

Studies of cadavers have shown that the levator ani and pubococcygeal muscles receive innervation directly from sacral nerve roots S2–S4 before the formation of the pudendal nerve trunk [52], so that theoretically these muscles
should not contract with stimulation of the pudendal nerve at the level of the
ischial spine. However, Smith [3] and subsequently Allen [42] were both able to
record the latency of pelvic floor responses with stimulation at this point (Figure
9.17). The pudendal terminal motor latency has been found to increase with age
in some studies [29, 53] but not in others [54].

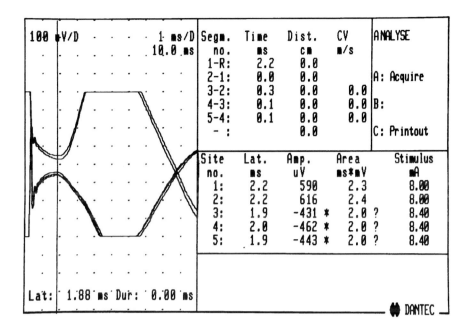

Figure 9.17 Traces recorded using the St. Mark's stimulator. Stimulation was given transvaginally, with two consecutive stimulations performed on the right and two on the left. (Amp = amplitude; CV = conduction velocity; D = division; Dist = distance; Dur = duration; Lat = latency; Segm = segment.)

The initial studies by the group from St. Mark's Hospital showed that perineal latency was abnormally prolonged in patients with urinary stress incontinence [55]—a finding that was confirmed by the Manchester group [3]. Working on the hypothesis that the pudendal nerve was stretched and injured during childbirth, several studies looked at the pudendal or perineal latency immediately postpartum. Although Allen et al. [42], using a concentric needle electrode, were able to demonstrate damage to the innervation of the pubococcygeal muscle in some women, they did not find a prolongation of the latency to stimulation of that muscle (when women were examined 2 months postpartum). Snooks et al. [56] found a significant increase in the mean pudendal nerve terminal motor latency 48–72 hours after vaginal delivery, but in 60% of cases this latency had returned to normal 2 months later. A follow-up study of 14 multiparous women from this group was conducted 5 years later [57]; the mean pudendal motor latency was found to be prolonged on both sides, fiber density of the anal sphincter was increased, and anal manometry showed that a reduction in anal canal pressure had occurred during maximal squeeze contraction. From these findings, the researchers concluded that occult damage to the pudendal innervation of the external anal sphincter had persisted and worsened over the 5-year period and had possibly been exacerbated by abnormal straining patterns of defecation. Sultan et al. [58] demonstrated a small (0.1 millisecond) but statistically significant increase in pudendal nerve latency after vaginal delivery; using anal endosonography, they demonstrated a defect of the internal or external anal sphincter or both in 35% of women after vaginal delivery. A strong association was found between these defects and the development of bowel symptoms. This association was thought to reflect a traumatic cause common to both rather than a causal relation between them. No correlation of pudendal nerve terminal latency to parity was found in another study [29].

The pudendal terminal latency has been found to be prolonged in women with pelvic floor prolapse [41, 59], with a further lengthening of the latency after vaginal dissection for repair or suspension procedures [59].

The term *pudendal neuropathy* is now established in the literature and is used particularly by coloproctologists. Those who have written about the pudendal motor latency are careful to avoid claiming that they are measuring denervation of the muscles innervated by the pudendal nerve, but others less familiar with clinical neurophysiology theory tend to equate a prolongation of pudendal motor latency with pelvic floor denervation. This supposition is mistaken, however, as prolongation of latency is a poor measure of denervation. Even if a delay occurs, a pathologic process affecting a nerve that causes an increase in latency of less than 1 millisecond over a 5-cm distance is unlikely to interfere significantly with the timing of reflex responses such as are involved with the recruitment of motor units on coughing or sneezing—that is, with maneuvers that cause stress incontinence.

An abnormality of this latency must indicate some sort of pathology of the pudendal nerve, and knowing what this might be is intriguing, because no relevant morphologic studies have yet been done. The full significance of these findings remains to be explained; perhaps, in patients with neurogenic lesions affecting the innervation of the pelvic floor, damage to the nerve occurs distally at sites where the motor nerve is branching within the muscle, unlike in carpal tunnel syndrome, in which conduction slowing is in the main trunk [42].

In the authors' laboratories, this test is used in conjunction with a needle EMG examination only if a proximal block of conduction in the motor axons is suspected, or if a motor lesion of the sacral reflex has to be differentiated from a sensory lesion in a patient with an absent sacral reflex response.

Stimulation of the Anterior Sacral Root (Cauda Equina)

Transcutaneous stimulation of deeply situated nervous tissue became possible with the development of special electrical [60] and magnetic [61] stimulators. When applied over the spine, these devices stimulate mainly the roots at the exit from the vertebral canal [62]. Various applications of these techniques to the sacral roots have been reported [63, 64]. Whether parasympathetic efferents can be stimulated using magnetic stimulation remains controversial. Although some have claimed that MEPs from the detrusor can be produced after magnetic stimulation of the cauda equina [65], others have demonstrated inhibition of detrusor hyperreflexia after sacral root stimulation [66].

Needle electrodes, rather than nonselective surface electrodes, should be used to record motor responses to electrical or magnetic stimulation (Figure 9.18), because both depolarize underlying neural structures in a nonselective fashion,

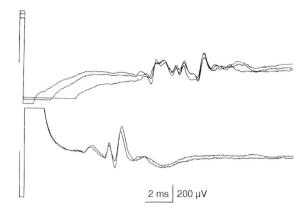

2 ms | 200 µV

Figure 9.18 Concentric needle electrode electromyographic recording from the anal sphincter of the same patient as in Figure 9.15, showing responses elicited by strong electrical stimulation with surface electrodes over the back (upper trace at level L1; lower trace at level S3). A Digitimer stimulator (Hertfordshire, UK) was used. Stimulus duration, 0.5 second; stimulus amplitude, 50% of maximum output. Three and two consecutive responses are superimposed, respectively.

and several muscles innervated by lumbosacral segments may be activated. Responses from gluteal muscles have been shown sometimes to contaminate attempts to record from the sphincters and to lead to error [67].

Recording of MEP with magnetic stimulation, at least with standard coils [68, 69], has been less successful than recording with electrical stimulation, and often large stimulus artifacts occur. Stimulation of the roots may be used to obtain a peripheral conduction time so that a central conduction time (i.e., conduction in central motor pathways from the motor cortex) can be calculated [68]. Positioning of the ground electrode between the recording electrodes and the stimulating coil should decrease the artifact [70].

Demonstrating the presence of a perineal MEP on stimulation over the lumbosacral spine via recording with a concentric needle electrode EMG may occasionally be helpful, but an absent response must be evaluated with caution, and the clinical value of the test has yet to be established.

Assessment of Central Motor Pathways

It is possible to stimulate the motor cortex using the same magnetic or electrical stimulation and to record a response from the pelvic floor. Magnetic stimulation is less unpleasant to the subject, and cortical electrical stimulation has been abandoned for use in awake subjects.

Electrical stimulation over the motor cortex of healthy subjects has been reported to produce MEPs in anal [67, 71] and urethral [71] sphincters, and the bulbocavernosus muscle [67]. The mean latencies were between 30 and 35 milliseconds if no "facilitatory maneuver" was used. If, however, stimulation was performed during a period of slight voluntary contraction of the muscle of interest, the latencies of MEPs shortened significantly (by up to 8 milliseconds).

A central conduction time can be obtained by applying stimulation both over the scalp and in the back (at level L1; see Figure 9.18) and subtracting the latency of the respective MEPs. Central conduction times of approximately 22 milliseconds without facilitation (i.e., slight voluntary contraction) and approximately 15 milliseconds with facilitation have been reported [68].

Substantially longer central conduction times have been found in patients with multiple sclerosis and spinal cord lesions than in healthy controls [72], but because all those patients had clinically recognizable cord disease, the diagnostic value of the method remains doubtful.

Because of the significant influence of voluntary contraction, the variability of both total conduction times and central conduction times makes the method somewhat unreliable. Obtaining a well-formed sphincter MEP with a normal latency in a patient with a functional disorder or in a medicolegal case may occasionally be helpful, but no established clinical use exists for this type of testing.

NEUROPHYSIOLOGY OF THE SACRAL SENSORY SYSTEM

Electroneurography of the Dorsal Penile Nerve

By placing a pair of stimulating electrodes across the glans and a pair of recording electrodes across the base of the penis, one can record a compound nerve action potential (with an amplitude of approximately 10 µV). The sensory conduction velocity of the dorsal penile nerve has been reported as 27 m per second; if the penis is stretched by a weight of 1 lb, the calculated velocity increases to approximately 33 m per second [73]. The method was claimed to be helpful in diagnosing neurogenic erectile dysfunction caused by sensory penile neuropathy [73], but the measurement of conduction distance poses considerable practical difficulties, and the test is not routinely used.

Electroneurography of Dorsal Sacral Roots

Compound sensory root action potentials with stimulation of the dorsal penile or clitoral nerve may be recorded intraoperatively when the sacral roots are exposed [74]. This procedure has been found helpful in preserving roots relevant for perineal sensation in spastic children undergoing dorsal rhizotomy and possibly decreasing the incidence of postoperative voiding dysfunction [75]. Root potentials in response to stimulation of the dorsal penile nerve can be recorded using epidural electrodes [76].

At the level of the lower thoracic and upper lumbar vertebrae, a low-amplitude (<1 µV) spinal somatosensory evoked potential (SEP) can be recorded with surface electrodes. It is a monophasic negative potential with a mean peak latency of approximately 12.5 milliseconds [77–79] and is probably due to postsynaptic activity in the spinal cord [68, 77–79]. It may be difficult to record in healthy but obese male subjects [68, 77, 78] and in most female subjects, and it is therefore not used in routine testing.

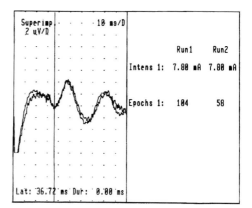

```
Superimp          · 18 ms/D
2 uV/D

                              Run1      Run2

                    Intens 1: 7.88 mA  7.88 mA

                    Epochs 1: 184        58




Lat: 36.72 ms Dur: 8.88 ms
```

Figure 9.19 Pudendal somatosensory evoked potential recorded after stimulation of the dorsal nerve of the penis. The trace shows the result of averaging twice superimposed. (D = division; Dur = duration; Intens = intensity; Lat = latency; Superimp = superimposed.)

With epidural electrodes, sacral root potentials in response to stimulation of the dorsal penile nerve could be recorded in only 13 subjects, and cord potentials in 9 out of 22 subjects [76]. Latencies of these spinal SEPs were 11.9 ± 1.8 milliseconds [76], substantiating the results obtained by surface recording [77, 78].

Cerebral Somatosensory Evoked Potential

The pudendal SEP is easily recorded after electrical stimulation of the dorsal penile or clitoral nerve [68, 77, 78, 80–82]. As a rule, this SEP is of highest amplitudes at the central recording site (Cz –2 cm : Fz of the International 10-20 System) [83] and is highly reproducible. Amplitudes of the P40 measure between 0.5 and 12 µV (Figure 9.19) [78]. The first positive peak at 41 ± 2.3 milliseconds [78] (called P1 or P40) is usually clearly defined in healthy subjects when a stimulus of two to four times sensory threshold current strength is used [78, 82]. A later negative wave (at approximately 55 milliseconds) and further positive and negative waves are quite variable in amplitude and expression from one individual to another and have little known clinical relevance.

Pudendal SEP recordings have been measured widely in patients with neurogenic erectile dysfunction, spinal cord lesions [81, 84], multiple sclerosis [85], and diabetes [86]. Such measurements were also once advocated in patients with neurogenic bladder dysfunction due to multiple sclerosis [72]; however, the tibial cerebral SEPs have been shown to be more often abnormal than the pudendal SEP [26]. Only in exceptional cases is the pudendal SEP abnormal but the tibial SEPs normal, pointing to an isolated conus involvement [26]. Measurement of cerebral SEPs in response to penile or clitoral stimulation was reported as a possibly valuable intraoperative monitoring method in patients with cauda equina or conus undergoing a surgical procedure [87, 88]. A study that used the pudendal SEP when investigating urogenital symptoms to detect relevant neurologic disease found it to be less valuable than did a clinical examination that looked for signs of spinal cord disease in the lower limbs (i.e., lower limb hyperreflexia and extensor plantar responses) [89].

The use of cerebral SEP recording in men with erectile dysfunction is discussed in Chapter 10. Under some circumstances, such as when a patient complains of loss of bladder or vaginal sensation, success in recording a normal pudendal evoked response may be reassuring.

Electrical Stimulation of Urethra, Bladder, and Anal Canal

A cerebral SEP can also be measured in response to stimulation of bladder mucosa [90]. When such measurements are made, use of bipolar stimulation in the bladder or proximal urethra is of utmost importance, because otherwise somatic afferents are depolarized [71, 91, 92]. These cerebral SEPs have been shown to have a maximum amplitude over the midline (Cz –2 cm : Fz) [92]; even so, the potential has a low amplitude (1 μV or less) and a variable configuration and may be difficult to identify in some control subjects [79, 92]. The typical latency of the most prominent negative potential (N1) is approximately 100 milliseconds [79, 92]. The responses are claimed to be more relevant to neurogenic bladder dysfunction than the pudendal SEP, because the A delta sensory afferents from the bladder and proximal urethra accompany the autonomic fibers in the pelvic nerves [92].

Another stimulation site in the perineal region is the anal canal. After stimulation of this area, cerebral SEPs with a slightly longer latency than those obtained with penis or clitoris stimulation have been reported [69], but this response cannot be recorded from all control subjects. The rectum and sigmoid colon have also been stimulated and cerebral SEPs of two types recorded. One was similar in shape and latency to the pudendal SEP, and the other to the SEP recorded in response to stimulation of the bladder and posterior urethra [93].

Mechanical Stimulation

Mechanical stimulation of the thumb and patella have been used to elicit SEPs and have been found to be more sensitive in disclosing neurogenic lesions in patients with multiple sclerosis [94]. The same principle has been used to elicit SEPs from the esophagus [95] and rectum [96]. Mechanical stimulation of the penis is obviously preferable to electrical stimulation when investigating children. Mechanical stimuli to elicit an SEP were delivered to the distal penis by a custom-designed electromechanical hammer triggered by an oscilloscope, and responses to 100 stimuli were averaged. The cerebral SEPs measured in response to such stimulation had the same shape and similar latency to those elicited by standard electrical stimulation [97].

MEASUREMENT OF SACRAL REFLEXES

Physiologic Background, Methods, and Terminology

The term *sacral reflexes* refers to electrophysiologically recordable responses of perineal and pelvic floor muscles to electrical stimulation in the urogenitoanal region. Two reflexes—the anal and the bulbocavernosus—are commonly elicited clinically in the lower sacral segments. Both have the afferent and efferent limbs of their reflex arc in the pudendal nerve and are centrally integrated at the S2–S4 cord levels. Electrophysiologic correlates of these reflexes have been described.

Electrical [49, 98–101], mechanical [102], or magnetic [69] stimulation can be used. Whereas the latter two modalities have been applied only to the penis and clitoris, electrical stimulation can be applied at various sites: to the dorsal penile nerve [49, 98–101, 103]; to the dorsal clitoral nerve [24, 49, 82, 104]; perianally [87, 105]; and at the bladder neck and proximal urethra using a catheter-mounted ring electrode [91, 106]. These reflexes are often referred to as "vesicourethral" and "vesicoanal" [107], depending on the muscle from which the reflex responses are recorded. The pudendal nerve itself may be stimulated by applying needle electrodes transperineally [102] or using the St. Mark's stimulator [108]; the term *deep pudendal reflex* was suggested for the reflex measured in response to such stimulation [108].

Reports of sacral reflexes measured after electrical stimulation of the dorsal penile or clitoral nerve cite consistent mean latencies of between 31.0 and 38.5 milliseconds [24, 49, 82, 98–104]. The latency of responses elicited by mechanical stimulation of the distal penis were reported to be either shorter [102] or longer [97] than the latency of those elicited by standard electrical stimulation. The latency with magnetic stimulation was reported to be longer [69]. These findings are probably related to technical aspects of the stimulators used [97].

Sacral reflex responses obtained after perianal stimulation or stimulation of the bladder neck or proximal urethra have latencies between 50 and 65 milliseconds [49, 105, 106]. This more prolonged response is thought to be due to the fact that the afferent limb of the reflex is conveyed by thinner myelinated nerves with slower conduction velocities than the thicker myelinated pudendal afferents.

The longer-latency anal reflex, the contraction of the anal sphincter on stimulation of the perianal region, may also have thinner myelinated fibers in its afferent limb because it is produced by a nociceptive stimulus. After perianal stimulation, a short-latency potential can also be recorded that results from depolarization of motor branches to the anal sphincter [21, 49]; this M wave or compound muscle action potential (CMAP) has been mistaken for a reflex response.

Sacral Reflex in Response to Electrical Stimulation of the Penis or Clitoris

The sacral reflex evoked by dorsal penile or clitoral nerve stimulation, the bulbocavernosus reflex, was shown to be a complex response, often forming two components [49, 101, 109]. The first component (with a typical latency of approximately 35 milliseconds) is the response that has been most often called the bulbocavernosus reflex (Figure 9.20). It is stable, does not habituate, and is thought to be an oligosynaptic reflex response, because the variability of single motor neuron discharges within this reflex is similar to that of the first component of the blink reflex [109]. The second component has a latency similar to that of the sacral reflexes evoked by perianal stimulation or stimulation from the proximal urethra. The variability of single motor neuron reflex responses within this component is much larger, as is typical for a polysynaptic reflex [109]. The

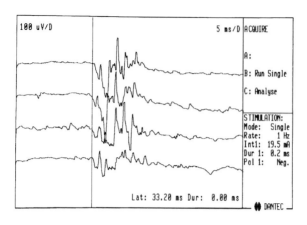

Figure 9.20 Bulbocavernosus reflex recorded after stimulation of the dorsal nerve of the penis and recorded from the bulbocavernosus muscle with a concentric needle electrode. (D = division; Dur = duration; Int = intensity; Lat = latency; Neg = negative; Pol = polarity.)

second component is not always demonstrable as a discrete response [102]. The two components of the reflex may behave somewhat differently in control subjects and in patients. In normal subjects, the first component usually has a lower threshold; in patients with partially denervated pelvic floor muscles, however, the first reflex component cannot be obtained with single stimuli, but on strong stimulation the later reflex component does occur [101]. This can cause confusion, as the investigator may record very "delayed" reflex responses in patients, not recognizing the possibility that the signal is not a delayed first component but an isolated second component of the reflex. The situation can be clarified by using double stimuli; this procedure facilitates the reflex response [102] and may reveal in such a patient the first component, which was not obvious on stimulation with a single stimulus [110].

Sacral reflex responses recorded with needle or wire electrodes can be analyzed separately for each side of the anal sphincter or each bulbocavernosus muscle [101]; such investigation is important, because unilateral or asymmetric lesions are common. Unilateral stimulation of the penis is not really possible, however, because in patients with sensory loss, the application of a stronger stimulus leads to electrical spread.

Measurement of sacral reflex responses elicited by stimulation of the dorsal penile and clitoral nerves has been proposed to be valuable in patients with cauda equina and lower motor neuron lesions [99], although measurement of a normal latency in a reflex does not exclude the possibility of an axonal lesion in its reflex arc. Most commonly, measurement of sacral reflex responses to stimulation of the penis has been proposed for evaluation of neurogenic erectile dysfunction (see also Chapter 10) [81, 99, 100]. However, many patients with probable neurogenic erectile dysfunction have been shown to have reflex latencies within the normal range [81, 111]; conversely, patients with hereditary motor and sensory demyelinating neuropathy who have normal bladder and sexual function have been found to have much-delayed sacral reflex responses [112]. Poor specificity of the abnormal sacral reflex has been reported by others [113], who have found normal nocturnal erections in patients with prolonged sacral reflex latencies. Also, in diabetic patients with suspected neurogenic impotence, the conduction velocity parameters in limbs have been found to be more sensitive in revealing peripheral neuropathy than sacral reflex latencies [86]. Others have proposed that testing for autonomic function is more sensitive than measurement of somatic parameters [114].

Most reports deal with abnormally prolonged sacral reflex latencies. Some contend that very short reflex latency suggests the possibility of a tethered cord [115]; the shorter latency is attributed in particular to the low location of conus. Shorter latencies of sacral reflexes in patients with suprasacral cord lesions have been reported as well [104].

Continuous intraoperative recording of sacral reflex responses elicited by stimulation of the penis or clitoris is feasible if double pulses [74, 116] or a train of stimuli is used.

Sacral reflex testing should be part of the diagnostic battery; concentric needle electrode EMG exploration of the pelvic floor muscles is the most important part of this testing. Measurement of sacral reflexes is established and carried out in laboratories worldwide and is the most time-honored uroneurophysiologic diagnostic procedure. However, the expectations of some authors that measurement of sacral reflexes could provide a single, easily learned test that could distinguish between neurogenic and non-neurogenic sacral dysfunction was unrealistic. Although testing reflex responses is a valid and useful method of assessing the integrity of reflex arcs, and although electrophysiologic assessment of sacral reflexes is a more quantitative, sensitive, and reproducible way of assessing the S2–S4 reflex arcs than any of the clinical methods, uncritical interpretation of results should be discouraged.

Sacral Reflex in Response to Mechanical Stimulation

Mechanical stimulation has been used to elicit the bulbocavernosus reflex in both sexes [117] and has been found to be a robust technique [102]. Either a standard, commercially available reflex hammer or a customized electromechanical hammer can be used [97]. Such stimulation is painless and can be used in children or patients with pacemakers for whom electrical stimulation is contraindicated. The latency of the bulbocavernosus reflex elicited mechanically is comparable to the latency of the electrically elicited reflex in the same patients, but it may be either slightly shorter [102] or longer [97] because of the particular electromechanical device used and variability in the actual onset of the mechanical stimulus compared with the electrical stimulus.

MEASUREMENT OF AUTONOMIC NERVOUS SYSTEM RESPONSES

All the uroneurophysiologic methods discussed so far assess the thicker myelinated fibers only, whereas the autonomic nervous system—the parasympathetic part, in particular—is most relevant for sacral organ function. Some have argued that local involvement of the sacral nervous system (as in cases of trauma and compression) usually involves somatic and autonomic fibers simultaneously; however, even some local pathologic conditions can result in purely isolated lesions (as in mesorectal excision of carcinoma or radical prostatectomy), so that methods allowing direct assessment of the parasympathetic and sympathetic nervous system innervating the pelvic viscera would be very helpful. Information on parasympathetic bladder innervation can be obtained to some extent by cystometry, but from a clinical neurophysiologic point of view, direct electrophysiologic testing would be desirable.

In cases in which a general involvement of thin fibers is expected, an indirect way to examine autonomic fibers is to assess thin sensory fiber function. Because unmyelinated afferent fibers transmit temperature sensation and pain, unmyelinated fiber neuropathy can be identified by testing thermal sensitivity. Diabetic patients with a presumed neurologic cause for their erectile dysfunction have been tested for thermal thresholds to both heating and cooling in the feet and have been found to have markedly impaired temperature sensitivity [118]. Thermal thresholds have also been tested in the penis in control subjects [119] and diabetic subjects [120].

Thin (visceral sensory) fibers are tested by stimulating the proximal urethra or bladder and recording sacral reflex responses or cerebral SEPs.

Sympathetic Skin Response

The sympathetic nervous system mediates sweat gland activity in the skin. Changes in sweat gland activity lead to changes in skin resistance. With stressful stimulation, a potential shift can be recorded with surface electrodes from the skin of palms and soles and has been reported to be a useful parameter in assessment of neuropathy involving unmyelinated nerve fibers [121]. This sympathetic skin response (SSR) can also be recorded from perineal skin and from the penis [122, 123] (Figure 9.21). The SSR is a reflex pathway that consists of myelinated sensory fibers, a complex central integrative mechanism, and a sympathetic efferent limb (with postganglionic nonmyelinated C fibers). The stimulus used in clinical practice is usually an electric pulse delivered to the upper or lower limb (to mixed nerves), but the genital organs can also be stimulated [122]. The latencies of the SSR on the penis after stimulation of a median nerve at the wrist have been reported to be between 1.5 [122] and 2.3 seconds [123] (Figure 9.22) and could be obtained in all normal subjects, although variability was high. The responses are easily habituated and depend on a number of endogenous and exogenous factors including skin temperature, which should be higher than 28°C. Only an absent SSR can be considered abnormal.

SSR recording in limbs was claimed to be more informative than somatic sacral reflex and SEP testing in patients with organic erectile dysfunction [114]; recording SSR also on the penis was reported to be even more informative [123], as it assesses local afferent innervation.

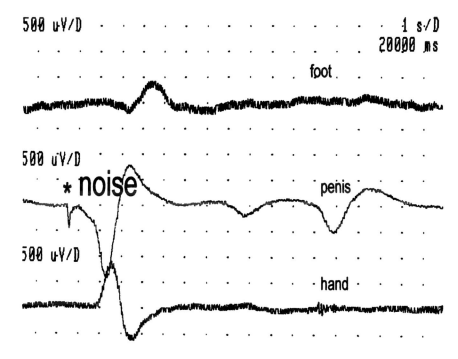

Figure 9.21 Sympathetic skin responses recorded with silver–silver chloride surface electrodes over foot, penis, and hand. A sudden noise evoked a response at all three sites. The latency to the response from the penis was similar to that from the hand; the response from the foot was considerably later (by approximately 2.5 seconds). (D = division.)

Figure 9.22 Sympathetic skin responses recorded from the foot and penis with silver– silver chloride surface electrodes in response to stimulation of the median nerve at the wrist. Responses occurred at 1.52 seconds (penis) and 2.3 seconds (foot) after stimulation. (D = division; HP = high pass; Int = intensity; LP = low pass; TR = trace.)

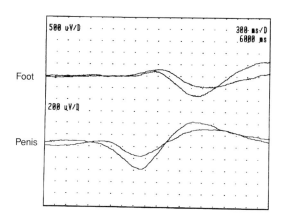

Corpus Cavernosum Electromyography

The EMG activity claimed to represent corpus cavernosum responses and its relationship to sympathetic skin responses is discussed in Chapter 10.

Although controversy remains about the nature of corpus cavernosum EMG, these recordings are acknowledged to represent a genuine advance, both by providing a direct measure of autonomic innervation of the genital region and by raising awareness of the inadequacies of former means of neurophysiologic testing in the investigation of erectile dysfunction.

CONCLUSIONS

Uroneurophysiologic techniques have been used most often in research. Neurophysiologic studies were valuable in substantiating the hypotheses that a proportion of patients with sacral dysfunctions—for instance, patients with erectile dysfunction [49, 99] or patients with stress urinary incontinence and idiopathic fecal incontinence [51, 56]—had involvement of the nervous system. The tests helped to establish the function of the sacral nervous system in patients with suprasacral spinal cord injury [124], to reveal the consequences of particular surgeries [125], to elucidate innervation of pelvic floor muscles [22, 126], and to describe activation patterns of pelvic floor muscles [1, 8]. The technique of intraoperative monitoring has been introduced, and evoked potential studies promise to help prevent lesions of the neural structures at risk from the surgical procedure [74, 87, 127]. Further research applications of uroneurophysiologic methods are expected, for many of the neurologic aspects of urologic, gynecologic, and proctologic problems have yet to be elucidated.

REFERENCES

1. Deindl F, Vodušek DB, Hesse U, Schüssler B. Pelvic floor activity patterns: comparison of nulliparous continent and parous urinary stress incontinent women. A kinesiological EMG study. Br J Urol 1994;73:413–417.
2. Lose G, Tanko A, Colstrup H, Andersen JT. Urethral sphincter electromyography with vaginal surface electrodes: a comparison with sphincter electromyography recorded via periurethral coaxial, anal sphincter needle and perianal surface electrodes. J Urol 1985;133: 815–818.
3. Smith A, Hosker G, Warrell D. The role of pudendal nerve damage in the aetiology of genuine stress incontinence in women. Br J Obstet Gynaecol 1989;96:29–32.
4. Nordling J, Meyhoff H, Walter S, Andersen J. Urethral electromyography using a new ring electrode. J Urol 1978;120:571–573.
5. Chantraine A, Leval J, Onkelinx A. Motor Conduction Velocity in the Internal Pudendal Nerves. In JE Desmedt (ed), New Developments in Electromyography and Clinical Neurophysiology (vol. 2). Basel, Switzerland: Karger, 1973;433–438.
6. Jesel M, Isch-Treussard C, Isch F. Electromyography of Striated Muscle of Anal Urethral Sphincters. In JE Desmedt (ed), New Developments in Electromyography and Clinical Neurophysiology (vol 2). Basel, Switzerland: Karger, 1973;406–420.
7. Vodušek DB. A Neurophysiological Study of Human Sacral Reflexes [master's thesis]. Ljubljana, Slovenia: University E. Kardelj, 1982;1–55.
8. Deindl FM, Vodušek DB, Hesse U, Schüssler B. Activity patterns of pubococcygeal muscles in nulliparous continent women. Br J Urol 1993;72:46–51.

9. Vereecken RL, Ketelaer P, Joossens J, Leruitte A. Frequency analysis of the electromyographic activity in striated pelvic floor muscles. Eur Neurol 1977;3:333–336.
10. Vereecken RL, Derluyn J, Verduyn H. Electromyography of the perineal striated muscles during cystometry. Urol Int 1975;30:92–98.
11. Blaivas JG, Sinha HP, Zayed AAH, Labib KB. Detrusor-external sphincter dyssynergia. J Urol 1981;125:542–544.
12. Rudy DC, Woodside JR. Non-neurogenic neurogenic bladder: the relationship between intravesical pressure and the external sphincter electromyogram. Neurourol Urodyn 1991;10:169–176.
13. Deindl FM, Vodušek DB, Bischof Ch, Hartung R. Zwei verschiedene Formen von Miktionsstörungen bei jungen Frauen: Dyssynerges Verhalten im Beckenboden oder Pseudomyotonie im externen urethralen Sphinkter? Akt Urol 1997;28:88–94.
14. Read NW. Functional Assessment of the Anorectum in Faecal Incontinence. In G Bock, J Whelan (eds), Neurobiology of Incontinence. Chichester, UK: Wiley, 1990;119–138. Ciba Foundation Symposium 151.
15. Mathers SE, Kempster PA, Law PJ, et al. Anal sphincter dysfunction in Parkinson's disease. Arch Neurol 1989;46:1061–1064.
16. Gosling JA, Dixon JS, Humperson JR. Functional Anatomy of the Urinary Tract. London: Churchill Livingstone, 1983:chap 5.
17. Lowe EM, Fowler CJ, Osborne JL, DeLancey JOL. Improved method for needle electromyography of the urethral sphincter in women. Neurourol Urodyn 1994;13:29–33.
18. Petersén I, Franksson C, Danielson CO. Electromyographic study of the muscles of the pelvic floor and urethra in normal females. Acta Obstet Gynecol Scand 1955;34:273–285.
19. Chantraine A. Electromyographie des sphincters striés ureal et anal humains. Rev Neurol (Paris) 1966;115:396–403.
20. Aanestad Ø, Flink R, Stålberg E. Interference pattern in perineal muscles: I. A quantitative electromyographic study in normal subjects. Neurourol Urodyn 1989;8:1–9.
21. Bartolo DCC, Jarratt JA, Read NW. The use of conventional electromyography to assess external anal sphincter neuropathy in man. J Neurol Neurosurg Psychiatry 1983;46:1115–1118.
22. Vodušek DB, Light JK. The motor nerve supply of the external urethral sphincter muscles. Neurourol Urodyn 1983;2:193–200.
23. Fowler CJ, Kirby RS, Harrison MJG, et al. Individual motor unit analysis in the diagnosis of disorders of urethral sphincter innervation. J Neurol Neurosurg Psychiatry 1984;47:637–641.
24. Varma JS, Smith AN, McInnes A. Electrophysiological observations on the human pudendo-anal reflex. J Neurol Neurosurg Psychiatry 1986;49:1411–1416.
25. Chantraine A, De Leval J, Depireux P. Adult female intra- and peri-urethral sphincter-electromyographic study. Neurourol Urodyn 1990;9:139–144.
26. Rodi Z, Vodušek DB, Denišlič M. External anal sphincter electromyography in the differential diagnosis of parkinsonism. J Neurol Neurosurg Psychiatry 1996;60:460–461.
27. Neill ME, Swash M. Increased motor unit fibre density in the external anal sphincter muscle in anorectal incontinence: a single fibre EMG study. J Neurol Neurosurg Psychiatry 1980;43:343–347.
28. Vodušek DB, Janko M. SFEMG in striated sphincter muscles [abstract]. Muscle Nerve 1981;4:252.
29. Jameson JS, Chia YW, Kamm MA, et al. Effect of age, sex and parity on anorectal function. Br J Surg 1994;81:1689–1692.
30. Stålberg E, Trontelj JV. Single Fiber Electromyography: Studies in Healthy and Diseased Muscle (2nd ed). New York: Raven Press, 1994.
31. Brown FW. The Physiological and Technical Basis of Electromyography. London: Butterworth, 1984.
32. Fowler CJ. Pelvic Floor Neurophysiology. In JW Osselton, Binnie CD, Cooper R, et al. (eds), Clinical Neurophysiology: EMG, Nerve Conduction and Evoked Potentials. Oxford, UK: Butterworth–Heinemann, 1995;233–252.
33. Trontelj J, Stålberg E. Bizarre repetitive discharges recorded with single fibre EMG. J Neurol Neurosurg Psychiatry 1983;46:310–316.
34. Fowler CJ, Kirby RS, Harrison MJG. Decelerating bursts and complex repetitive discharges in the striated muscle of the urethral sphincter associated with urinary retention in women. J Neurol Neurosurg Psychiatry 1985;48:1004–1009.
35. Palace J, Chandiramani VA, Fowler CJ. Value of sphincter EMG in the diagnosis of multiple system atrophy. Muscle Nerve 1997;20:1396–1403.
36. Beck RO, Betts CD, Fowler CJ. Genitourinary dysfunction in multiple system atrophy: clinical features and treatment in 62 cases. J Urol 1994;151:1336–1341.
37. Stocchi F, Carbone A, Inghilleri M, et al. Urodynamic and neurophysiological evaluation in Parkinson's disease and multiple system atrophy. J Neurol Neurosurg Psychiatry 1997;62:507–511.

38. Eardley I, Quinn NP, Fowler CJ, et al. The value of urethral sphincter electromyography in the differential diagnosis of parkinsonism. Br J Urol 1989;64:360–362.
39. Vallderiola F, Valls-Solè J, Tolosa ES, Marti MJ. Striated anal sphincter denervation in patients with progressive supranuclear palsy. Mov Disord 1995;9:117–121.
40. Anderson R. A neurogenic element to urinary genuine stress incontinence. Br J Urol 1984;91:41–45.
41. Smith ARB, Hosker GL, Warrell DW. The role of partial denervation of the pelvic floor in aetiology of genitourinary prolapse and stress incontinence of urine: a neurophysiological study. Br J Obstet Gynaecol 1989;96:24–28.
42. Allen R, Hosker G, Smith A, Warrell D. Pelvic floor damage and childbirth: a neurophysiological study. Br J Obstet Gynaecol 1990;97:770–779.
43. Siroky M, Krane R. Functional Voiding Disorders in Women. In R Krane, M Siroky (eds), Clinical Neuro-Urology. Boston: Little, Brown, 1991;445–457.
44. Fowler CJ, Christmas TJ, Chapple CR, et al. Abnormal electromyographic activity of the urethral sphincter, voiding dysfunction, and polycystic ovaries: a new syndrome? BMJ 1988;297: 1436–1438.
45. Fowler CJ, Kirby RS. Electromyography of the urethral sphincter in women with urinary retention. Lancet 1986;i:1455–1456.
46. Caress J, Kothari M, Bauer S, Shefner J. Urinary dysfunction in Duchenne muscular dystrophy. Muscle Nerve 1996;19:819–822.
47. Dixon PJ, Christmas TJ, Chapple CR. Stress incontinence due to pelvic floor muscle involvement in limb-girdle muscular dystrophy. Br J Urol 1990;65:653–660.
48. AAEE glossary of terms used in clinical electromyography. Muscle Nerve 1987;10:G1–G60.
49. Vodušek DB, Janko M, Lokar J. Direct and reflex responses in perineal muscles on electrical stimulation. J Neurol Neurosurg Psychiatry 1983;46:67–71.
50. Pedersen E, Klemar B, Schroder HD, et al. Anal sphincter responses after perianal electrical stimulation. J Neurol Neurosurg Psychiatry 1982;45:770–773.
51. Kiff ES, Swash M. Normal proximal and delayed distal conduction in the pudendal nerves of patients with idiopathic (neurogenic) faecal incontinence. J Neurol Neurosurg Psychiatry 1984;47:820–823.
52. Jünemann K-P, Lue T, Schmidt R, Tanagho E. Clinical significance of sacral and pudendal nerve anatomy. J Urol 1988;139:74–80.
53. Laurberg S, Swash M. Effects of aging on the anorectal sphincters and their innervation. Dis Colon Rectum 1989;32:737–742.
54. Barret JA, Brocklehurst JC, Kiff ES, et al. Anal function in geriatric patients with faecal incontinence. Gut 1989;30:1244–1251.
55. Snooks SJ, Badenoch DF, Tiptaft RC, Swash M. Perineal nerve damage in genuine stress incontinence. Br J Urol 1985;57:422–426.
56. Snooks SJ, Swash M, Setchell M, Henry MM. Injury to the pelvic floor sphincter musculature in childbirth. Lancet 1984;ii:546–555.
57. Snooks SJ, Swash M, Mathers SE, Henry MM. Effect of vaginal delivery in the pelvic floor: a 5-year follow-up. Br J Surg 1990;77:1358–1360.
58. Sultan A, Kamm M, Hudson C, et al. Anal-sphincter disruption during vaginal delivery. N Engl J Med 1993;329:1905–1911.
59. Benson T, McClellan E. The effect of vaginal dissection on the pudendal nerve. Obstet Gynecol 1993;82:387–389.
60. Merton PA, Morton HB. Stimulation of the cerebral cortex in the intact human subject. Nature 1980;285:227.
61. Barker AT, Jalinous R, Freeston IL. Non-invasive magnetic stimulation of the human motor cortex. Lancet 1985;i:1106–1107.
62. Mills KR, Murray NMF. Electrical stimulation over the human vertebral column: which neural elements are excited? Electroencephalogr Clin Neurophysiol 1986;63:582–589.
63. Swash M, Snooks SJ. Slowed motor conduction in lumbosacral nerve roots in cauda equina lesions: a new diagnostic technique. J Neurol Neurosurg Psychiatry 1986;49:809–816.
64. Vodušek DB. Electrophysiology. In B Schüßler, J Laycock, P Norton, S Stanton (eds), Pelvic Floor Re-Education, Principles and Practice. London: Springer-Verlag, 1994;83–97.
65. Bemelmans BLH, Van Kerrebroeck PEV, Debruyne FMJ. Motor bladder responses after magnetic stimulation of the cauda equina. Neurourol Urodyn 1991;10:380–381.
66. Sheriff MKM, Shah PJR, Fowler CJ, et al. Neuromodulation of detrusor hyper-reflexia by functional magnetic stimulation of the sacral roots. Br J Urol 1996;78:39–46.

67. Vodušek DB, Zidar J. Perineal motor evoked responses. Neurourol Urodyn 1988;7:236–237. (Proceedings of the 18th Annual Meeting of the International Continence Society, Oslo, Norway.)
68. Opsomer RJ, Caramia MD, Zarola F, et al. Neurophysiological evaluation of central-peripheral sensory and motor pudendal fibres. Electroencephalogr Clin Neurophysiol 1989;74:260–270.
69. Loening-Baucke V, Read NW, Yamada T, Barker AT. Evaluation of the motor and sensory components of the pudendal nerve. Electroencephalogr Clin Neurophysiol 1994;93:35–65.
70. Jost WH, Schimrigk K. A new method to determine pudendal nerve motor latency and central motor conduction time to the external anal sphincter. Electroencephalogr Clin Neurophysiol 1994;93:237–239.
71. Thiry AJ, Deltenre PF. Neurophysiological assessment of the central motor pathway to the external urethral sphincter in man. Br J Urol 1989;63:515–519.
72. Eardley I, Nagendran K, Lecky B, et al. The neurophysiology of the striated urethral sphincter in multiple sclerosis. Br J Urol 1991;67:81–88.
73. Bradley WE, Lin JTY, Johnson B. Measurement of the conduction velocity of the dorsal nerve of the penis. J Urol 1984;131:1127–1129.
74. Vodušek DB, Deletis V, Abbott R, et al. Intraoperative Monitoring of Pudendal Nerve Function. In M Rother, U Zwiener (eds), Quantitative EEG Analysis—Clinical Utility and New Methods. Jena, Germany: Universitätsverlag Jena, 1993;309–312.
75. Deletis V, Vodušek DB, Abbott R, et al. Intraoperative monitoring of dorsal sacral roots: minimizing the risk of iatrogenic micturition disorders. Neurosurgery 1992;30:72–75.
76. Ertekin Ç, Mungan B. Sacral spinal cord and root potentials evoked by the stimulation of the dorsal nerve of penis and cord conduction delay for the bulbocavernosus reflex. Neurourol Urodyn 1993;12:9–22.
77. Haldeman S, Bradley WE, Bhatia N. Evoked responses from the pudendal nerve. J Urol 1982;128:974–980.
78. Vodušek DB. Pudendal somatosensory evoked potential and bulbocavernosus reflex in women. Electroencephalogr Clin Neurophysiol 1990;77:134–136.
79. Gänzer H, Madersbacher H, Rumpl E. Cortical evoked potentials by stimulation of the vesicourethral junction: clinical value and neurophysiological considerations. J Urol 1991;146:118–123.
80. Haldeman S, Bradley WE, Bhatia N, Johnson BK. Cortical evoked potentials on stimulation of pudendal nerve in women. Urology 1983;6:590–593.
81. Tackmann W, Vogel P, Porst H. Somatosensory evoked potentials after stimulation of the dorsal penile nerve: normative data and results from 145 patients with erectile dysfunction. Eur Neurol 1987;27:245–250.
82. Vodušek DB. Pudendal somatosensory evoked potentials. Neurologija 1990;39(suppl 1):149–155.
83. Guérit JM, Opsomer RJ. Bit-mapped images of somatosensory evoked potentials after stimulation of the posterior tibial nerves and dorsal nerve of the penis/clitoris. Electroencephalogr Clin Neurophysiol 1991;80:228–237.
84. Ertekin Ç, Akyürekli O, Gürses AN, et al. The value of somatosensory-evoked potentials and bulbocavernosus reflex in patients with impotence. Acta Neurol Scand 1985;71:48–53.
85. Kirkeby HJ, Poulsen EU, Petersen T, Dorup J. Erectile dysfunction in multiple sclerosis. Neurology 1988;38:1366–1371.
86. Vodušek DB, Ravnik-Oblak M, Oblak C. Pudendal versus limb nerves electrophysiologic abnormalities in diabetics with erectile dysfunction. Int J Impotence Res 1993;2:37–42.
87. Vodušek DB, Deletis V, Abbott R, Turndorf H. Prevention of iatrogenic micturition disorders through intraoperative monitoring. Neurourol Urodyn 1990;9:444–445. Proceedings of the ICS 20th Annual Meeting; September 12–15, 1990; Århus, Denmark.
88. Cohen BA, Major MR, Huizenga BA. Pudendal nerve evoked potential monitoring in procedures involving low sacral fixation. Spine 1991;16(suppl 8):375–378.
89. Delodovici ML, Fowler CJ. Clinical value of the pudendal somatosensory evoked potential. Electroencephalogr Clin Neurophysiol 1995;96:509–515.
90. Badr GG, Carlsson CA, Fall M, et al. Cortical evoked potentials following the stimulation of the urinary bladder in man. Electroencephalogr Clin Neurophysiol 1982;54:494–498.
91. Sarica Y, Karacan I. Bulbocavernosus reflex to somatic and visceral nerve stimulation in normal subjects and in diabetics with erectile impotence. J Urol 1986;138:55–58.
92. Hansen MV, Ertekin Ç, Larsson LE. Cerebral evoked potentials after stimulation of the posterior urethra in man. Electroencephalogr Clin Neurophysiol 1990;77:52–58.
93. Loening-Baucke V, Read NW, Yamada T. Further evaluation of the afferent nervous pathways from the rectum. Am J Physiol (Gastrointest Liver Physiol) 1992;25:G927–G933.

94. Prevec TS, Denišlič M. Diagnostic value of somatosensory cerebral evoked potentials to electrical and mechanical stimulation in multiple sclerosis. Neurologija 1990;39(suppl 1):59–67.
95. Smout AJPM, De Vore MS, Castell DO. Cerebral potentials evoked by esophageal distention in humans. Am J Physiol (Gastrointest Liver Physiol) 1990;259:G955–G959.
96. Collett L, Menuier P, Duclaux R, et al. Cerebral electrical potential after anorectal mechanical stimulation in humans. Am J Physiol (Gastrointest Liver Physiol) 1988;254:G477–G482.
97. Podnar S, Vodušek DB, Tršinar B, Rodi Z. A method of uroneurophysiological investigation in children. Electroencephalogr Clin Neurophysiol 1997;104:389–392.
98. Rushworth G. Diagnostic value of the electromyographic study of reflex activity in man. Electroencephalogr Clin Neurophysiol 1967;(suppl 25):65–73.
99. Ertekin Ç, Reel F. Bulbocavernosus reflex in normal men and patients with neurogenic bladder and/or impotence. J Neurol Sci 1976;28:1–15.
100. Vacek J, Lachman M. The bulbocavernosus reflex in diabetics with erectile dysfunction: a clinical and EMG study. Cas Lek Cesk 1977;33:1014–1017.
101. Krane RJ, Siroky MB. Studies on sacral evoked potentials. J Urol 1980;124:872–876.
102. Vodušek DB. Neurophysiological Study of Bulbocavernosus Reflex in Man [doctoral thesis]. University of Ljubljana, Ljubljana, Slovenia, 1988;1–129.
103. Vereecken RI, De Meirsman J, Puers B, et al. Electrophysiological exploration of the sacral conus. J Neurol 1982;227:135–144.
104. Bilkey WJ, Awad EA, Smith AD. Clinical application of sacral reflex latency. J Urol 1983;129: 1187–1189.
105. Pedersen E, Harving H, Klemar B, et al. Human anal reflexes. J Neurol Neurosurg Psychiatry 1978;41:813–818.
106. Bradley WE. Urethral electromyelography. J Urol 1972;108:563–564.
107. Fowler CJ, Betts CD. Clinical Value of Electrophysiological Investigations of Patients with Urinary Symptoms. In AR Mundy, TP Stephenson, AJ Wein (eds), Urodynamics: Principles, Practice and Application (2nd ed). Edinburgh, UK: Churchill Livingstone, 1994;165–181.
108. Contreras Ortiz O, Bertotti AC, Rodriguez Nuñez JD. Pudendal reflexes in women with pelvic floor disorders. Zentralbl Gynakol 1994;116:561–565.
109. Vodušek DB, Janko M. The bulbocavernosus reflex: a single motor neuron study. Brain 1990;113:813–820.
110. Rodi Z, Vodušek DB. The sacral reflex studies: single versus double pulse stimulation. Neurourol Urodyn 1995;14:496–497. Proceedings of the 25th Annual Meeting of the International Continence Society; October 17-20, 1995; Sydney, Australia.
111. Desai KM, Dembny K, Morgan H, et al. Neurophysiological investigation of diabetic impotence. Are sacral response studies of value? Br J Urol 1988;61:68–73.
112. Vodušek DB, Zidar J. Pudendal nerve involvement in patients with hereditary motor and sensory neuropathy. Acta Neurol Scand 1987;76:457–460.
113. Lavoisier P, Proulx J, Courtois F, De Carnfel F. Bulbocavernosus reflex: its validity as a diagnostic test of neurogenic impotence. J Urol 1989;141:311–314.
114. Kunesch E, Reiners K, Müller-Mattheis V, et al. Neurological risk profile in organic erectile impotence. J Neurol Neurosurg Psychiatry 1992;55:275–281.
115. Hanson P, Rigaux P, Gilliard C, Bisset E. Sacral reflex latencies in tethered cord syndrome. Am J Phys Med Rehabil 1993;72:39–43.
116. Deletis V, Vodušek DB. Intraoperative recording of the bulbocavernosus reflex. Neurosurgery 1997;40:88–92.
117. Dystra D, Sidi A, Cameron J, et al. The use of mechanical stimulation to obtain the sacral reflex latency: a new technique. J Urol 1987;137:77–79.
118. Fowler CJ, Ali Z, Kirby RS, Pryor JP. The value of testing for unmyelinated fibre, sensory neuropathy in diabetic impotence. Br J Urol 1988;61:63–67.
119. Yarnitsky D, Sprecher E, Vardi Y. Penile thermal sensation. J Urol 1996;156:391–393.
120. Robinson LQ, Woodcock JP, Stephenson TP. Results of investigation of impotence in patients with overt or probable neuropathy. Br J Urol 1987;60:583–587.
121. Shahani BT, Halperin JJ, Boulu P, Cohen J. Sympathetic skin response—a method of assessing unmyelinated axon dysfunction in peripheral neuropathies. J Neurol Neurosurg Psychiatry 1984;47:536–542.
122. Opsomer RJ, Pesce Fr, Abi Aad A, et al. Electrophysiologic testing of motor sympathetic pathways: normative data and clinical contribution in neurourological disorders. Neurourol Urodyn 1993;12:336–338. Proceedings of the 23rd Annual Meeting of the International Continence Society; Rome.

123. Daffertshofer M, Linden D, Syren M, et al. Assessment of local sympathetic function in patients with erectile dysfunction. Int J Impotence Res 1994;6:213–225.
124. Koldewijn EL, van Kerrebroeck PEV, Bemelmans BLH, et al. Use of sacral reflex latency measurements in the evaluation of neural function of spinal cord injury patients: a comparison of neuro-urophysiological testing and urodynamic investigations. J Urol 1994;152:463–467.
125. Liu S, Christmas TJ, Nagendran K, et al. Sphincter electromyography in patients after radical prostatectomy and cystoprostatectomy. Br J Urol 1992;69:397–403.
126. Percy JP, Neill ME, Swash M, et al. Electrophysiological study of motor nerve supply of pelvic floor. Lancet 1981;1:16–17.
127. Gearhart JP, Burnett A, Owen JH. Measurement of pudendal evoked potentials during feminizing genitoplasty: technique and applications. J Urol 1995;153:486.

10
Investigation of Male Erectile Dysfunction

Rupert O. Beck

Male sexual dysfunction occurs when a problem exists with libido, erectile function, or ejaculation. The underlying cause may be psychological, pathologic, or both.

Although this chapter is concerned primarily with the diagnosis of neurogenic male erectile dysfunction (MED), the investigations used in the detection of vasculogenic and psychogenic erectile failure are also reviewed. However, the advent of simple, quick, and reliable symptomatic treatments for MED (see Chapter 13) has meant that only a few men experiencing from erectile dysfunction undergo detailed investigation. The available tests are summarized in Table 10.1, but most of these, both neurophysiologic and otherwise, are of debatable value.

A good history and examination often point toward the cause of the condition. A patient with severe arteriopathy is likely to have vasculogenic impotence; a patient with myelopathy is likely to have neurogenic impotence. Important clues pointing to a psychological cause may be contained in the history: A man who has a normal erection with one partner but not another, or can achieve a normal erection during masturbation but not during intercourse, is unlikely to have an organic cause for his symptoms. In fact, the first objective approach used in the diagnosis of MED was the attempt to differentiate between psychogenic and organic impotence using nocturnal penile tumescence monitoring.

In 1977, Karacan et al. [1] suggested that, in men with erectile dysfunction, the presence of full, sustained erections during sleep was indicative of psychogenic impotence, and the absence of turgid nocturnal erections indicated organic impotence. Nocturnal penile tumescence testing quickly became accepted as a way of eliminating an organic cause for the erectile dysfunction. Various techniques to assess nocturnal activity are described. Some centers have elaborate sleep laboratories and monitor electroencephalograms and nocturnal penile tumescence activity as well as performing video monitoring of erections; others use simpler snap gauge devices for home evaluation. Some investigators have reported that dreams with a high anxiety content have little or no associated nocturnal tumescence and may even cause detumescence. However, some patients with abnormal

Table 10.1   Investigations that may be performed in the diagnosis of male erectile dysfunction

Vasculogenic
    Arterial flow
        Penile/brachial pressure index
        Color duplex ultrasonography flow studies
        Doppler ultrasonography with intracavernosal injection
        Penile angiography
    Venous leak
        Cavernosography and cavernosometry
        Color duplex ultrasonography
Psychogenic
    Nocturnal penile tumescence
    Snap gauge testing
    Psychological profile
Neurologic
    Urethral sphincter electromyography
    Sacral reflex latencies
    Somatosensory evoked potentials
    Corpus cavernosum electromyography
Endocrine
    Testosterone, prolactin, follicle-stimulating hormone, luteinizing hormone levels
    Glucose, thyroid function tests

nocturnal penile tumescence tests have normal coital activity. Moreover, the neurologic pathways needed to initiate and maintain nocturnal erections are probably different from those involved in both psychogenic and reflexogenic erections, so that in some neurologic diseases, especially multiple sclerosis, one type of erection may be present, whereas another may be absent. Nocturnal penile tumescence testing in these patients may produce misleading results.

MED is a common complaint in men with established neurologic disease; it is an almost inevitable part of spinal cord disease and is also a common feature of any generalized peripheral neuropathy, particularly if autonomic pathways are affected. The neural pathways involved in the initiation and maintenance of an erection are described in Chapter 5. To diagnose neurogenic impotence—or often, more importantly, to rule out a neurologic cause for erectile dysfunction—the clinician must evaluate all the pathways involved. To date, this has proved impossible to achieve, so that currently the neurophysiologic assessment of suspected neurogenic MED relies almost exclusively on tests of the somatic nervous system. Therefore, failure to detect an abnormality in autonomic innervation is not surprising.

The first section of this chapter covers the methodology and the advantages and disadvantages of each of the neurophysiologic techniques in current use. It is divided into subparts covering sacral reflex latencies, cortical somatosensory evoked potentials, sphincter electromyography (EMG), and tests that attempt to measure autonomic function, including the somewhat controversial corpus cavernosum EMG. Figure 10.1 illustrates the parts of the nervous system that are

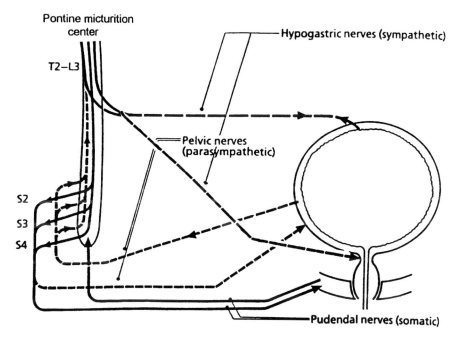

Figure 10.1 Diagrammatic representation of the innervation of the genitourinary tract from pons to bladder. Only transmission in the somatic nervous system (*bold continuous line*) can be assessed by the following current neurophysiologic techniques:

a. Sacral reflex testing
   Pudendal afferent → sacral cord → pudendal efferent → bulbocavernosus muscle
b. Pudendal evoked potentials
   Pudendal afferent → sacral cord → spinal cord → frontal cortex
c. Sphincter electromyography
   Onuf's nucleus → pudendal nerve → striated urethral/anal sphincter

tested by neurophysiologic investigations. The latter part of the chapter provides a short resumé of the investigations used in the diagnosis of vasculogenic MED.

NEUROGENIC ERECTILE FAILURE

Sacral Reflex Testing

Sacral reflexes are reflex contractions of parts of the pelvic floor that occur in response to a stimulus applied either to the perineum, genitalia, or mucosa of the lower urinary tract. The finding of no response or a response at a prolonged latency is taken as evidence of neuronal damage either in the afferent or efferent pathways of the reflex arc, or in the conus itself, because the spinal segments that serve these reflexes are S2–S4. The reflexes that have been investigated are the

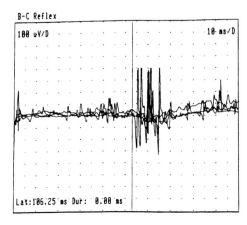

B-C Reflex

100 uV/D · · · · · · · · · 10 ms/D

Lat: 106.25 ms Dur: 0.00 ms

Figure 10.2   Prolonged bulbocavernosus reflex response from a patient with erectile dysfunction after an acute L5–S1 central disk prolapse. Four consecutive responses have been superimposed so that the latency of the reflex is easily recognizable. (D = division; Dur = duration; Lat = latency.)

bulbocavernosus reflex and the pudendoanal, vesicourethral, and vesicoanal reflexes, although only the bulbocavernosus reflex has been used extensively for the diagnosis of neurogenic erectile dysfunction. Details of how this reflex is recorded are given in Chapter 9.

The bulbocavernosus reflex has two components. The first response, at approximately 35 milliseconds (see Chapter 9), is the result of conduction in an oligosynaptic pathway [2] and is the response used clinically. A second, more variable response is often found at approximately 70 milliseconds. Most investigators have used a concentric needle electrode to record from the bulbocavernosus muscles and report the minimum latency of a number of consecutive raw EMG responses [3].

Theoretically, neurophysiologic investigation of the bulbocavernosus reflex might identify both peripheral neuropathic damage to the pudendal nerve and lesions of the cauda equina. In early studies, many patients with neurogenic impotence due to either cauda equina or lower motor neuron lesions were found to have abnormally prolonged or absent bulbocavernosus reflex responses (Figure 10.2) [4]. However, in other patients with cauda equina lesions, the response was normal [5, 6], so the sensitivity of the test cannot be regarded as high. In patients with an advanced peripheral neuropathy, latency measurements may be increased or the amplitude of the response decreased. This latter finding is of little clinical significance in the individual patient, however, because the amplitude of a response depends to a large extent on the site of the recording electrode relative to the motor unit, and large variations in amplitude can occur with small changes of needle position.

Bulbocavernosus reflex testing has been used to test diabetic patients with erectile dysfunction [7–11]. Although a delay of the response can be shown in some patients, especially those with a severe peripheral neuropathy, the response in others who also have presumed neurogenic impotence can be normal [11, 12]. Furthermore, the response may be prolonged in some men who have normal sexual function but a generalized neuropathy, as shown by Vodušek and Zidar when testing patients with hereditary motor and sensory neuropathy [13].

The value of testing sacral reflexes in patients with suspected neurogenic MED remains doubtful [14]. The test is useful clinically in confirming the suspicion of a cauda equina lesion either in patients with otherwise mild neurologic signs or in those with MED and an atonic bladder of previously unknown etiology. It is a poor test of peripheral neuropathy and does not assess conduction in autonomic fibers at all.

Pudendal Evoked Responses

An objective assessment of the integrity of the sensory pathways from the periphery to the cortex can be made by recording somatosensory evoked potentials. Details of recording techniques are given in Chapter 9.

The waveform of the pudendal evoked potential is similar in shape and latency to that of the tibial evoked potential and consists of a series of consecutive peaks and troughs (Figure 10.3) [15, 16]. The relative delay in conduction of the pudendal response is thought to occur at both the peripheral and spinal cord levels, where the sensory information ascends in slower pathways than in the tibial nerves. Difficulty in interpretation can occur, because the investigator can very easily miss the small initial response and measure the latency to the second negative deflection. A latency of 60 milliseconds or longer would be expected only in a patient who had clinically obvious spinal cord disease. If this is not the case, either the result has been misinterpreted or further detailed tests of spinal cord function are appropriate. Such abnormally prolonged latencies are not found in patients with peripheral neuropathy [17].

Some urologists have used pudendal evoked response testing as part of their screening tests in the investigation of erectile dysfunction. Several studies have reported that the latency of the pudendal evoked potential is prolonged in patients with impotence of spinal cord origin. Kirkeby et al. [18] found the response abnormal in 26 out of 29 impotent men with multiple sclerosis, whereas Betts et al. [19] found that 38 out of 46 impotent men with multiple sclerosis had prolonged latencies. However, the sensitivity of the test in assessing spinal cord dis-

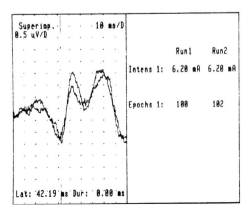

Figure 10.3   Pudendal evoked response. Two consecutive responses superimposed to make identification of latency (P40) easily recognizable. (D = division; Dur = duration; Intens = intensity; Lat = latency; Superimp = superimposed.)

ease is uncertain, as six of the eight patients with normal responses studied by Betts et al. had clinical evidence of definite spinal cord pathology.

A further area of controversy is whether the test adds any specific information to what can be obtained by careful clinical examination or measurement of the lower limb evoked potentials, which are of larger amplitude and are therefore easier to interpret. Bemelman et al. [20] found that the pudendal evoked potential was delayed or unrecordable in 21 out of 123 patients (17%) with no clinically demonstrable neurologic disorder. In only four of these patients was the tibial evoked potential also abnormal. They concluded that subclinical peripheral neuropathies were important in the etiology of impotence. However, one would not expect to find significant abnormalities in evoked potentials in patients with no clinical signs of a sensory neuropathy or myelopathy, and measurement of pudendal evoked responses may have a low specificity because of difficulties in identifying a small P40 deflection. Another study that examined the value of the pudendal evoked potential in a large group of unselected men attending an erectile dysfunction clinic found that most abnormalities of the test could be predicted from a knowledge of pre-existing neurologic disease or diabetic status, thereby rendering the test of little clinical significance [21].

Electromyography of the Anal or Urethral Sphincter

Analysis of sphincter EMG has been used to identify somatic nerve injury between the sacral cord and pelvic sphincters. Lesions causing neuronal damage between Onuf's nucleus [22] and the sphincter muscles supplied by those cells result in denervation of the sphincter muscle. Changes of denervation and reinnervation in the urethral or anal sphincter are indicative of lower motor neuron lesions affecting the S2–S4 myotomes. The damage may occur in the conus medullaris, the cauda equina, or peripherally in the pelvis.

Damage to the cauda equina commonly results in erectile failure, because both the sacral parasympathetic and pudendal nerves may be affected. Clinically, partial damage to the cauda equina may be difficult to diagnose; the resultant sensory loss may be very minor and anal sphincter tone only slightly reduced, yet MED may still occur. Single motor unit analysis reveals abnormalities in both urethral and anal sphincter EMGs with these lesions, and sphincter EMG is considered a useful contributory test in these situations.

Major pelvic surgery, such as radical prostatectomy or cystoprostatectomy, carries a significant risk to sexual function because the neurovascular bundle that contains the cavernous nerves runs along the posterolateral border of the prostate. Liu et al. showed that the response duration of motor units as identified by sphincter EMG is significantly longer in men with erectile dysfunction who have had this type of surgery than in a control group [23].

Sphincter Electromyography in the Diagnosis of Multiple System Atrophy

Multiple system atrophy is a condition characterized by cell loss and gliosis in certain well-defined central nervous system structures [24]; one of the earliest symptoms of the disorder is erectile or ejaculatory failure [25]. Sphincter EMG is now recognized to be a useful investigation in the diagnosis of this disorder, because Onuf's nucleus is one of the areas frequently affected [26, 27]. The result is dener-

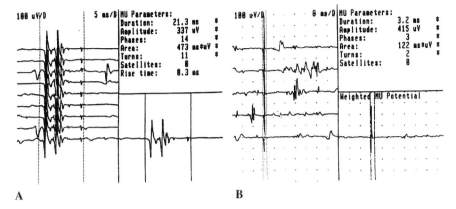

Figure 10.4 Abnormal motor unit (MU) response **(A)** from a patient with multiple system atrophy. The MU response is prolonged and polyphasic compared with that of a normal subject **(B)**. (D = division.)

vation of both the urethral and anal sphincters with subsequent changes of reinnervation that are recordable on sphincter EMG (Figure 10.4; see Chapter 9) [28, 29].

Autonomic Function Testing

Clinically, the integrity of the autonomic nervous system is assessed by measuring the responses to parasympathetic or sympathetic activation rather than by measuring conduction along the nerves themselves.

In neurologic practice, autonomic function testing is used in the diagnosis of generalized autonomic failure and only rarely in the identification of purely localized abnormalities. Most investigations relate either to the general control of circulation or to sweat production.

Cardiovascular autonomic function tests measure changes in heart rate variability and blood pressure in response to deep breathing, alteration of posture from lying to standing, cold stimuli, isometric exercise, sudden inspiratory gasps, or Valsalva's maneuver. These maneuvers alter autonomic activity, so that failure to respond adequately to them is indicative of autonomic impairment. When a combination of tests is used, generalized cardiovascular sympathetic and parasympathetic failure can be differentiated.

The sympathetic nervous system also regulates sweat gland activity, which can be evaluated using techniques that gauge sweat production. One such technique measures the change in voltage on the skin surface secondary to sweat production, known as the sympathetic skin response (SSR). This response was first described by Tarchanoff at the end of the nineteenth century [30]. The SSR has been used in the investigation of male erectile dysfunction, and it is described in more detail in the discussion of cavernosal EMG.

A correlation exists between the results of certain autonomic function tests and neurogenic male erectile dysfunction, although a wide range of variability is reported among different studies. Kunesch et al. [31] found that, of 30 selected patients with impotence, 53% had abnormal heart rate variability to both deep

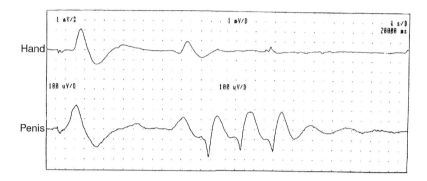

Figure 10.5   Corpus cavernosum electromyographic recording from surface electrodes placed on the penile skin. The time base is set at 1 second per division; 40 seconds of the recording is illustrated and compared with recordings of the sympathetic skin response from the hand. (D = division.)

inspiration and standing, indicating generalized parasympathetic impairment. In a larger study involving 542 impotent men with various risk factors, 14% showed reduced heart rate variability [32]. In patients with diabetes, the number showing abnormality rose to over 20%. Quadri et al. [33] reported abnormal cardiovascular responses to deep breathing in 21 of 38 men (55%) with diabetic impotence, but 26% of potent diabetic patients also had abnormal results. Robinson et al. [34] found that cardiovascular autonomic function testing was not accurate or predictive in identifying neuropathy as a cause of MED in a series of 50 men.

These tests investigated only generalized cardiovascular autonomic failure and overlook possible focal or regional abnormalities in peripheral or central autonomic nerve function. Therefore, it is not surprising that abnormal cardiovascular results are found in some patients with normal erectile function and vice versa.

Corpus Cavernosum Electromyography and Sympathetic Skin Responses

In 1988, Wagner et al. [35] showed that electrical activity could be recorded from the corpus cavernosum using concentric needle electrodes. The measurement of this bioelectric activity was termed *corpus cavernosum electromyography* (CCEMG). A compressed time base made analysis of individual electrical potentials difficult. An overall decrease in activity was noted in normal subjects in response to visual sexual stimulation; the conclusion was that this represented a reduction in sympathetic activity in the penis, allowing for smooth muscle relaxation and penile erection. Stief et al. [36] extended the time base and analyzed what originally was thought to be individual cavernosal smooth muscle potentials. This form of recording was given the acronym SPACE—*s*ingle *p*otential *a*nalysis of *c*avernosal *E*MG. In 1992, Stief et al. [37] recorded CCEMG with surface electrodes placed on the penile skin overlaying the corpora cavernosa (Figure 10.5). In seven of eight patients, surface electrical activity was synchronous with that measured by needle

CCEMG and of similar shape, amplitude, and duration. These findings were corroborated by Merckx et al. [38]; together with Stief, they concluded that SPACE recordings were an important part of the armamentarium in the diagnosis of neurogenic impotence. It soon became apparent, however, that the reported bioelectric activity could not represent single cavernosal smooth muscle potentials, and therefore the acronym SPACE was abandoned at the first international workshop on CCEMG in 1993 [39]. Studies on CCEMG by both Stief et al. and Merckx et al. have recognized that the recorded potentials are sympathetically mediated [36, 38]. Stief et al. showed that mental stimulation increased the frequency of the potentials—a feature known to occur with the sympathetic skin response. Merckx et al. commented that the initial 10 minutes of a CCEMG recording after cavernosal needle insertion showed excessive activity because of the pain and stress experienced by the subject, and related this result to a high degree of sympathetic activity.

Other investigators have shown that potentials similar to those found in CCEMG can be recorded from surface electrodes placed on the limb of a patient [40, 41]. The duration, amplitude, and shape of the SPACE waveforms recorded with surface electrodes on the penis were found to be very similar to those obtained when recording perineal, penile, and limb SSRs (Figure 10.6). In these studies, identical recording parameters (i.e., filter, amplitude, and time-base settings) were used. The concept that CCEMG and SSR are related bears further discussion.

The changes in skin resistance that occur after various internally generated or externally applied arousal stimuli result from an increase in sweat gland activity mediated by the sympathetic nervous system and lead to changes in skin voltage that can be recorded using two surface electrodes. As noted above, this response is called the *sympathetic skin response* [42]. Stimuli used to elicit an SSR have included deep inspiration, startling or painful stimuli, and electrical impulses applied to peripheral nerves [43]. When recorded on neurophysiologic apparatus, the response appears as a slow depolarization of the skin. This depolarization is thought to originate from synchronized activation of sweat glands in response to a volley discharge in efferent sympathetic nerve fibers. SSR responses recorded from the limbs can be used in the detection of mixed axonal neuropathies [44]. Ertekin et al. [45]

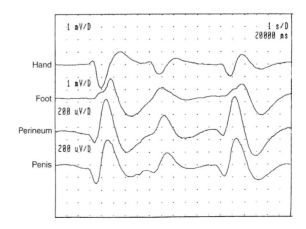

Figure 10.6 Potentials recorded from the limbs are recognized as standard sympathetic skin responses. Simultaneous recordings of electrical activity with surface electrodes on the penile skin, perineum, and both limbs are shown. (D = division.)

were the first to measure the SSR on the genital skin. The recording electrodes were placed on the mons pubis (active) and the dorsum of the penis (reference), and a variety of different stimuli were used to elicit a response, including electrical stimuli to the median nerve at the wrist, the peroneal nerve at the knee, and the dorsal nerve of the penis. The SSR could be recorded from the genitalia in normal subjects, but the response was absent in some diabetic patients with erectile dysfunction, both with and without a previously diagnosed polyneuropathy [46].

Did the CCEMG recordings made with surface electrodes actually represent sympathetic sudomotor sweat gland activity, or were two different types of sympathetically induced electrical activity possibly being recorded on the penile skin simultaneously? On some occasions, potentials were present only on the genital skin and no electrical activity was recorded elsewhere [40]. However, these potentials still bore a striking resemblance to the SSR. However, an argument in favor of CCEMG response being a separate entity from the SSR is that CCEMG activity is abolished after intracavernosal injection of the smooth muscle relaxant prostaglandin E_1, whereas penile SSR is still elicitable [47].

In the author's mind, doubts still exist about the neurophysiologic origin of recordings made with surface electrodes and, by inference, those made by needle electrodes as well. However, good evidence is found that these recordings represent some form of autonomic activity from the genitalia; thus, they are a significant improvement on many of the other neurophysiologic tests that have been used to evaluate MED.

VASCULOGENIC ERECTILE FAILURE

For the penis to become erect, more blood must flow into the cavernosal tissue than flows out. Poor arterial inflow or excessive venous leakage therefore results in erectile failure. Despite this straightforward concept, the investigation of blood flow to and from the penis has been surrounded by controversy and confusion.

Evaluation of Arterial Inflow

A good history and examination give the first clue to the state of the arterial inflow. Patients who have normal, firm erections at some time—either at night, during masturbation, or with one partner but not another—are very unlikely to have a significant vascular problem. However, patients who report a steady decline in erectile strength and duration, who have lost nocturnal erections, and who have other signs of arterial disease (peripheral vascular disease, angina, hypertension) probably have reduced flow through the penile arteries during stimulation. A brief description of the various methods that have been used to assess arterial supply follows.

Penile/Brachial Index

To measure the penile/brachial index, a neonatal blood pressure cuff is placed around the base of the penis when it is in a flaccid state. The penile arteries are localized by Doppler ultrasonography, and penile systolic pressure is measured in the same way that blood pressure is measured in the arm. The brachial systolic blood pressure is also measured, and the ratio of penile to brachial pressure is calculated. A relative ratio of less than 0.75 is reported as abnormal, and certainly a value of less than 0.6 is highly suggestive of arterial insufficiency [48]. Unfortunately, Gerstenberg et al. [49] found that 66% of patients with erectile failure and a normal penile/brachial index were considered to have arterial insufficiency after more detailed vascular investigations.

Intracavernosal Injection Test

In this test, either papaverine hydrochloride or prostaglandin E_1 is injected into the corpora cavernosum, and the erectile response is assessed 10 minutes after injection. Diagnostically, if a poor response is obtained using a high dose, the cause of the erectile failure is likely to be vascular, whereas if a good response is obtained from a low-dose injection, the cause is likely to be neurogenic, psychogenic, or endocrine [50]. However, the sensitivity of this test is rather low; many studies show a significant false-negative response to intracavernosal injection [51]. Psychological inhibition, often caused by the anxiety of having a penile injection in such an impersonal setting as a hospital clinic, is likely to be responsible for these inaccuracies [52]. This inhibited response to intracavernosal injection can persist in a substantial proportion of cases even when maximum doses of intracavernosal drug are administered.

Color Duplex Ultrasonography with Intracavernosal Injection

Since color duplex ultrasonography was first introduced by Lue et al. in 1985 [53], it has become a widespread tool in the investigation of vasculogenic impotence. Color duplex ultrasonography is performed in conjunction with cavernosal injection therapy to maximize smooth muscle relaxation and hence blood flow through the corpora. When a 7–10 MHz probe is used, all components of the penis, including the corpora cavernosa, corpus spongiosum, septum, urethra, cavernous artery, and dorsal vein, can be visualized. The flaccid penis is first examined, and the cavernosal artery's diameter and peak systolic velocity noted. Ten minutes after intracavernosal injection, repeat measurements are taken. The artery should increase in diameter from 0.3 to 1.0 mm, and mean peak systolic velocity should reach 35–60 cm/second. A mean peak systolic velocity of 25–35 cm/second indicates mild arterial insufficiency, whereas a mean flow less than 25 cm/second corresponds to severe arterial insufficiency [54]. Nevertheless, no uniform agreement exists regarding what constitutes normal and abnormal penile artery flow. For instance, Gilbert et al. [55] found a cutoff for severe arterial insufficiency of 28 cm/second to be more accurate, whereas Benson et al. [56] set a much higher limit of 40 cm/second, above which arterial flow was thought to be normal.

However, color duplex ultrasonography is widely acknowledged to be an ideal screening imaging modality for both functional and anatomic evaluation of penile arterial blood flow. It is not expensive and involves no radiation exposure, unlike pudendal arteriography. However, it is extremely operator dependent, and its accuracy has been questioned in a number of studies. Rajfer et al. [57] reported poor correlation between mean peak systolic velocity as an indicator of arterial disease and the findings on selective pudendal angiography. Meuleman et al. [58] found no difference in the arterial response measured by color duplex ultrasonography in men with MED and in healthy controls. Mills and Sethia [59] showed the test to be poorly reproducible, with 60% of patients showing at least a 20% variation in mean peak systolic velocity when measured in sessions 2 weeks apart. In addition, 4 of the 58 patients in the study obtained a full erection after injection despite having a mean peak systolic velocity of less than 16 cm/second.

As with the more straightforward intracavernosal injection test, the crucial factor allowing for proper evaluation of the arterial inflow is the degree of smooth muscle relaxation. This cannot be standardized and is dependent on factors such as the patient's anxiety, so the results are often variable.

Selective Pudendal Arteriography

Selective pudendal arteriography is invasive, time consuming, and expensive, and is rarely used, although it does give the best anatomic demonstration of the entire hypogastric and pudendal arterial supply. The test is mainly used to evaluate men with erectile failure secondary to pelvic trauma, in whom pudendal arterial reconstruction is a possibility.

Evaluation of Venous Leakage

Failure of the veno-occlusive mechanism to trap arterial blood within the penis results in venous leak erectile failure The underlying cause, diagnosis, and treatment of venous leakage remains controversial. Many different pathologic processes have been described, which are listed in Table 10.2 [60]. The majority of patients with "venous leak" actually have normal venous anatomy but experience failure to adequately compress the emissary veins as they exit from the cavernosal bodies, as described in the following paragraphs.

Smooth muscle degeneration, such as occurs in diabetes, may result in inadequate sinusoidal relaxation with inadequate inflow and failure of the intracavernosal pressure to rise sufficiently to occlude the emissary veins. A healthy tunica

Table 10.2   Classification of venous leak erectile dysfunction

	Disease process
A. Inadequate compression of normal venous system leading to excess venous leakage	
Cavernosal	Smooth muscle degeneration, as in diabetes
Tunica albuginea	Peyronie's disease
Inadequate inflow	Arterial insufficiency or neurologic damage
B. Primary excess venous outflow	
Venous	Large abnormal veins draining corpora
Acquired venous shunts	Postpriapism surgery

albuginea that stretches and kinks the emerging emissary veins as the penis engorges is also necessary for veno-occlusion. In Peyronie's disease, firm fibrous plaques form at random on the tunica, preventing full elongation of the penis; the consequence is penile curvature and venous leak in some patients.

Primary abnormalities of the venous system itself are rarer. Obviously, the desired creation of a fistula between spongiosal tissue and the corpora in the treatment of priapism must predispose to the later phenomenon of venous leak. The origin of venous leak in patients who have large abnormal veins draining the cavernosal vessels remains obscure.

Color Doppler ultrasonography studies, cavernosometry, and cavernosography are all used in the diagnosis of venous leak. After injection of a vasodilator (e.g., prostaglandin E_1, 20 µg), peak systolic velocity should rise to higher than 35 ml per second in the cavernosal arteries. Flow should stop in diastole or even reverse if the veno-occlusive mechanism is functioning adequately. Excessive forward flow in the cavernosal arteries during diastole with failure to obtain a firm erection is taken as evidence of a venous leak.

To diagnose venous leak erectile dysfunction conclusively, intracavernosal pressure must be measured in response to corporeal perfusion—a technique known as *cavernosometry*—and abnormal venous outflow must be seen radiologically after contrast agent perfusion—called *cavernosography* [61].

To perform cavernosometry, both cavernosa are cannulated with 19-gauge needles; one needle is used to monitor intracavernosal pressure and the other to infuse fluid. Maximal smooth muscle relaxation is important so that recorded pressure and flow measurements are akin to those found during erection. Relaxation is obtained by injection of prostaglandin E_1. Ten minutes after injection, normal saline is infused using an infusion pump capable of maintaining flow at a constant rate irrespective of intracavernosal pressure until the pressure rises to 150 mm Hg. The flow required to maintain this intracavernosal pressure is then calculated. The pump is switched off, and the drop in pressure after 5 minutes is recorded. In venous leak, excessive flows are needed to maintain a pressure of 150 mm Hg within the cavernosal bodies, and the drop in pressure after cessation of infusion is quicker than in potent control subjects. Immediately after cavernosometry, a mixture of saline and contrast solution is infused into the corpora to achieve a pressure greater than 150 mm Hg. Fluoroscopy is then performed for radiologic evidence of venous leak. Unfortunately, normal and abnormal findings overlap, and the exact criteria to establish venous leak have not been defined [62].

The treatment of erectile dysfunction secondary to venous leak is not straightforward, because the underlying pathogenesis is often unclear. Attempts to reduce leakage by dividing draining veins show some short-term success, but the longer-term results are poor.

CONCLUSIONS

1. Neurophysiologic testing is useful in certain well-selected men with erectile dysfunction who have other symptoms or signs suggestive of neurologic disease.
2. Normal neurophysiologic investigations do not rule out a neurologic cause for erectile failure, because autonomic pathways are not tested.

3. Direct autonomic function testing on the penis, such as CCEMG, remains experimental and controversial.
4. Vasculogenic impotence may be either arterial or venous in origin and is best evaluated by color duplex ultrasonographic imaging with intracavernosal injection and cavernosometry, respectively, although the sensitivity and specificity of these tests remain speculative.
5. Full nocturnal penile tumescence monitoring is time-consuming and expensive, and snap gauge testing is frequently unreliable. The relationship between nocturnal erections and physiologic sexual function remains undetermined.
6. The advent of effective therapies has revolutionized the treatment of erectile dysfunction so that the investigations described in this chapter are now performed only on a selected group of patients in specialist centers.

REFERENCES

1. Karacan I, Williams RL, Thornby JI, Salis PJ. Sleep-related tumescence as a function of age. Am J Psychiatry 1975;132:932–937.
2. Vodušek DB, Janko M. The bulbocavernosus reflex. Brain 1990;113:813–820.
3. Hassouna M, Lebel M, Abdel-Rahman M, Elhilali M. Evoked potential of the sacral arc reflex: technical aspects. Neurourol Urodyn 1986;5:543–553.
4. Ertekin C, Reel F. Bulbocavernosus reflex in normal men and in patients with neurogenic bladder and/or impotence. J Neurol Sci 1976;28:1–15.
5. Bilkey WJ, Awad EA, Smith AD. Clinical application of sacral reflex latency. J Urol 1983;129:1187–1189.
6. Blaivas JG, Zayed AAH, Labib KB. The bulbocavernosus reflex in urology: a prospective study of 299 patients. J Urol 1981;126:197–199.
7. Sarica Y, Karacan I. Bulbocavernosus reflex to somatic and visceral nerve stimulation in normal subjects and in diabetics with erectile impotence. J Urol 1987;138:55–58.
8. Ertekin C, Akyurekli O, Gurses AN, Turgut H. The value of somatosensory-evoked potentials and bulbocavernosus reflex in patients with impotence. Acta Neurol Scand 1985;71:48–53.
9. Kaneko S, Bradley WE. Penile electrodiagnosis: value of bulbocavernosus reflex latency versus nerve conduction velocity of the dorsal nerve of the penis in diagnosis of diabetic impotence. J Urol 1987;137:933–935.
10. Tackmann W, Porst H, Van Ahlen H. Bulbocavernosus reflex latencies and somatosensory evoked potentials after pudendal nerve stimulation in the diagnosis of impotence. J Neurol 1988;235:219–225.
11. Desai K, Dembny K, Morgan H, et al. Neurophysiological investigation of diabetic impotence: are sacral response studies of value? Br J Urol 1988;61:68–73.
12. Siracusano S, Aiello I, Sau GF, et al. Bulbocavernosus reflex and somatosensory evoked potential of the pudendal nerve in diabetic impotence. Arch Esp Urol 1992;45:549–551.
13. Vodušek DB, Zidar J. Pudendal nerve involvement in patients with hereditary motor and sensory neuropathy. Acta Neurol Scand 1987;76:457–460.
14. Nogueira MC, Herbaut AG, Wespes E. Neurophysiological investigations of two hundred men with erectile dysfunction. Eur Urol 1978;18:37–41.
15. Haldeman S, Bradley WE, Bhatia N. Evoked responses from the pudendal nerve. J Urol 1982;128:974–980.
16. Opsomer RJ, Guerit JM, Wese FX, Van Gangh PJ. Pudendal cortical somatosensory evoked potentials. J Urol 1986;135:1216–1218.
17. Ziegler D, Muhlen H, Dannehl K, Gries FA. Tibial somatosensory evoked potentials at various stages of peripheral neuropathy in insulin dependant diabetic patients. J Neurol Neurosurg Psychiatry 1993;56:58–64.
18. Kirkeby HJ, Poulsen EU, Petersen T, Dorup J. Erectile dysfunction in multiple sclerosis. Neurology 1988;38:1366–1371.

19. Betts CD, Jones S, Fowler CG, Fowler CJ. Erectile dysfunction in multiple sclerosis; associated neurological and neurophysiological deficits, and treatment of the condition. Brain 1994;117: 1303–1310.
20. Bemelmans BLH, Meuleman EJH, Anten BWM, et al. Penile sensory disorders in erectile dysfunction. J Urol 1991;146:777–780.
21. Pickard RS, Powell PH, Schofield IS. The clinical application of dorsal penile nerve cerebral evoked response recording in the investigation of impotence. Br J Urol 1994;74:231–235.
22. Onufrowicz B. On the arrangement and function of the cell groups of the sacral region of the spinal cord in man. Arch Neurol Psychopathol 1900;3:387.
23. Liu S, Christmas TJ, Nagendran K, Kirby RS. Sphincter electromyography in patients after radical prostatectomy and cystoprostatectomy. Br J Urol 1992;69:397–403.
24. Oppenheimer DR, Graham JG. Orthostatic hypotension and nicotine sensitivity in a case of multiple system atrophy. J Neurol Neurosurg Psychiatry 1969;32:28–34.
25. Beck RO, Betts CD, Fowler CJ. Genito-urinary dysfunction in multiple system atrophy: clinical features and treatment in 62 cases. J Urol 1994;151:1336–1341.
26. Sakuta M, Nakanishi T, Toyokura Y. Anal muscle electromyograms differ in amyotrophic lateral sclerosis and the Shy-Drager syndrome. Neurology 1978;28:1289–1293.
27. Eardley I, Quinn NP, Fowler CJ. The value of urethral sphincter electromyography in the differential diagnosis of parkinsonism. Br J Urol 1989;64:360–362.
28. Kirby R, Fowler CJ, Gosling J, Bannister R. Urethro-vesical dysfunction in progressive autonomic failure with multiple system atrophy. J Neurol Neurosurg Psychiatry 1986;49:554–562.
29. Sung JH, Mastri AR, Segal E. Pathology of the Shy-Drager syndrome. J Neuropathol Exp Neurol 1978;38:253–268.
30. Tarchanoff G. Über die galvanischen Erschienung an der Haut des Menschen bei Reizung der Sinnesorgane und bei verschiedenen Formen der physischen Thatigheit. Pflugers Arch Ges Physiol 1890;46:46–55.
31. Kunesch E, Reiners K, Muller-Mathias V, et al. Neurological risk profile in organic erectile impotence. J Neurol Neurosurg Psychiatry 1992;55:275–281.
32. Nisen HO, Larsen A, Lindstrom BC, et al. Cardiovascular reflexes in the neurological evaluation of impotence. Br J Urol 1993;71:199–203.
33. Quadri R, Veglio M, Flechia D, et al. Autonomic neuropathy and sexual impotence in diabetic patients: analysis of cardiovascular reflexes. Andrologia 1989;21:346–352.
34. Robinson LQ, Woodcock JP, Stephenson TP. Results of investigation of impotence in patients with overt or probable neuropathy. Br J Urol 1987;60:583–587.
35. Wagner G, Gerstenberg T, Levin RJ. Electrical activity of corpus cavernosum during flaccidity and erection of the human penis: a new diagnostic method? J Urol 1989;142:723–725.
36. Stief CG, Djamilian M, Schaebsdau, et al. Single potential analysis of cavernous electric activity— a possible diagnosis of autonomic impotence? World J Urology 1990;8:75–79.
37. Stief CG, Thon WF, Djamilian M, et al. Transcutaneous registration of cavernous smooth muscle electrical activity: noninvasive diagnosis of neurogenic autonomic impotence. J Urol 1992; 147:47–50.
38. Merckx LA, De Bruyne RM, Keuppens FI. Electromyography of cavernous smooth muscle during flaccidity: evaluation of technique and normal values. Br J Urol 1993;72:353–358.
39. Junemann KP, Burhle CP, Stief CG. Current trends in corpus cavernosum EMG. Int J Impotence Res 1993;5:105–108.
40. Yarnitsky D, Sprecher E, Barilan Y, Vardi Y. Corpus cavernosum electromyogram: spontaneous and evoked electrical activities. J Urol 1995;153:653–654.
41. Beck RO, Fowler CJ. Neurophysiology of Urogenital Dysfunction. In D Rushton (ed), Handbook of Neuro-Urology. New York: Marcel Dekker, 1994;151–181.
42. Schondorf R. The Role of the Sympathetic Skin Response in the Assessment of Autonomic Function. In P Low (ed), Clinical Autonomic Disorders. Evaluation and Management. Boston: Little, Brown, 1993;231–241.
43. Elie B, Guihenec P. Sympathetic skin response: normal results in different experimental conditions. Electroencephalogr Clin Neurophysiol 1990;76:258–267.
44. Shahani BT, Halperin JJ, Boulu P, Cohen J. Sympathetic skin response—a method of assessing unmyelinated axon dysfunction in peripheral neuropathies. J Neurol Neurosurg Psychiatry 1984;47:536–542.
45. Ertekin C, Ertekin N, Mutlu S, et al. Skin potentials recorded from the extremities and genital regions in normal and impotent subjects. Acta Neurol Scand 1987;76:28–36.

46. Opsomer RJ, Boccasena P, Traversa R, Rossini PM. Sympathetic skin responses from the limbs and genitalia: normative study and contribution to the evaluation of neuro-urological disorders. Electroencephalogr Clin Neurophysiol 1996;101:25–31.
47. Derouet H, Jost WH, Osterhage J, et al. Penile sympathetic response in erectile dysfunction. Eur Urol 1995;28:314–319.
48. Lue TF. Physiology of Erection and Pathophysiology of Impotence. In PC Walsh, AB Retik, TA Stamey, E Darracott Vaughan (eds), Campbell's Urology. Philadelphia: Saunders, 1992;709–728.
49. Gerstenberg TC, Nordling J, Hald T, Wagner G. Standardised evaluation of erectile dysfunction in 95 consecutive patients. J Urol 1989;141:857–862.
50. Buvat J, Buvat-Herbaut M, Dehaene JL, Lemaire A. Is intracavernous injection of papaverine a reliable screening test for vascular impotence? J Urol 1986;135:476–478.
51. Gutierrez P, Pye S, Bancroft J. What does duplex ultrasound scanning add to sexual history, nocturnal penile tumescence monitoring and intracavernosal injection of smooth muscle relaxant, in the diagnosis of erectile dysfunction? Int J Impot Res 1993;5:123–131.
52. Allen RP, Engel RME, Smolev JK, Brendler CB. Comparison of duplex ultrasonography and nocturnal penile tumescence in evaluation of impotence. J Urol 1994;151:1525–1529.
53. Lue TF, Hricak H, Marich KW, Tanagho EA. Evaluation of arteriogenic impotence with intracorporal injection of papaverine and duplex ultrasound scanner. Semin Urol 1985;3:43–48.
54. Muller SC, Lue TF. Evaluation of vasculogenic impotence. Urol Clin North Am 1998;15:65–76.
55. Gilbert HW, Desai KM, Gingell JC. Non-invasive assessment of arteriogenic impotence: a comparative study. Br J Urol 1991;67:512–516.
56. Benson CB, Vickers MA. Sexual impotence caused by vascular disease: diagnosis with duplex sonography. Am J Radiol 1989;153:1149–1153.
57. Rajfer J, Canan V, Dorey FJ, Mehringer MC. Correlation between penile angiography and duplex scanning of cavernous arteries in impotent men. J Urol 1990;143:1120–1130.
58. Meuleman EJH, Bemelmans BLH, van Asten WNJC, et al. Assessment of penile blood flow by duplex ultrasonography in 44 men with normal erectile potency in different phases of erection. J Urol 1992;147:51–56.
59. Mills RD, Sethia KK. Reproducibility of penile arterial colour doppler ultrasonography. Br J Urol 1996;78:1109–1112.
60. Carrier S, Brock G, Kour NW, Lue TF. Pathophysiology of erectile dysfunction. Urology 1993;42: 468–481.
61. Wespes E, Schulman C. Venous impotence: pathophysiology, diagnosis and treatment. J Urol 1995; 149:1238–1245.
62. Vickers MA, Benson C, Dluhy R, Ball RA. The current cavernosometric criteria for corporovenous dysfunction are too strict. J Urol 1991;147:614–617.

III
TREATMENTS

11
Treatment of Neurogenic Bladder Dysfunction

Prokar Dasgupta and Collette Haslam

The term *neurogenic bladder* encompasses vesical dysfunction occurring as a result of a suprapontine, suprasacral, sacral, or peripheral nerve lesion. Detrusor hyperreflexia (Figure 11.1) is seen in cases of suprasacral or suprapontine lesion because the normal inhibitory control of the higher centers on micturition is lost or diminished. With detrusor sphincter dyssynergia, the external urethral sphincter contracts at the same time as the detrusor, so that the bladder is unable to empty to completion.

Lesions at or below the level of the sacral cord, on the other hand, cause hypocontractile or acontractile bladders with incomplete emptying and large postvoid residual volumes.

This chapter deals with the principles behind the management of detrusor hyperreflexia and incomplete bladder emptying, either in association with hyperreflexia or as seen in areflexic bladders. It also describes the practical management of incontinence in neurologically disabled patients.

INITIAL ASSESSMENT

The simplest way of assessing a patient with neurogenic voiding dysfunction is to perform a flow rate test followed by a postvoid residual scan by ultrasonography (see Chapter 8). Because a normal bladder would empty completely, a postvoid residual of more than 100 ml should be regarded as significant. In a patient with a combination of detrusor hyperreflexia and incomplete emptying, the residual volume may exacerbate the hyperreflexia, stimulating bladder contraction and thus causing urgency and frequency to occur soon after the last attempt at bladder emptying. Although medication aimed at lessening detrusor hyperreflexia will be of benefit if frequency and urgency are due only to bladder overactivity, it will not suppress symptoms if the bladder activity is due to a persistent high residual. For this reason, it is essential to measure the postmicturition residual before instigating treatment such as anticholinergics and to follow the management algorithm shown in Figure 11.2. In a patient with established neurologic disease, such as multiple sclerosis (MS), complaining of urgency and frequency, full cys-

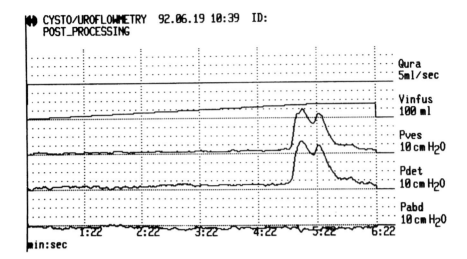

Figure 11.1   Detrusor hyperreflexia in a woman with multiple sclerosis during cystometry. The patient reported a feeling of imminent voiding as the detrusor pressure started to rise. She was not incontinent on this occasion. The rise in detrusor pressure occurred when the bladder contained just over 100 ml. (Pabd = abdominal [rectal] pressure; Pdet = detrusor pressure [Pves – Pabd]; Pves = intravesical pressure; Qura = flow of urine; Vinfus = volume infused.)

tometry is not essential, because detrusor hyperreflexia can be assumed to be the underlying problem. However, the patient's history often does not give a true indication of the extent of incomplete bladder emptying, and for this reason, measurement of the postmicturition residual must be made either using ultrasound or by "in-out" catheterization.

A further potential problem is that, although drugs such as anticholinergics effectively lessen hyperreflexia, they may also impair bladder emptying, which may already be compromised for neurologic reasons, and thus increase the postmicturition residual and worsen symptoms of hyperreflexia. For this reason, the postmicturition residual must be checked if a patient starts on anticholinergic medication and fails to respond (see Figure 11.2).

TREATMENT OF DETRUSOR HYPERREFLEXIA

Drugs

Anticholinergics

Most patients with detrusor hyperreflexia respond well to therapy with oral anticholinergics, which act by blocking the effect of acetylcholine on muscarinic receptors. Although the majority of muscarinic receptors in the human bladder are of the M2 subtype, the M3 category is the type that is pharmacologically important, and research over the last few years has focused on the development of bladder-specific antimuscarinics.

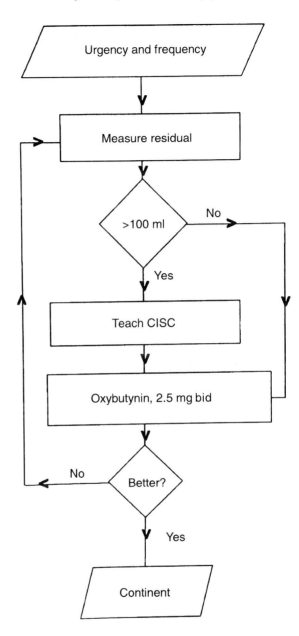

Figure 11.2 Algorithm for management of neurogenic incontinence. (CISC = clean intermittent self-catheterization.) (Reprinted with permission from CJ Fowler. Investigation of the neurogenic bladder. J Neurol Neurosurg Psychiatry 1996;60:6–13.)

The most common nonspecific antimuscarinic is oxybutynin chloride, which is started at a low dosage of 2.5 mg twice daily (see Figure 11.2). Oxybutynin chloride was initially reported in 1965 as a drug with clinical efficacy against gastrointestinal spasms in children [1]. Its urologic benefits as an anticholinergic were soon recognized [2]. Thompson and Lauvetz reported its therapeutic efficacy in bladder spasm, neurogenic bladder, and enuresis [3]. Many years later, the drug continues to be the first-line treatment for detrusor hyperreflexia. The dosage can be increased as necessary, but higher dosages can cause troublesome antimuscarinic side effects, primarily dry mouth, dry skin, constipation, and blurring of vision. Dry mouth is reported even at low dosages, and a patient who does not experience this side effect is probably not achieving therapeutic concentrations. Approximately 42% of patients on oxybutynin chloride develop mild to moderate hyposialosis; another 26% have severe hyposialosis requiring treatment with sialagogues and occasionally with artificial saliva [4]. The drug is contraindicated in persons with acute angle-closure glaucoma [5]. A dose of 2.5 mg of oxybutynin chloride given when needed is believed to be adequate in some patients. This dosage prevents the onset of severe side effects while maintaining clinical efficacy.

Treatment with oral oxybutynin chloride, if initiated early, results in an increase in bladder capacity, decrease in detrusor pressure at maximal capacity, and improvement in bladder compliance in children with myelomeningocele and detrusor hyperreflexia [6].

Propantheline bromide in a dosage of 15 mg three times daily can be prescribed for patients who are unable to tolerate the side effects of oxybutynin chloride. In a controlled trial in patients with multiple sclerosis, oxybutynin chloride was found to be effective in 67%, whereas propantheline bromide was effective in 36%. The former drug was also more effective in increasing cystometric capacity in these patients [7]. The addition of imipramine, a tricyclic antidepressant with antimuscarinic properties, is sometimes helpful in patients who fail to respond to oxybutynin chloride alone [8].

The search for new anticholinergics with fewer side effects has led to the introduction of tolterodine tartrate, which has been shown to possess a high affinity and specificity for muscarinic receptors in in vitro studies [9]. Although it is as potent as oxybutynin chloride in the bladder [10], its affinity for salivary gland receptors is eight times lower than that of oxybutynin chloride [9]. A phase I study in healthy volunteers showed that the drug is well tolerated and markedly inhibits bladder function after a single oral dose [11]. In a phase II randomized, placebo-controlled study involving 81 patients, tolterodine tartrate was found to be effective in reducing the symptoms of detrusor instability at optimal dosages of 1–2 mg twice daily. Although improvements in subjective and objective variables were more marked at a dosage of 4 mg twice daily, this dosage increased residual urinary volume by a mean of 143 ml, and one patient in this treatment group developed urinary retention. At its optimal dosage, no serious adverse side effects were observed, and no significant impact was seen on electrocardiographic or laboratory findings [12].

Desmopressin Acetate

Desmopressin acetate is an analog of antidiuretic hormone that increases reabsorption of water at the collecting tubule of the kidney, thereby reducing urine formation. It is used in the form of nasal spray or tablets to reduce troublesome nocturia in patients not responding to anticholinergics alone. Because of the risk of dilutional hyponatremia, a safe procedure may be to monitor serum sodium levels [13] and to stop the drug periodically to allow the pituitary to recover. Although

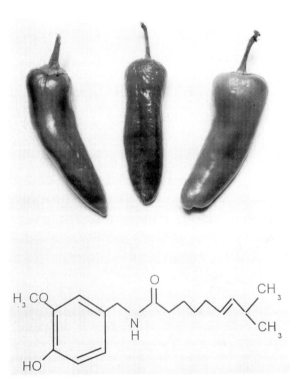

Figure 11.3 Chili peppers—plant source of capsaicin. (Courtesy of Dr. Clare Fowler.)

some studies point to its safety [14], the drug should be used with caution in patients with compromised renal or cardiovascular function, and it should be avoided in the elderly. A double-blind, placebo-controlled, crossover trial has found that desmopressin acetate significantly decreases urinary frequency in multiple sclerosis if given during the daytime [15].

Capsaicin

Capsaicin (8-methyl-N-vanillyl-6-nonenamide) is the pungent ingredient in red-hot chili peppers (Figure 11.3) used for medicinal purposes for hundreds of years [16]. The application of capsaicin either in the fluid for cystometrography or on the outer surface of the rat bladder was shown to stimulate reflex micturition [17]. A vanilloid receptor, thought to be the site of action of capsaicin, has been identified in the rat bladder [18]. Caterina et al. have isolated the complementary DNA encoding the receptor protein that binds capsaicin and have named it *vanilloid receptor subtype 1* [19].

The first use of intravesical capsaicin in hypersensitive bladders in humans was reported in 1989 [20]. Reports followed of its benefits in treating detrusor hyperreflexia at doses of 1 mmol/liter in 30% alcohol in saline [21]. The scientific rationale for this treatment was experimentation in spinal cats. Capsaicin given subcutaneously did not block the A-delta-evoked bladder reflex in normal cats, but in spinal cats it abolished the C-fiber-evoked long-latency micturition reflex [22]. Capsaicin was therefore tried in patients with intractable detrusor hyperreflexia unresponsive to anticholinergics, to test whether a similar C-afferent-mediated vesical reflex became active in patients with spinal cord disease like multiple sclerosis.

Capsaicin (1 mmol/liter) increases bladder capacity and reduces the amplitude of hyperreflexic contractions [23–26]. The benefit lasts for an average of 3–4 months, after which the instillations are repeated using 2 mmol/liter. Over a 5-year period, the beneficial effect of these repeated instillations has been found to be sustained [27], and the treatment is safe in humans and has no permanent adverse effects [28]. This treatment also decreases autonomic dysreflexia in patients with spinal cord injury [29]. A randomized study of capsaicin versus its solvent (30% alcohol in saline) has shown capsaicin to be effective, independent of its vehicle [30].

Lidocaine is routinely instilled in the bladder before capsaicin to reduce any suprapubic discomfort during treatment [31]. Dasgupta et al. have shown that the suprapubic pain is negligible if electromotive administration of lidocaine is used before capsaicin instillations [32].

Immunohistochemical studies of bladder biopsy tissue obtained with a flexible cystoscope [33] have demonstrated a reduction in suburothelial nerve densities 6 weeks after intravesical capsaicin treatment in humans. These nerves are thought to have a sensory function, and a reduction in their densities might explain the prolonged beneficial effect observed after a single intravesical dose of capsaicin [34].

Resiniferatoxin

Resiniferatoxin (RTX), an extract from the latex of *Euphorbia resinifera*, is an ultrapotent capsaicin analog. Cruz et al. showed that RTX could desensitize bladder sensory fibers in rats and reported the use in humans of 50–100 nmol/liter RTX, demonstrating clinical efficacy at dosages that do not cause initial symptomatic deterioration like capsaicin [35]. Using 10-nmol solutions of RTX in 15 human subjects (6 with detrusor hyperreflexia), Lazzeri et al. demonstrated an increase in mean bladder capacity without the initial warm or burning suprapubic sensation produced by capsaicin [36]. RTX seems to be an attractive alternative to capsaicin, but it will be a few years before its effectiveness and safety are established in human subjects.

Subtrigonal Phenol Injection

After initial enthusiasm, the simple endoscopic technique of subtrigonal phenol injection appears to have fallen out of favor, as the benefits are not sustained and the incidence of complications is high. It is contraindicated in male patients because erectile dysfunction almost always occurs afterward [37]. Its main benefits are in a selected group of patients with pericatheter leakage due to severe detrusor hyperreflexia. A single procedure can result in improved continence for a period of approximately 6 months, when the injections are repeated.

Magnetic Stimulation

External application of low magnetic fields to the brain has been found to improve bladder control in approximately 70% of patients with MS. This result is possibly mediated by melanin release by the pineal gland [38].

Functional magnetic stimulation of the sacral nerve roots can also markedly reduce hyperreflexic contractions in patients with spinal cord injury [39]. The disadvantage of this treatment is the large size of the magnet required and its lack of portability. Until a hand-held device becomes available, such treatment, although effective, remains experimental.

Electrical Stimulation

Although various studies report benefits from different techniques of electrical stimulation, the results are conflicting, and such procedures should be performed only in appropriately equipped centers. The methods used include intravaginal stimulation, transcutaneous nerve stimulation [40], percutaneously inserted spinal cord electrical stimulation, spinal electrostimulation, dorsal spinal cord stimulation, and epidural spinal electrostimulation [41, 42].

Surgical Options

Clam Ileocystoplasty

Clam ileocystoplasty is occasionally indicated in a fit patient with severe hyperreflexia in whom available conservative treatments have produced no response. Before performing this procedure, the surgeon should make sure that the patient is able to perform clean intermittent self-catheterization, as up to 50% of patients have incomplete bladder emptying postoperatively [43]. Follow-up is lifelong, because the incidence of malignancy after enterocystoplasty is unknown. Tumors arise from the bladder rather than the bowel segment. Carcinogenicity is associated with elevated levels of urinary nitrosamines and angiogenic growth factors. Surgery is indicated in only a minority of patients with neurogenic bladders.

Detrusor Myectomy

The evidence regarding the use of detrusor myectomy to treat resistant detrusor overactivity is controversial [44]. However, Swami et al. have found the procedure beneficial in up to 50% of patients with neurogenic bladders, with a minimum follow-up of 1 year [45].

TREATMENT OF INCOMPLETE BLADDER EMPTYING AND PRACTICAL MANAGEMENT OF INCONTINENCE

In patients with detrusor hyperreflexia and significant postvoid residual, the treatment of incomplete bladder emptying takes precedence, for any intervention to reduce detrusor overactivity is unlikely to be effective in the presence of large residual volumes. In patients with sacral lesions or peripheral neuropathy, promoting bladder emptying remains the mainstay of management.

Medical or surgical management is not successful in some patients; these individuals then require practical help with their continuing continence problems. Before deciding which of a number of continence aids should be recommended, the physician should take into consideration the patient's lifestyle, mobility, manual dexterity, and mental awareness, so that an informed choice can be made [46].

Voiding Techniques

Many neurologic patients with voiding problems develop their own methods of assisting bladder emptying. Patients such as those with MS or spinal cord injury may find trigger points that initiate voiding when stimulated; for example, tapping the abdomen, stroking the inner thigh, pulling pubic hair, using digital stimulation, standing up then sitting down again, or even rubbing the upper sternum may prove effective. Patients should be encouraged to experiment with finding a maneuver that helps them with bladder emptying [47].

Intermittent Catheterization

Intermittent catheterization involves inserting a catheter into the bladder to drain the residual urine and then removing it. This technique was first described in 1966 by Guttman and Frankel as a sterile procedure for the management of incomplete bladder emptying in patients with spinal cord injuries [48]. In 1972, Lapides et al. promoted the practice as a clean procedure, and it is now regarded as the primary management method in assisting bladder emptying [49]. Intermittent catheterization should be a clean procedure when carried out by the patient in his or her own environment. Studies have shown no disadvantage of this method over a sterile procedure [50]. Intermittent catheterization can be carried out as necessary, usually one to six times a day depending on the residual urine and symptoms. A patient in complete retention would need to catheterize every 4–6 hours depending on fluid intake, whereas someone who has a residual of 100 ml in 24 hours would perhaps need to catheterize only once a day.

Intermittent insertion of a catheter rather than placement of an indwelling catheter reduces the problems that can be associated with long-term catheterization (see the following section, Indwelling Catheters). Intermittent catheterization also allows patients to be more independent in managing their bladders and general lifestyle. Many patients with night-time frequency find that catheterization before going to bed allows them to get a good night's sleep, and their general condition improves because they are not so tired. The benefit may also extend to their caregivers, who formerly may have had disturbed sleep.

With intermittent self-catheterization, the patient carries out his or her own catheterization, but some neurologically impaired patients are unable to do this.

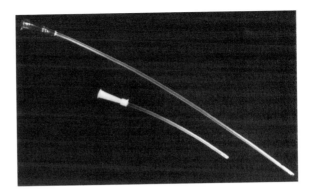

Figure 11.4 Nelaton (Narang Enterprises, New Delhi, India) catheters (for intermittent self-catheterization)— for men (top) and women (bottom).

Many patients can manage after repeated lessons and with various appliances to aid catheter insertion, such as mirrors, catheter holders, and leg abductors. For others, a caregiver may undertake the procedure. This approach, however, requires a special relationship between patient and caregiver; some patients may feel that the procedure is too intimate or that it diminishes their sexuality.

Motivation, mobility, manual dexterity, and mental awareness must be considered in assessing the suitability of a patient for intermittent self-catheterization. One or all of these can be compromised by neurologic disease. Follow-up is very important to ascertain continuity of correct procedure and patient compliance.

Choosing the type of catheter suitable for a given individual requires careful consideration. Catheters for intermittent use are made in various materials by different manufacturers. The most commonly used catheters (Nelaton; Narang Enterprises, New Delhi, India) are made from polyvinyl chloride (Figure 11.4). These are fairly flexible and are available in female (20–23 cm) and male (40.0–40.5 cm) lengths in sizes 6–24 Ch (Ch, a Charrière unit, is the outer circumference of the catheter in millimeters and is equivalent to approximately three times the diameter). The usual size for patients with neurogenic bladders is 10–12 Ch for women and 10–14 Ch for men. These catheters are classed as semidisposable and, depending on the manufacturers' instructions, can be reused for up to 7 days with careful washing after each use. If a patient is prone to urinary tract infections, more frequent changing of the catheter is advised. Disposal is as normal household waste.

Other Nelaton catheters are available that are coated with a hydrophilic film, which is activated by immersion in water for 30 seconds within the packet. These are for single use only. Patients who are prone to frequent urinary tract infections may need to use them despite their considerable extra expense. Patients with reduced manual dexterity may find this type of catheter too slippery to hold, although a device to assist is available. Some patients prefer to use a Scott catheter (SIMS Portex, Keene, NH; Figure 11.5), which is a slightly curved, semirigid catheter. This type is available for women only.

Also available for women only are metal catheters made from stainless steel or silver that can be sterilized chemically or with heat. These may be easier to handle and insert because they are rigid. To help people with reduced dexterity, catheters are available with a mirror or handle attached (Figure 11.6).

The continence advisor, be it the nurse or physician, may have a preference; however, to encourage patient compliance, a selection of catheters that patients

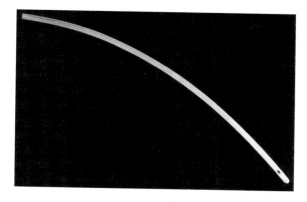

Figure 11.5 The Scott catheter (SIMS Portex, Keene, NH) is a semirigid, slightly curved catheter for use in women only.

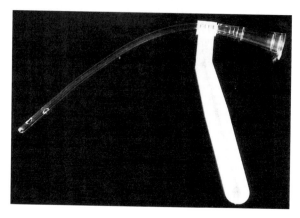

Figure 11.6 The Intex catheter (EMS Medical, Gloucestershire, UK) features a handle to make insertion easier for women who have reduced manual dexterity.

can try on their own should be provided. In the United Kingdom, most catheters are available by prescription.

Indwelling Catheterization

For the majority of patients with neurogenic bladders, an indwelling catheter is usually the last option. The benefits and drawbacks of long-term catheterization must be discussed with the patient. Some patients choose to have an indwelling catheter when they feel they can no longer manage intermittent self-catheterization due to their increasing disability or feel that their quality of life would improve if they did not have to worry about frequent toileting or struggle with intermittent self-catheterization or other continence aids, such as pads.

Problems with catheterization—such as infection, catheter blockage, urinary leakage, and expulsion—are common, and most people with an indwelling catheter experience one, if not all, of these problems at some stage. Other possible complications of urethral catheters, such as urethral destruction, are well known [51].

Many people with neurologic disease remain sexually active, and although intercourse is possible with an indwelling urethral catheter, the catheter undoubt-

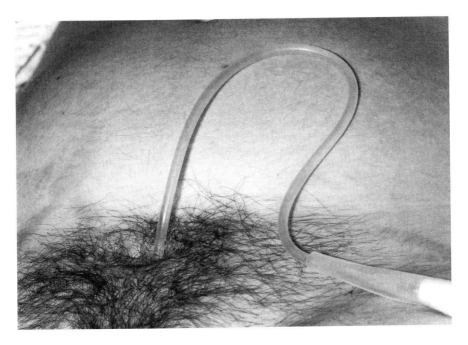

Figure 11.7   Suprapubic catheterization.

edly has an adverse effect. This is just one of the reasons why many such patients are choosing to have a long-term suprapubic catheter.

Suprapubic Catheterization

With suprapubic catheterization, a catheter is inserted into the bladder through the lower abdominal region (Figure 11.7). This procedure should be planned and performed by a urologist under general or local anesthetic. After the first catheter change, the patient or caregiver can be instructed in how to perform further catheter changes if they choose; otherwise, a nurse carries out the changes. One of the benefits of this type of catheterization is ease of changing, especially for women who, due to spasticity, may have difficulty in abducting their legs. Catheter hygiene is also easier to maintain in both sexes. Urethral damage, especially in patients with hyperreflexic bladders who are at risk of expelling the catheter with the balloon still inflated, or trauma due to pulling on the catheter by a heavy, over-filled urine bag is diminished. Sexual activity can be facilitated by taping the catheter to the side of the abdomen. Several studies have shown the benefits of suprapubic catheterization for neurologic patients, and this intervention should be considered a favorable option for long-term bladder drainage [52, 53].

Over the years, catheters have been made from a variety of materials, including reeds, palm leaves, onion stalks, and metals such as bronze, gold, and even silver. The self-retaining catheter, introduced by Frederic Foley in the 1930s, remains the blueprint for the catheter design of today (Figure 11.8). The most common catheter

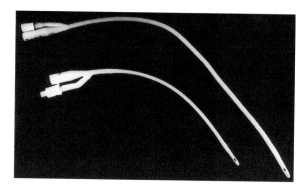

Figure 11.8   Foley indwelling catheters— for men (top) and women (bottom).

in general use has a double-lumen shaft, one for urine drainage and the other for inflation or deflation of a balloon that acts to retain the catheter in the bladder. Many different indwelling catheters are now manufactured, and the choice of which to insert is determined by the length of time for which it is to be used. For short-term use (up to 14 days), catheters made from latex are recommended; for medium-term use (28 days), a catheter covered by siliconized latex, plastic (polyvinyl chloride), or latex coated with Teflon or polytetrafluoroethylene is recommended. For the long term (up to 3 months), catheters made from silicon or coated silicon, or hydrogel-coated catheters are preferred. Bull et al. found fewer catheter-related problems when hydrogel-coated catheters were used [54]. Catheters are made in both female and male lengths (approximately 26 cm for women and 43 cm for men), in sizes varying from 8 to 24 Ch. Catheters of 12–14 Ch are usually adequate.

Some wheelchair-bound women who have a urethral catheter in situ prefer to use a male-length catheter, because it makes positioning of the catheter and bag easier when they are sitting in their chairs.

Drainage Bags

Various drainage bags are available for use with an indwelling catheter. Thought should be given to bag selection, because this choice can make all the difference in patient compliance. Drainage bags are available with a range of capacities from 350 to 800 ml. The choice depends on type of use and fluid volume. Bags are usually supplied with leg straps made from Velcro, rubber, latex, or elastic. These can cause some discomfort if applied too tightly or can cause urethral trauma due to catheter dragging if the bag is allowed to fill excessively and becomes too heavy for the straps. Body-worn attachments are available, such as net sleeves or a "sporran." The length of the bladder outlet tube should be carefully considered. Most bags are manufactured with a selection of inlet tubing that varies from 5 to 40 cm, and some can be cut to the preferred length. This is important to the patient in terms of ease of emptying and use with clothing. For patients with reduced manual dexterity, the type of drainage outlet tap is very important, because some taps are easier to open and close with one hand than others. Bags are usually made of plastic, and some have a soft material backing for comfort. The use of a sterile bag with a nonreturn valve is essential to reduce the risk of ascending infection [54].

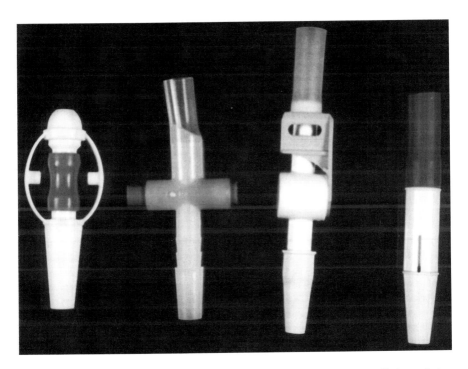

Figure 11.9 A selection of catheter valves with different outlet mechanisms, offering a choice to patients who have reduced manual dexterity.

Catheter Valves

The introduction of catheter valves has allowed patients with adequate storage capacity to use a catheter valve instead of attaching a drainage bag. Before the development of such valves, some people used a spigot instead of a drainage bag; however, this practice increased the risk of ascending infection due to frequent removal of the spigot for bladder drainage. The valve, which is connected to the catheter, enables the bladder to fill and be emptied at a convenient time, as would occur with normal bladder function. Use of a valve is suitable for patients who have a stable, reasonable capacity bladder (over 300 ml); anything less than this capacity would require too-frequent opening of the valve and would increase the risk of contamination. Patients must be able to sense the need to empty the bladder for the valve to be safely used and, as with the catheter bags, must be able to manipulate the outlet mechanism. Valves are designed to be used for 1 week to 3 months, depending on manufacturers' guidelines [55]. Little research has been carried out comparing the use of catheter valves to drainage bags. An article by German et al. found that patient preference determined how to use the valve in the most convenient way. Using the valve during the day and attaching a free drainage bag system at night is recommended, although some valves do not have this facility (Figure 11.9) [56, 57].

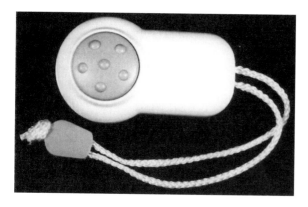

Figure 11.10   Queen Square bladder stimulator (buzzer).

Other Voiding Aids

Little published data exist on the use of noninvasive aids to enhance voiding in patients with neurogenic bladders. In 1977, Nathan described a method of emptying the neurogenic bladder by applying vibration to the abdominal wall between the umbilicus and the symphysis pubis [58]. This idea was not developed for another 20 years, until Dasgupta et al. [59] described the use of a small, hand-held vibrating device placed on the lower abdomen. Use of this device helped to reduce the postvoid residual in a number of patients with MS (Figure 11.10). The most promising response occurred in patients with detrusor hyperreflexia and incomplete emptying who were still relatively mobile and were able to feel the vibrating stimulus in the suprapubic region. An improvement in flow and a reduction in residual volume were seen. The device is portable and is easy to use, even by patients with poor hand function who may find it difficult to perform clean intermittent self-catheterization. The mechanism of action has been debated. Some have suggested that it is a form of tapping (as used by some patients with spinal cord disease to help aid bladder emptying), but the technique appears to differ from tapping in that it does not work unless the patient perceives the stimulus, and blockade of cutaneous afferent nerves with local anesthetic abolishes its effect. Vibration has been postulated to act not directly, by stimulating the bladder muscle, but by stimulating a medullary reflex mechanism. A vibration stimulus is known to induce a tonic reflex of the somatic muscles via spindle input to alpha motor neurons at the spinal level; the idea behind applying vibration to aid bladder emptying was to see if a similar reflex might be functional in relation to the detrusor in patients with neurologic disease. Suprapubic vibration is a cheap, effective, and noninvasive alternative to intermittent self-catheterization for some patients with relatively mild neurologic disability. It is ineffective in those with acontractile bladders. As the search for less invasive alternatives to clean intermittent self-catheterization goes on, further controlled studies using vibration in selected patients are needed [59].

Pelvic Floor Exercises

Many studies have reported the effectiveness of pelvic floor exercises in the management of genuine stress incontinence with or without urge incontinence. However, little is known about the use of pelvic floor exercises in the management of patients with voiding dysfunction due to a neurologic condition. These exercises require motivation and cognitive awareness, and the general fatigue felt by many neurologic patients can make pelvic floor exercises extremely hard to maintain. Therefore, the selection of suitable patients is very important. Pelvic floor exercises must be taught by a knowledgeable teacher, and many continence advisors and physiotherapists have been trained to do this. In some areas, special clinics led by physiotherapists offer neuromuscular stimulation, which is used for biofeedback to teach the patient to use the correct group of muscles to control bladder symptoms.

Controlled studies are required to ascertain the effectiveness of pelvic floor exercises in cases of neurogenic bladder. One such study in patients with MS indicated that those with low postvoid residuals can benefit from combined electrical stimulation and pelvic floor exercises [60].

Bladder and Behavioral Retraining

Many patients develop a habit of going to the toilet "just in case." Timing toileting and building confidence in the bladder's ability to hold urine can help to alleviate some bladder symptoms of frequency and urgency. Bladder or behavioral retraining has been shown to be of some benefit if the patient is aware of the principle and is committed to participating in the program. However, patients with neurologic disease may find this difficult due to their cognitive impairment and loss of voluntary control. Accurate record-keeping, guided education, and support from family and nursing staff are important for this method to have any success [61].

Surgical Options

Nerve Root Stimulation

Two different treatment modalities are available for nerve root stimulation. In patients with spinal cord injury, posterior sacral root rhizotomies with implantation of Brindley stimulators on the anterior sacral roots produces excellent results (see Chapter 18). In patients with urge incontinence and voiding dysfunction, sacral nerve root stimulation with an implantable system is gradually gaining popularity [62].

Many articles have focused on the effects of sacral rhizotomies, eventually in combination with sacral anterior root stimulation. Long-term follow-up data from a single center using this technique have shown improvement in quality of life for patients with spinal cord injury [63]. A smaller study using intradural anterior sacral root stimulation has demonstrated marked improvement in continence [64]. The Dutch study group on sacral rhizotomies and electrical bladder stimulation reported complete continence in 73% of patients during the day and in 86% at night with this procedure. The incidence of urinary tract infection was lower due to improved bladder emptying. Although the initial costs were high, they were recouped in approximately 8 years [65]. The problem with stimulating sacral roots is that the external urethral sphincter can contract at the same time as the detrusor. The urethral sphincter can now be prevented from contracting by using anodal blocking [66].

Sacral nerve root neuromodulation involves a two-stage procedure. The initial phase is a percutaneous nerve evaluation of the S3 root using a temporary electrode inserted under local anesthetic. Permanent implantation of a sacral nerve root stimulator is carried out as the second phase in patients demonstrating at least 50% improvement in their voiding symptoms after placement of the temporary lead. The exact mechanism of action is still unclear, but potentiation of the afferent limb of the micturition reflex probably occurs [67].

Reduction Cystoplasty and Vesicoplication

The results of reduction cystoplasty and vesicoplication are generally disappointing [68], and cystoreduction is not associated with a return to normal voiding function.

Urinary Diversion

A select group of patients unable to perform clean intermittent self-catheterization by urethra benefit from urinary diversion using the Mitrofanoff principle. A catheterizable umbilical appendicovesicostomy was effective in patients with quadriplegia [69]. However, some of these patients needed revision surgery, which may be detrimental in those who are already neurologically compromised. Some hopelessly incontinent patients could be treated by simply diverting the urine into an ileal conduit.

Myoplasties

The vesical cap operation, in which the acontractile detrusor is strengthened by ileal seromuscular patch grafts, has been used successfully in animal and human experiments [70]. Latissimus dorsi myoplasty has been used in dog experiments and works on the principle of using skeletal muscle contraction to facilitate bladder emptying. The transposed muscle can evacuate up to 50% of a bladderlike reservoir; however, a residual volume of 50% still necessitates the use of intermittent catheterization [71]. Further human research in this field is currently under way.

Prostheses

Endourethral stents have been used in selected patients with external sphincter dyssynergia [72]. A new intraurethral prosthesis containing a small valve and pump, controlled by a battery-operated remote control unit, has been reported effective in emptying the acontractile bladder [73].

MISCELLANEOUS APPLIANCES FOR INCONTINENCE

At some stage, many patients require advice about or need to use appliances or aids to improve continence. Reduced mobility, reduced manual dexterity, and cognitive problems must be considered in selecting the most suitable appliance to maintain patients' dignity and self-esteem in carrying out their daily activities. Individual patients may have their own personal requirements as to what they want

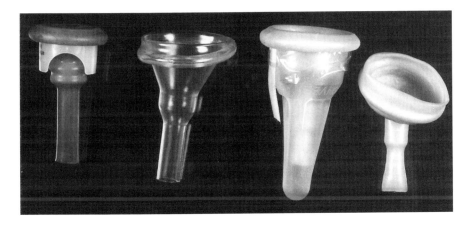

Figure 11.11   Selection of penile sheaths.

or require from a product, but in general their first priority is usually containment of any possible leakage.

The following subsections discuss appliances that may aid in the management of urinary leakage. They are not presented in any order of effectiveness, as the patient's preference is what is important.

Appliances for Women

A few devices are available for the management of stress or urge incontinence, including Femassist (an external device that supports the tissue around the urethra; Insight Medical Corporation, Bolton, MA), Reliance (a small intraurethral insert with balloon; AstraTech Ltd., Gloucestershire, England), and the Conveen Continence Guard (a vaginal insert that supports the neck of the bladder; Coloplast Group, Humlebeck, Denmark). Unfortunately, no device has been tested for the containment of incontinence in female patients with neurologic bladder symptoms.

Appliances for Men

Although intermittent self-catheterization is the method of choice in managing incomplete emptying in men, some neurologically impaired male patients may be unable or unwilling to use an intermittent catheter or indwelling catheter. In men who have urge incontinence or postmicturition dribbling, a penile sheath system may be the most beneficial method of management.

A penile sheath (also known as a condom urinal, external catheter, or incontinence sheath) is a soft rubber sleeve that fits over the penis (Figure 11.11). It is designed to fit onto a nonsterile drainage bag for the collection of urine and should be changed daily for skin washing and inspection. Sheaths vary in size and materials. Unfortunately, the sheath system is unsuitable for some men, such as those with a very small or retracted penis, cognitively impaired individuals who tend to pull the device off, men with skin sensitivity to the materials used, and those with reduced manual dexterity. Proper use of the appliance must be taught

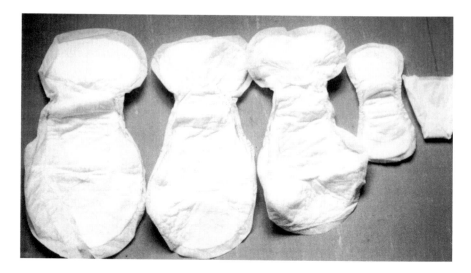

Figure 11.12   Selection of absorbent incontinence pads for use with net pants.

to the patient or caregiver for best compliance. For men who are unable to use the sheath system, body-worn urinals are available. However, these are not easy to use, and proper fitting and instruction on use must be provided by a specialist.

Absorbent Products

Most patients with urinary incontinence have tried some form of absorbent pad. These are quite popular with patients because they can be bought from local shops as are sanitary pads, and the need for patients to tell someone of their problem is avoided. A range of specially designed pads exists, and the choice of pad depends on comfort and absorbency (amount and type of incontinence).

Four types of basic design are available:

1. Insert pads with waterproof backing—used with net pants for correct fitting (Figure 11.12).
2. Insert pads without backing—used with pants that have waterproofing.
3. Male disposable pouches—used with net pants, Y fronts, or pants with waterproof pouches (see Figure 11.12).
4. All-in-one disposables—usually used for heavy incontinence.

All products are available in various absorbencies. Some are made of washable materials, and these are becoming more popular for economic and ecologic reasons.

CONCLUSIONS

The symptoms of most patients with neurogenic bladders can be managed conservatively. Medical management in the form of anticholinergic therapy is effective in approximately 70% of patients with detrusor hyperreflexia, and the introduction of new drugs with minimal side effects provides hope that fewer patients will need other interventions. Some patients fail to respond to first-line treatment and may benefit from intravesical administration of capsaicin. Further research into pharmacotherapy is in progress, particularly involving methods of decreasing afferent activity using RTX. Surgery is restricted to selected patients who are minimally disabled but do not respond satisfactorily to medical management.

Intermittent self-catheterization is an effective way of improving bladder emptying in those able to master the technique. For incapacitated patients, an indwelling catheter may be the only option. Current evidence indicates that these patients are prone to develop upper urinary tract damage, and they should be closely monitored. Nerve root stimulation is becoming increasingly popular in selected patient groups, and the concerns about the initial high cost appear to be allayed when long-term cost-effectiveness is considered.

REFERENCES

1. Garcia Herrera E, Avrutzki FK. Clinical usefulness of the compound oxybutynin chloride in gastrointestinal spasm in children. Medicina (Mex) 1965;45:179–189.
2. Diokno AC, Lapides J. Oxybutynin: a new drug with analgesic and anticholinergic properties. J Urol 1972;108:307–309.
3. Thompson IM, Lauvetz R. Oxybutynin in bladder spasm, neurogenic bladder, and enuresis. Urology 1976;8:452–454.
4. Arango Toro O, Nohales Taurines G, Cortadellas Angel R, et al. Management of hyposalivation caused by oxybutynin chloride in the treatment of the unstable bladder. Actas Urol Esp 1998;22:124–130.
5. Sung VC, Corridan PG. Acute-angle closure glaucoma as a side-effect of oxybutynin. Br J Urol 1998;81:634–635.
6. Goessl C, Knispel HH, Fiedler U, et al. Urodynamic effects of oral oxybutynin chloride in children with myelomeningocele and detrusor hyperreflexia. Urology 1998; 51:94–98.
7. Gajewski JB, Awad SA. Oxybutynin versus propantheline in patients with multiple sclerosis and detrusor hyperreflexia. J Urol 1986;135:966–968.
8. Rabey JM, Moriel EZ, Farkas A, et al. Detrusor hyperreflexia in multiple sclerosis: alleviation by a combination of imipramine and propantheline, a clinico-laboratory study. Eur Neurol 1979;18:33–37.
9. Nilvebrant L, Glas G, Jönsson Å, Sparf B. The in vitro pharmacological profile of tolterodine—a new agent for the treatment of urinary urge incontinence. Neurourol Urodyn 1994;13:433–435.
10. Hills CJ, Winter SA, Balfour JA. Tolterodine. Drugs 1998;55:813–820.
11. Stahl MMS, Ekström B, Sparf B, et al. Urodynamic and other effects of tolterodine: a novel antimuscarinic drug for the treatment of detrusor over-activity. Neurourol Urodyn 1995;14:647–655.
12. Rentzhog L, Stanton SL, Cardozo L, et al. Efficacy and safety of tolterodine in patients with detrusor hyperreflexia: a dose ranging study. Br J Urol 1998;81:42–48.
13. Eckford SD, Carter PG, Jackson SR, et al. An open, in-patient incremental safety and efficacy study of desmopressin in women with multiple sclerosis and nocturia. Br J Urol 1995;76:459–463.
14. Kinn AC, Larsson PO. Desmopressin: a new principle for symptomatic treatment of urgency and incontinence in patients with multiple sclerosis. Scand J Urol Nephrol 1990;24:109–112.
15. Hoverd PA, Fowler CJ. Desmopressin in the treatment of daytime frequency in patients with multiple sclerosis. J Neurol Neurosurg Psychiatry 1998;65:778–780.
16. Dasgupta P, Fowler CJ. Chillies: from antiquity to urology. Br J Urol 1997;80:845–852.
17. Maggi CA, Santicioli P, Meli A. The effects of topical capsaicin on rat urinary bladder motility in vivo. Eur J Pharmacol 1984;103:41–50.
18. Szallasi A, Conte B, Goso C, et al. Characterization of a peripheral vanilloid (capsaicin) receptor in the urinary bladder of the rat. Life Sci 1993;52:PL221–PL226.
19. Caterina MJ, Schumacher MA, Tominaga M, et al. The capsaicin receptor: a heat-activated ion channel in the pain pathway. Nature 1997;389:816–824.

20. Maggi CA, Barbanti G, Santicioli P, et al. Cystometric evidence that capsaicin-sensitive nerves modulate the afferent branch of micturition reflex in humans. J Urol 1989;142:150–154.
21. Fowler CJ, Jewkes D, McDonald WI, et al. Intravesical capsaicin for neurogenic bladder dysfunction. Lancet 1992;339:1239.
22. De Groat WC, Kawatani M, Hisamitsu T, et al. Mechanisms underlying the recovery of urinary bladder function following spinal cord injury. J Auton Nerv Syst 1990;30(suppl):S71–S78.
23. Fowler CJ, Beck RO, Gerrard S, et al. Intravesical capsaicin for treatment of detrusor hyperreflexia. J Neurol Neurosurg Psychiatry 1994;57:169–173.
24. Geirsson G, Fall M, Sullivan L. Clinical and urodynamic effects of intravesical capsaicin treatment in patients with chronic traumatic spinal detrusor hyperreflexia. J Urol 1995;154:1825–1829.
25. Cruz F, Guimaraes M, Silva C, et al. Desensitization of bladder sensory fibres by intravesical capsaicin has long lasting clinical and urodynamic effects in patients with hyperactive or hypersensitive bladder dysfunction. J Urol 1997;157:585–589.
26. Chancellor MB. Should we be using chili pepper extracts to treat the overactive bladder? J Urol 1997;158:2097.
27. DeRidder D, Chandiramani V, Dasgupta P, et al. Intravesical capsaicin as a treatment for refractory detrusor hyperreflexia: a dual center study with long-term follow-up. J Urol 1997;158:2087–2092.
28. Dasgupta P, Chandiramani VA, Parkinson MC, et al. Treating the human bladder with capsaicin: is it safe? Eur Urol 1998;33:28–31.
29. Igawa Y, Komiyama I, Nishizawa S, Ogawa A. Intravesical capsaicin inhibits autonomic dysreflexia in patients with spinal cord injury. Neurourol Urodyn 1996;4:374–376.
30. Wiart L, Joseph PA, Petit H, et al. The effects of capsaicin on the neurogenic hyperreflexic detrusor: a double blind placebo controlled study in patients with spinal cord disease. Preliminary results. Spinal Cord 1998;36:95–99.
31. Chandiramani VA, Peterson T, Duthie GS, Fowler CJ. Urodynamic changes during therapeutic intravesical instillations of capsaicin. Br J Urol 1996;77:792–797.
32. Dasgupta P, Fowler CJ, Stephen RL. Electromotive drug administration of lidocaine to anesthetize the bladder before intravesical capsaicin. J Urol 1998;159:1857–1861.
33. Dasgupta P, Chandiramani V, Beckett A, et al. Flexible cystoscopic biopsies for nerve density evaluation of the suburothelium of the human urinary bladder. Br J Urol 1997;80:490–492.
34. Dasgupta P, Chandiramani V, Fowler CJ, et al. Intravesical capsaicin: its effects on nerve densities in the human urinary bladder. Neurourol Urodyn 1996;15:373–374.
35. Cruz F, Guimaraes M, Silva C, Reis M. Suppression of bladder hyperreflexia by intravesical resiniferatoxin. Lancet 1997;350:640–641.
36. Lazzeri M, Beneforti P, Turini D. Urodynamic effects of intravesical resiniferatoxin in humans: preliminary results in stable and unstable detrusor. J Urol 1997;158:2093–2096.
37. Blackford HN, Murray K, Stephenson TP, Mundy AR. Results of transvesical infiltration of the pelvic plexuses with phenol in 116 patients. Br J Urol 1984;56:647–649.
38. Sandyk R, Iacono RP. Improvement by picoTesla range magnetic fields of perceptual-motor performance and visual memory in a patient with chronic progressive multiple sclerosis. Int J Neurosci 1994;78:53–66.
39. Sheriff MK, Shah PJ, Fowler C, et al. Neuromodulation of detrusor hyper-reflexia by functional magnetic stimulation of the sacral roots. Br J Urol 1996;78:39–46.
40. Flanigan RC, August HM Jr, Young B, et al. Cutaneous stimulation of the bladder in multiple sclerosis: a case report. J Urol 1983;129:1047–1048.
41. Hawkes CH, Myke M, Desmond A, et al. Stimulation of dorsal column in multiple sclerosis. BMJ 1980;280:889–891.
42. Young RF, Goodman SJ. Dorsal spinal cord stimulation in the treatment of multiple sclerosis. Neurosurgery 1979;5:225–230.
43. Shah J, Dasgupta P, Selim A. A twelve-year experience with "clam" ileocystoplasty: a safe and successful procedure. Eur Urol 1996;30(suppl 2):769A.
44. Kennelly MJ, Gormley EA, McGuire EJ. Early clinical experience with adult auto-augmentation. J Urol 1994;152:303–306.
45. Swami KS, Feneley RCL, Hammonds JC, Abrams P. Detrusor myectomy for detrusor overactivity: a minimum 1-year follow-up. Br J Urol 1998;81:68–72.
46. Continence Products Directory. The Continence Foundation. London: 1997.
47. O'Hagan M. Neurogenic Bladder Dysfunction. In C Norton (ed), Nursing for Continence. Bucks, UK: Beaconsfield Publishers, 1996.
48. Guttman L, Frankel H. The value of intermittent catheterisation in the management of traumatic paraplegia and tetraplegia. Paraplegia 1966;4:63–78.

49. Lapides J, Diokno C, Silber SJ, Lowe BS. Clean intermittent self catheterisation in the treatment of urinary tract disease. J Urol 1972;107:458–461.
50. Webb RJ, Lawson AL, Neal DE. Clean intermittent catheterisation in 172 adults. Br J Urol 1990;65:20–23.
51. Getliffe K. Catheter and Catheterization. In K Getliffe, M Dolman (eds), Promoting Continence— A Clinical and Research Resource. London: Bailliere Tindall, 1997;281–341.
52. Eckford SD, Swami KS, Jackson SR, Abrams PH. Long-term follow up of transvaginal urethral closure and suprapubic cystostomy for urinary incontinence in women with multiple sclerosis. Br J Urol 1994;74:733–735.
53. MacDiarmid SA, Arnold EP, Palmer NB, Anthony A. Management of spinal cord injured patients by indwelling suprapubic catheterisation. J Urol 1995;154:492–494.
54. Bull E, Chilton CP, Gould CA, Sutton TM. Single-blind, randomised, parallel study of the Bard Biocath and a silicone elastomer-coated catheter. Br J Urol 1991;68:394–399.
55. Mulhall AB, King S, Lee K, Wiggington E. Maintenance of closed urinary drainage systems: are practitioners aware of the dangers? J Clin Nurs 1993;2:135–140.
56. Disability Equipment Assessment. Catheter Valves—A Multi-Centre Comparative Evaluation. London: Medical Device Agency, September 1997.
57. German K, Rowley P, Stone D, et al. A randomised cross-over study comparing the use of a catheter valve and a leg bag in urethrally catheterised male patients. Br J Urol 1997;79:96–98.
58. Nathan P. Emptying the paralysed bladder. Lancet 1977;1:377.
59. Dasgupta P, Haslam C, Goodwin R, Fowler CJ. The "Queen Square bladder stimulator": a device for assisting emptying of the neurogenic bladder. Br J Urol 1997;80:234–237.
60. Vahtera T, Haaranen M, Viramo-Koskela AL, Ruutiainen J. Pelvic floor rehabilitation is effective in patients with multiple sclerosis. Clin Rehabil 1997;11:211–219.
61. Watson R. Mostly Men. In K Getliffe, M Dolman (eds), Promoting Continence—A Clinical and Research Resource. London: Bailliere Tindall, 1997;107–137.
62. Van Kerrebroeck PE. The role of electrical stimulation in voiding dysfunction. Eur Urol 1998;34(suppl 1):27–30.
63. Wielink G, Essink-Bot ML, Van Kerrebroeck PE, Rutten FF. Sacral rhizotomies and electrical bladder stimulation in spinal cord injury. 2. Cost-effectiveness and quality of life analysis. Dutch Study Group on Sacral Anterior Root Stimulation. Eur Urol 1997;31:441–446.
64. Schurch B, Rodic B, Jeanmonod D. Posterior sacral rhizotomy and intradural anterior sacral root stimulation for treatment of the spastic bladder in spinal cord–injured patients. J Urol 1997;157: 610–614.
65. Van Kerrebroeck EV, vander Aa HE, Bosch JL, et al. Sacral rhizotomies and electrical bladder stimulation in spinal cord injury. Part I: clinical and urodynamic analysis. Dutch Study Group on Sacral Anterior Root Stimulation. Eur Urol 1997;31:263–271.
66. Rijkhoff NJ, Hendrikx LB, van Kerrebroeck PE, et al. Selective detrusor activation by electrical stimulation of human sacral nerve roots. Artif Organs 1997;21:223–236.
67. Elabbady AA, Hassouna MM, Elhilahi MM. Neural stimulation for chronic voiding dysfunctions. J Urol 1994;152:1–5.
68. Klarskov P, Holm Bentzen M, Larsen S, et al. Partial cystectomy for the myogenic decompensated bladder with excessive residual urine. Scand J Urol Nephrol 1988;22:251–256.
69. Sylora JA, Gonzalez R, Vaughn M, Reinberg Y. Intermittent self-catheterization by quadriplegic patients via a catheterizable Mitrofanoff channel. J Urol 1997;157:48–50.
70. Mraz J, Michek J, Sutory M, Zerhau P. Surgical treatment of the atonic bladder ("vesical cap"). Urol Res 1992;20:241–245.
71. Von Heyden B, Anthony J, Kaula N, et al. The latissimus dorsi muscle for detrusor assistance: functional recovery after nerve division and repair. J Urol 1994;151:1081–1087.
72. Joseph AC, Juma S, Niku SD. Endourethral prosthesis for treatment of detrusor sphincter dyssynergia: impact on quality of life for persons with spinal cord injury. Sci Nurs 1994;11:95–99.
73. Monga AK, Beyar M, Nativ O, Stanton SL. A new intraurethral sphincter prosthesis for retention: preliminary clinical results. Neurourol Urodyn 1996;15:406–407.

12
Investigation and Treatment of Bowel Problems

Christine Norton and Michael Henry

Although considerable literature exists on the prevalence and pathophysiology of bowel dysfunction in neurologic disease or injury, remarkably little work has been done on practical management. In particular, very few controlled trials of interventions exist, and many articles finish their review of causes with rather vague advice on the importance of a good fluid intake and balanced diet. For example, although 30–40% of stroke patients are fecally incontinent on admission, 18% are incontinent at discharge, and 7–9% are incontinent 6 months later, a review found no studies on treatment of fecal incontinence after stroke [1].

Many patients with neurologic problems tread a fine dividing line between constipation and fecal incontinence. Great care is needed to assure that in treating one, the other is not precipitated [2, 3]. For example, when sensation is imperfect, leading to a diminished call to stool and eventual drying of the stool and constipation, treatment with laxatives may cause incontinence, especially if that diminished sensation is associated with impaired mobility and inability to cope with urgent defecation. Many patients prefer constipation to incontinence because it is more socially acceptable, but care is needed that side effects of constipation, such as exacerbation of bladder symptoms [4] like bladder instability or limb spasticity [2] or fecal impaction with overflow diarrhea, do not in turn cause problems. In patients with high spinal lesions, impaction can precipitate autonomic dysreflexia, making it potentially life-threatening [5]. Many patients with neurologic problems need to actively plan bowel evacuation rather than wait until problems develop.

In the colorectal literature, *neurogenic incontinence* often denotes fecal incontinence presumed to be secondary to damage to the pudendal nerve during childbirth, rather than that associated with major neurologic disease. This can make the literature very confusing.

It is also clear from the literature on bowel management in neurologic conditions that very little cross-fertilization has occurred in the treatment of different patient groups. Some techniques that have been found highly effective in one patient group have never been reported at all in treating patients with similar lesions due to different causes (e.g., the spinal injury literature and spina bifida literature almost never make reference to each other). This chapter reviews the rather limited literature available to enable those working with a given group of patients to consider whether techniques that have been found helpful elsewhere might be transferable.

PREVALENCE OF BOWEL PROBLEMS

One should not forget how common are both fecal incontinence and constipation in the general population. Fecal incontinence affects more than 1% of community-dwelling adults, and flatus incontinence a further 1% [6]. Approximately 5% of people in Western populations report fewer than three bowel actions per week [7]. Childbirth is probably the single most common cause of incontinence [8], and patients with neurologic problems are not exempt from bowel problems due to other causes. For example, Swash et al. found coincidental pelvic nerve lesions after childbirth in 12 patients with multiple sclerosis [9]. Not uncommonly, patients with neurologic disease have been told that their bowel symptoms are inevitable with their disease, and so no investigation or specific treatment is undertaken. Acceptance of bowel symptoms seems to be common among patients and professionals alike.

More than one-third of people who have a stroke have fecal incontinence on admission to hospital. The number falls to 10% at 6 months, with older patients, women, and those with the most severe strokes, diabetes, or another disabling disease being most at risk [10]. This fecal incontinence may be more a product of immobility and dependency than of neurologic damage [11].

Spinal cord injury (SCI) commonly causes major bowel dysfunction, with 11% reporting fecal incontinence weekly or more, and only 39% having reliable bowel continence [12]. Many people with neurologic problems are dependent on others for toileting needs. Half of SCI patients need help to manage their bowels; 53% use digital anal stimulation and two-thirds use manual removal of feces. One-half take more than 30 minutes for a bowel routine; one in five needs more than 1 hour [12]. Thirty-eight percent of those with SCI subjectively report their bowel function as a moderate or severe problem [13].

Sixty-five percent of 424 members of the Danish Paraplegic Association use digital stimulation [14]. Only 19% feel a normal desire to defecate; 38% have no desire; 37% can sense a need by abdominal discomfort and 25% by headache, uneasiness, or perspiration. Seventy-five percent have some fecal incontinence, but for the majority this is rare (56% have a few episodes per year); 39% feel that bowel function places restrictions on their lives.

Parkinson's disease can lead to both slow transit and evacuation-difficulty-type constipation in up to 50% of patients [15]. Multiple sclerosis is associated with constipation in more than 40% and with fecal incontinence in more than 50%; those with the greatest disability are most affected by both [16].

Many other disabling conditions are associated with either fecal incontinence, constipation, or both. Some conditions show clear pathophysiologic changes affecting bowel function and the ability to control it voluntarily. But in many individual cases, the results of nerve damage can be difficult to disentangle from the results of immobility and dependence on others for what most people see as a very private and embarrassing bodily function.

EFFECTS OF BOWEL PROBLEMS

As was seen in Chapter 6, lack of bowel control can have personally devastating effects on individuals and those around them. These patients often have very damaged self-esteem and confidence, and may severely restrict their lives to avoid the embarrassment of a public accident. Fecal incontinence need not happen often to make someone very reluctant to take the risk again. Many people have difficulty talking about their bowels, and many do not have a vocabulary to describe what is happening. Even those in contact with medical care often do not tell their physicians about fecal incontinence because of embarrassment or pessimism about the prospects for improvement [17].

With careful individual assessment and multidisciplinary care planning, however, acceptable management methods can be found for most patients, and some do adapt successfully and cope well with disordered bowel function. For example, Kannisto and Rintala found that people who had sustained SCI in childhood were generally continent and content [18]. Although many of these patients have to spend considerable amounts of time with bowel routines and may need help from others, the majority should be able to find effective and acceptable defecation without complications such as incontinence [19].

INVESTIGATION OF BOWEL PROBLEMS

Many patients can be managed symptomatically without recourse to sophisticated investigations. When management is not leading to satisfactory bowel control, however, investigation may be useful to precisely define the pathophysiology and also to exclude the non-neurologic causes of fecal incontinence or constipation that can affect anyone. Rectal bleeding or a sudden change in bowel habit unrelated to major changes in neurologic condition always warrants urgent colonoscopy or barium enema study to exclude malignancy (bowel cancer is the second most common malignancy in the developed world [20]). A wide variety of other tests may be indicated, such as thyroid function tests to exclude hypothyroidism as a cause of constipation and investigation of diarrhea. A sigmoidoscopy should be considered for all patients with disordered defecation.

Anorectal Physiology Tests

A number of anorectal physiology tests are usually done in the same laboratory session [21, 22].

Anal manometry assesses the resting pressure (a marker for the function of the smooth muscle internal anal sphincter, responsible for 80% of resting tone and therefore passive retention of stool) and squeeze pressure (a test of the striated voluntary external anal sphincter, which is responsible for the ability to resist the urge to defecate when the rectum fills).

Balloon distension involves slowly filling a rectal balloon with air or water and noting first sensation, urge, and maximum tolerated volumes. This test assesses whether the patient has normal sensitivity to rectal contents and evaluates for the presence of a megarectum.

The *rectoanal inhibitory reflex* can be elicited by distending the rectum with an air-filled balloon and measuring the consequent drop in anal pressure. Absence of this reflex is usually diagnostic of Hirschsprung's disease, occasionally missed until adult life, but the reflex can also be impaired in other neurologic conditions.

Balloon expulsion tests can assess the degree of pelvic floor coordination on attempted defecation using surface electromyographic electrodes. Normally, the anal sphincter should relax with expulsion of the balloon. Any paradoxical contraction or "anismus" can be clearly observed. The presence of this paradoxical contraction can effectively obstruct defecation and has been described in cases of multiple sclerosis [23] and in Parkinson's disease [24].

Electrosensitivity thresholds can be measured in the anus and rectum. Rectal sensation to electrical stimulation is a good marker for detecting hindgut denervation.

Other tests include measurement of pudendal terminal motor latencies, single fiber electromyography of the anal sphincter (see Chapter 9), saline retention tests, and assessment of rectal compliance to distension.

Radiology

Anal ultrasonography using an intra-anal ultrasound probe gives a very clear view of the structural integrity of the internal and external anal sphincters [25]. Childbirth-related defects or scarring are very common but are not always immediately symptomatic [8]. Only when mobility or neurologic function is also impaired may urgency become overt urge fecal incontinence. Other common causes of sphincter damage include anal surgery, such as hemorrhoidectomy or sphincterotomy; anal stretch; and direct trauma.

Evacuating proctography assesses the ability of the rectum to retain barium paste, the integrity of the sphincters, and coordination of pelvic floor relaxation with attempted emptying, as well as the presence of any megarectum, prolapse, or rectocele [26].

Transit studies [27] require the patient to take a capsule of radiopaque markers on three successive days; a plain abdominal radiograph is taken on day 5. Normal ranges are available. Eighty percent of markers should have been passed by day 5. Slow transit constipation, as well as inefficient evacuation (all markers in the rectum) can be diagnosed. Radioisotope studies can also be used to assess gut transit times.

INDIVIDUAL ASSESSMENT

In addition to the sophisticated tests outlined here, an assessment should include inquiries regarding symptoms, toilet abilities, environment, diet, and the effects on the individual and any caregivers involved. Table 12.1 suggests the most important areas for assessment.

Bowel problems in these patients are often multifactorial, with defects in neurologic control often exacerbated by physical difficulties with defecation, immobility, and inappropriate toilet facilities.

Table 12.1   Areas to address in assessment of bowel problems

Usual bowel pattern
Usual stool consistency
Presence of blood or mucus
Ability to sense bowel fullness
Pain before or with defecation
Urgency and ability to defer defecation
Urge incontinence
Evacuation difficulties: straining, sense of incomplete emptying, digital stimulation or
   extraction of stool, use of evacuants
Passive soiling (loss of stool without a prior urge to defecate)
Ability to control flatus and distinguish flatus from stool
Use of pads
Obstetric history
Bladder control
Ability to use toilet independently
Toilet adaptations
Attitude and availability of caregivers
Effect on lifestyle and relationships
Psychological factors

SELECTION OF MANAGEMENT OPTIONS

The importance of conducting a multidisciplinary assessment to identify and minimize impairments, disabilities, and handicaps related to bowel dysfunction, and
of setting person-centered goals in line with desired postrehabilitation lifestyle,
is often emphasized [28]. Any bowel schedule has to fit with other activities of
the patient and of any caregiver involved.

Bowel control is often easier to manipulate than bladder control because, if
complete evacuation can be achieved, the rectum is normally empty, mass movements are an infrequent event, and stool consistency can be regulated by diet or
medication. With careful planning of a bowel regime, most patients should be
able to achieve bowel continence and adequate evacuation. Often, this involves
a package of care rather than a single intervention—attention to diet, bowel
habit, evacuation techniques, and, in selected cases, use of medication or surgery.
As so little research is available, trial and error often are required to find the best
regime for any individual patient.

DRUG TREATMENT

The two main approaches in drug treatment are the use of laxatives to stimulate
more effective evacuation of the bowel and the use of antidiarrheal agents to slow
an overactive bowel or to enable planned evacuation with rectal preparations.

Table 12.2   Commonly used laxatives

Category	Comments and contraindications	Examples
Bulking agents	Introduce gradually, only after impaction cleared. Avoid if patient has loss of rectal sensation or terminal reservoir syndrome. Ensure sufficient fluid intake.	Natural bran Ispaghula husk Methylcellulose Sterculia
Stool softeners	Avoid general use of liquid paraffin (risk of paraffinomas).	Castor oil Dioctyl sodium sulfo-succinate (osmotic also)
Stimulant/chemical	Use minimum effective dose.	Senna Bisacodyl
Osmotics	Flatus may be a problem.	Milk of magnesia Lactulose Polyethylene glycol Dioctyl sodium sulfosucci-nate (softener also)
Rectally admin-istered aids	Some patients may need assis-tance or fail to retain.	Suppositories (e.g., glyc-erin, bisacodyl) Enemas (e.g., phosphate, sodium-based micro-enemas)

Treatment of Constipation

Different approaches are indicated for different types of constipation. Bulk-forming laxatives may be useful for those on an inadequate oral diet and to soften the stool and stimulate peristalsis when the bowel is a little sluggish. However, the use of bulking agents can be counterproductive if peristalsis is impaired, and it can merely add to the tendency to impaction in frail, immobile individuals [29]. Stool softeners may help when the main problem is difficult evacuation, whereas stimulants may help with slow transit. Table 12.2 summarizes the most widely used preparations [30].

Very few controlled trials have been performed of laxatives in general, and almost none specific to neurologic patients. Some experts recommend the same regime of stimulant laxatives or enemas as is used for chronic idiopathic constipation and cast doubt on the idea that long-term use may lead to myenteric plexus damage [31]. They provide an algorithm for drug treatment of constipation (Figure 12.1). However, some suggestion exists of an association between long-term use of anthraquinone and colorectal cancer [32].

Stimulant laxatives should be used with extreme caution if the patient is suspected to be fecally impacted. One of the few comparative trials of laxatives in the literature has found that a senna-fiber combination is more effective than the commonly used lactulose in increasing bowel frequency, improving stool consistency, and easing evacuation in continent frail older people, and the cost is lower [33]. Small-scale studies have found that oral polyethylene glycol can be effective in relieving impaction [34].

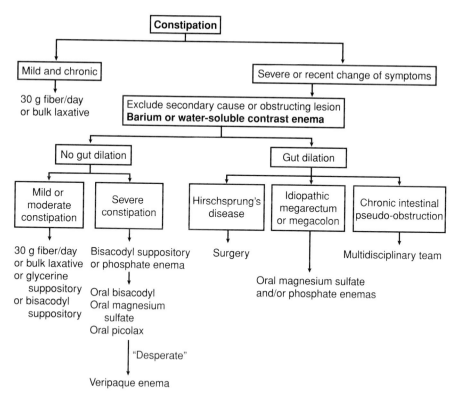

Figure 12.1 Outline of drug treatment in constipated patients. (Reprinted with permission from JM Gattuso, MA Kamm. Review article: the management of constipation in adults. Aliment Pharmacol Ther 1993;7:497.)

An extensive systematic review of the treatment of constipation in older adults has been conducted [35]. The authors recommend the use of bulk laxatives for ambulatory people, the use of sorbitol if this fails, and the uses of glycerine suppositories if straining is the predominant symptom. Frail older people need extra fluid if bulk laxatives are used; they can be given sorbitol if this treatment fails or senna if slow transit problems exist. Tap water enemas are suggested as a safer alternative to phosphate enemas, which may cause damage to the rectal mucosa or hyperphosphatemia [35]. Many of the same recommendations may apply to neurologic patients.

Dunn and Galka have compared Therevac (Jones Pharma, Inc., St. Louis, MO) microenemas (5-ml stimulant enemas) to bisacodyl suppositories in SCI patients and have found that patients need more than 45 minutes to respond to the suppositories. The microenemas reduced both digital stimulation time and evacuation time and, although much more expensive, could potentially reduce caregiver time by up to 1 hour per day, with obvious cost savings [36]. Another two randomized studies found that the carrier is important for suppositories. Hydrogenated vegetable oil bisacodyl takes longer to work than polyethylene-glycol-based bisacodyl; the shorter time for the latter is assumed to be the result of quicker bioavailability, as the former has to dissolve in body heat [37, 38]. Clinical experience suggests that many laxatives and evacuants take longer to work in patients with neurologic damage.

Patient compliance is often poor with prescribed medication. In a study of 114 rehabilitation patients, 66% were discharged taking bowel medication; only 42% were found to be taking it 1 month later in telephone interviews [39]. Whether this result indicates overprescribing and appropriate cessation at home or failure to comply with needed medication is unclear.

When suppositories are used, they are easier to insert and more effective if applied blunt end first [40]. People with limited dexterity who need to use suppositories may find the Spinal Injuries Association (76 St. James Lane, London N10 3DF) suppository inserter helpful.

Cisapride is used to stimulate distal colonic motility, but reports are equivocal as to its effect. Early studies reported reduced transit time and increased intraluminal tone and decreased capacity in the rectum [41]; however, later placebo-controlled studies showed little effect [42], and isolated reports exist of fatal cardiac arrhythmias linked to its use [43].

Apomorphine hydrochloride administration has been reported to improve defecation and lessen paradoxical puborectalis contraction in five patients with Parkinson's disease [44]. The authors recommend evaluation of other, more easily available dopamine agonists for this problem.

Weber reported that treatment with nonirritant laxatives and daily suppositories or "manual maneuvers" is sufficient, without a special diet, to restore fecal autonomy in 80% of SCI subjects, but no details were given [45]. He also reported this regime to be successful in patients with multiple sclerosis if the delay in transit is in the transverse or left colon; however, if delay is right-sided, the condition is difficult to treat, and patients have frequent pseudo-obstructive episodes.

In a cohort study of patients with multiple sclerosis in Norway, only 58.7% were found to manage their bowels without any medication or dietary manipulation [46]. The need for intervention increases with time and with progress of the disease. Assistance from others in managing evacuation or fecal incontinence was required by 8.7%.

Constipating Agents

Patients who experience urge incontinence of feces associated with loose stool or who have a passive anal seepage of soft stool may benefit from taking low dosages of constipating medication [47], although no data exist on its use in patients with neurologic problems. Use of loperamide hydrochloride has been found to reduce fecal incontinence, improve stool consistency, and reduce stool weight compared to placebo. Continence to rectally infused saline improved on dosages of 4 mg three times a day in 26 patients with chronic diarrhea, and a small increase in resting anal pressure was also seen [48]. The authors suggested that stools might have been loose as a response to a weak anal sphincter. Loperamide oxide has a similar effect [49]. Also, some evidence exists that loperamide hydrochloride increases water absorption by slowing colonic transit and, based on an animal model, that it decreases internal anal sphincter relaxation in response to rectal distension [50] and increases mucosal fluid uptake [51]. The use of codeine phosphate is also effective for some patients [29]. These drugs need to be taken before eating and the dose individually titrated. Loperamide hydrochloride is available as a syrup when the capsules are too constipating.

Some patients may choose to effectively stop spontaneous evacuation by using these agents and then perform evacuation at a convenient time by using suppositories or a microenema. Although not ideal, this regime can at least give the patient an element of control and predictability to enable a reasonable quality of life. This practice has been found to be effective in a nursing home environment, even when staff compliance with prescribed regimes is not good [52].

BIOFEEDBACK

Fecal incontinence is a widely reported clinical indication for biofeedback, and several studies of its efficacy in patients with neurologic disease have been undertaken. Many other studies have included a mixed group of consecutive patients presenting with fecal incontinence to a colorectal service, but information about the specific group with neurologic disease cannot be extracted. Early uncontrolled studies suggested benefit of biofeedback in cases of spina bifida. Six of eight patients with myelomeningocele reduced incontinence after two to six sessions of training to contract the external anal sphincter in response to internal sphincter relaxation on rectal distension [53]. In a selected group of eight spina bifida patients, ability to contract the gluteals and recognize rectal sensation enabled a reduction of 75% or more in soiling episodes for one-half of the patients [54]. Rectal sensation was found to be a determinant of outcome in 15 patients; those with lower thresholds of sensation did best [55]. Another group who administered urodynamic biofeedback training for urinary incontinence to eight children found no improvement in bladder control; however, four of eight improved bowel control, presumably in response to training of external anal sphincter contractions [56].

Later controlled studies, however, have shown no benefit of biofeedback training over well-monitored conventional therapy, including the use of behavior modification techniques and medication [57], and no objective improvement in any of the parameters that the biofeedback was intended to modify in their 12 subjects (no increase in anal squeeze pressure, no lowering of the threshold of rectal discrimination of distension, and no improvement in the volume of rectally infused saline that could be held continently). Whitehead et al. likewise found little additional benefit of biofeedback over conventional therapy in 33 children, except in those patients with myelomeningocele lesions at L2 or below [58]. One study of five patients after head injury reported benefit, but minimal data were given [59].

Patients with SCI may lose rectal sensation but maintain a deep nonspecific pelvic sensation of rectal contents [60]. In patients with infrequent peristalsis and a spastic external anal sphincter, the potential for teaching patients to discriminate this sensation by biofeedback and then stimulate reflex emptying (see following section, Bowel Training Programs) merits further exploration.

Patients with multiple sclerosis are documented as having reduced voluntary anal squeeze increment compared to controls (e.g., Jameson et al. [61] and Caruana et al. [62]). However, whether this sphincter function can be improved by biofeedback and sphincter exercises in the same way that it can in non-neurologic patients with fecal incontinence is not known.

The role of biofeedback in treating paradoxical puborectalis contraction in the constipated adult patient with neurologic impairment remains to be investigated. This paradoxical contraction, effectively obstructing successful defecation, has been described in multiple sclerosis [23, 63] and in Parkinson's disease [24]. Research has established that patients with this "anismus" in the absence of neurologic cause respond well to biofeedback training [31]. Biofeedback has been used with mixed success as part of a package of care for children with spina bifida who suffer from constipation [64].

Nearly all of the studies described here have been very small in scale and have involved a highly selected patient population. Larger-scale studies are needed.

BOWEL TRAINING PROGRAMS

Many different interventions have been tried in the name of bowel training [65]. Most extol the virtues of a high fiber diet, adequate fluid intake, as much exercise as feasible, and a regular toileting regime to capitalize on the gastrocolic reflex. When this regime fails to establish a habit, use of a suppository or digital stimulation is often advocated. In practice, many patients resort to evacuation by Valsalva's maneuver or straining. However, this practice can eventually lead to problems with hemorrhoids or even rectal prolapse.

Children with spina bifida have been found to respond to behavior modification, a regular toilet habit, and dietary manipulation, with use of laxative medication or evacuants as indicated [66]. Most programs stress the importance of teaching the child to self-initiate toileting after each meal, rewarding successful defecation, and using suppositories or an enema if no self-initiated bowel motion occurs in 2 days.

Table 12.3   Protocol for progressive steps in bowel program in patients with spina bifida

1. Bowel cleanout if hard stool is present in the rectal vault or palpable above the descending colon.
2. Appropriately soft stool consistency with diet (fiber or trigger foods) and bulking agents.
3. Glycerin suppository 20 minutes after meal. Ten minutes later on toilet, limited to less than 40 minutes, relieving skin pressure every 10 minutes (especially emphasized if child is heavier than 50 lb).
4. Dulcolax suppository in place of glycerin.
5. Digital stimulation—20 minutes postsuppository every 5 minutes × 3.
6. Timed oral medications—Peri-Colace, Senokot, Dulcolax tablets timed so that the bowel movement would otherwise result 0.5–1.0 hour after the anticipated triggered bowel timing.

Source: Reprinted with permission from JC King, DM Currie, E Wright. Bowel training in spina bifida: importance of education, patient compliance, age, and anal reflexes. Arch Phys Med Rehabil 1994;75:244.

A protocol for a stepwise program for bowel management in spina bifida, with a strong emphasis on patient education, has been developed [67] (Table 12.3). Forty patients with spina bifida were entered in a prospective evaluation of this protocol. Social continence (defined as one or fewer episodes of fecal incontinence per month) was increased in 13% to 60% of subjects. Success was associated with younger age at onset of the program, compliance with the prescribed regime, and presence of the anocutaneous reflex. Of those who had been previously incontinent and who complied, 79% achieved continence.

After a cerebrovascular accident, patients developed a consistent elimination pattern by a program of daily digital rectal stimulation [68]. Daily stimulation was more effective than alternate-day stimulation, with 24 of 25 patients achieving success. Patients with a right hemiplegia took longer to develop an established elimination pattern than did those with a left hemiplegia; those with less mobility also took longer.

Many people with neurologic problems are dependent on others for toileting needs. The most developed protocols for bowel management tend to be for SCI patients. Upper motor neuron lesion patients are usually taught to stimulate reflex emptying every 1–3 days by gently rotating a gloved finger in the anus until the rectal wall is felt to relax or flatus is passed and the stool comes down. This procedure is seldom performed for more than 1 minute at a time and is repeated every 10 minutes until the internal anal sphincter is felt to close off again or no stool has been passed after the last two stimulations. Many can sense when defecation is complete. Whether these techniques would be helpful to other populations is not known. Lower motor neuron lesion patients often need to manually evacuate the rectum one or more times per day to stay continent. Tight pants or a gel cushion may help support a lax perineum [28].

In a nursing home population, frequency of defecation and number of continent stools was increased significantly in a trial of prompted voiding for urinary incontinence [69]. The authors suggested that this incidental finding may relate to increased opportunity to sit on the toilet, together with improved mobility and fluid intake. Thus dependent individuals may increase bowel frequency simply by being able to access a toilet more frequently. This finding has particular relevance for people with a urinary catheter who may seldom be offered use of the toilet.

BOWEL WASHOUT REGIMES

Bowel washouts are used much more frequently in Europe than in the United Kingdom. Research on optimal regimes and techniques and on which fluids are the most effective is limited. Gattuso et al. found that colostomy irrigation with water produced high-pressure-propagated waves of colonic contraction and effective evacuation without subsequent breakthrough when the volume was 500 ml or more (but not 250 ml) [70]. Patients preferred 500 ml to larger volumes. This work was done with anal irrigation. Some patients find it impossible to retain fluid instilled rectally.

Shandling has developed an enema continence catheter incorporating an inflatable balloon and reported 100% success with 40% of 112 children with spina bifida; however, selection criteria were not made clear and length of follow-up was not stated [71]. Others are more cautious in their appraisals. Thirty-one children aged 3–19 years (mean age, 9 years) with spina bifida who were dissatisfied with current bowel management started using the catheter, instilling 20 ml/kg of saline every 24 or 48 hours [72]. Six children dropped out immediately, and nine more had stopped using the catheter at 30 months. Among those who continued to use the catheter, the percentage of continent stools rose from 28% to 94%, and the percentage with constipated stools dropped from 55% to 15%. Potential adverse effects include bowel perforation, allergic reaction to latex in the catheter, electrolyte disturbances, and bacteremia, but none of the papers reviewed here has reported these.

One group reported that 83 of their 190 patients with spina bifida performed irrigation daily or on alternate days via a cone in the anus, with good compliance to the regimen [73]. Water in the amount of 20 ml per kilogram of body weight was used, with evacuation within 30 minutes. The importance of having a specialist nurse oversee the program was stressed. The irrigation did not help with bladder compliance or instability, however. Details of the technique were given by Scholler-Gyure et al., who used 20 ml/kg of tap water 1 hour after the evening meal, ran in half the volume, allowed 5 minutes without the cone, and then ran in the rest of the water, allowing up to 20 minutes for defecation afterward [74]. They stated that the volume needed was very individual and often found only by trial and error. Of 41 patients with spina bifida who had failed other bowel management programs, 66% were continent at a mean follow-up of 33 months. Seven had monthly incontinence and seven weekly incontinence; none had daily incontinence. Minor side effects included abdominal pain, headaches, and poor appetite, but these were rare. Parental satisfaction was high in 63% of cases and good in 37%. Sixty-six percent of the children rated continence as the most important advantage, but half felt that the procedure took up too much time and energy. Six found irrigation painful and three unpleasant; five were dependent on others to help.

Clinical experience suggests that response to rectal washout is very individual, and experimenting with volumes, temperatures, and fluids, with or without addition of enemas, is worthwhile to find the optimum for a given individual. A danger of autonomic dysreflexia exists in those with a thoracic-level lesion; in such cases, careful monitoring and patient teaching are required.

A mechanical pump that introduces 25 ml of warm water in pulses into the rectum has been described [75]. It was reported to clear fecal impaction on the first attempt in 24 of 37 procedures and was well tolerated by most patients.

When rectal washout is incomplete, a catheterizable continence conduit may be surgically constructed to achieve antegrade colonic irrigation (see the following section on Antegrade Continence Enema).

MANUAL EVACUATION

Considerable controversy has arisen in nursing about the use of manual rectal evacuation and its possible complications. Almost no research has been done on this practice, and no evidence of harmful effects has been reported. Undoubtedly, a group of patients exists who have little or no reflex activity in the lower colon (and so cannot stimulate peristalsis) and who have little alternative to planned manual evacuation, done by themselves or by a caregiver or nurse. The majority of SCI patients must use this method regularly [12]. The Royal College of Nursing [76] has reviewed manual evacuation and suggested a procedure and safety points.

SURGERY

Anal Sphincter Repair

When preoperative anal ultrasonography has demonstrated division of the external anal sphincter ring after trauma such as that caused by childbirth or previous anal fistula surgery, repair of the sphincter ring yields excellent results, with return to near-normal function in up to 80% of patients [77]. If preoperative investigation has revealed coexistent damage to the innervation of these sphincters, the postoperative results are less satisfactory, but patients whose physical disabilities have led to an inability to cope with urgency due to sphincter disruption may be considered for surgery.

In patients in whom the sphincter ring is intact but the underlying cause is denervation, some improvement in anal function can be expected from the procedure of postanal repair, in which the puborectalis muscle is plicated, thus increasing the anorectal angle and the length of the anal canal [78]. However, long-term results are often unsatisfactory, even in patients without neurologic problems [79].

Antegrade Continence Enema

Malone first described an operation to bring the appendix onto the abdominal surface as a small, continent, catheterizable stoma, which enables antegrade irrigation and evacuation of the colon [80]. The aim is to wash out the entire contents of the colon while sitting on the toilet, thus facilitating both evacuation and continence (Figure 12.2). The majority of reports on the use of this procedure relate to children, particularly those with spina bifida, of whom two-thirds are reported continent afterward [81]. A cecostomy tube has also been inserted for the same purpose [82]. Few such procedures have been reported in adults, but the technique may be helpful and warrants consideration, particularly for patients who have a combined evacuation difficulty and incontinence and who have insufficient anal tone to retain suppositories or enemas.

Sacral Nerve Stimulation

Anterior root stimulators have been implanted to regulate bladder function since 1976 and have more recently been tried for bowel function, either to induce evacuation or to maintain continence. MacDonagh et al. reported on 12 SCI patients who underwent such a procedure; 6 achieved complete rectal evacuation without manual removal, and 11 reduced the time needed for their bowel routine [83].

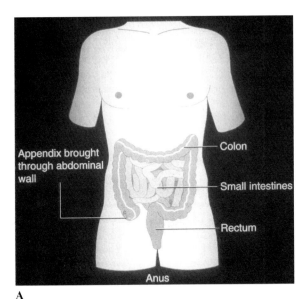

A

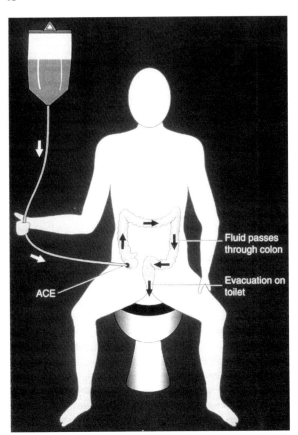

B

Figure 12.2   **(A)** Antegrade continence enema (ACE) procedure. **(B)** Irrigating the ACE.

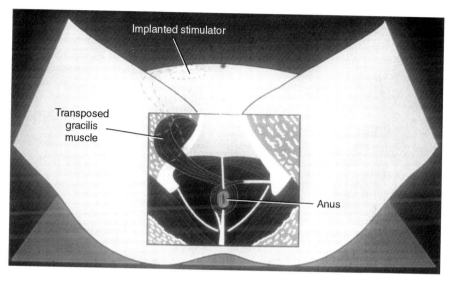

Figure 12.3 Dynamic gracioplasty operation.

Dynamic Gracioplasty

A damaged or absent anal sphincter may be reconstructed using the gracilis leg muscle (Figure 12.3). This procedure usually works best if combined with implantation of an electrical stimulator, which is programmed to gradually convert the muscle fibers from predominantly fast-twitch fibers to slow-twitch fibers capable of continuous activity as a sphincter [84]. Although the procedure is not without complications, in specialized centers more than 75% of carefully selected patients who undergo the operation are pleased with the results [85].

Artificial Bowel Sphincter

The artificial urinary sphincter (AMS Medical, Minnetonka, MN) has a proven track record. It has now been modified and enlarged for use as an artificial anal sphincter (Figure 12.4). This development is very recent, and the number of cases worldwide is under 100, so its efficacy and long-term results and problems cannot yet be predicted. Early results look promising, although sepsis can be a problem necessitating removal [86, 87]. In the future, replacing the function of both bladder and bowel sphincters in the same individual may become possible.

Stoma

Creation of a stoma may seem a drastic option, but it can make a dramatic contribution to quality of life in selected patients (our observations). If bowel function remains unpredictable and uncontrollable in the long term, the patient can

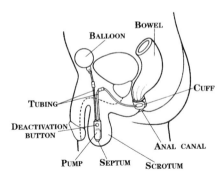

Figure 12.4　Artificial bowel sphincter.

find it very difficult to cope. As explained in the following section, Managing Intractable Fecal Incontinence, containment products are often unsatisfactory in enabling social continence for those with fecal incontinence, and chronic constipation can lead to chronic lethargy. People with severe physical disabilities often find that inability to cope independently with toileting severely restricts their scope for social, work, and personal activities. A person in a wheelchair has great difficulty managing an episode of fecal incontinence, or even defecation, alone in a public toilet. A stoma is much more accessible.

A colostomy or ileostomy, depending on the bowel dysfunction present, can at least give the individual containment and control over bowel management. For the person who cannot transfer independently and cannot manage to clean up after incontinence, a stoma may enable independence so that friends, lovers, and work colleagues are not asked to act as caregivers also. The amount of time spent on bowel care can also be reduced dramatically; one study found a reduction from 98.6 minutes per day to 17.8 minutes [88], and patients reported an improved quality of life.

The decision to follow this course must obviously be an individual one and should be taken only after the patient has been given full information on the benefits and possible disadvantages of the procedure.

GENERAL MEASURES AND ADVICE

Patients with bowel problems often need considerable psychological support, as well as teaching and information on the normal workings of the bowel (about which most people have little idea) and an understanding of what has gone wrong in their particular case. Knowledge about peristalsis, the gastrocolic reflex, and the normal coordination of internal and external anal sphincters can enable planning and development of coping strategies. For example, many patients with urgency mistakenly contract their abdominal muscles in a desperate attempt to "hang on." This maneuver exacerbates the tendency to urge incontinence if it is done when the internal sphincter is reflexively relaxed on rectal distension. Others who move only with great effort find that, if this exertion coincides with an urge to defecate and a relaxed internal sphincter, incontinence can be precipitated.

Sometimes, providing an explanation of the mechanism and advising the patient to contract the external sphincter until the urge diminishes and then go to the toilet can help. So can instruction on the best posture for effective defecation [89]. Patients with high spinal lesions also need to be aware of the dangers and signs of autonomic dysreflexia or impaction, because 10% of SCI fatalities may be ascribed to undiagnosed abdominal emergencies [90].

Exercise has been found to increase propagated colonic contractions [91], but it may not be feasible for people with mobility difficulties. Abdominal massage in the direction of colonic peristalsis is often recommended and may be an alternative [92], but its use has not been systematically evaluated in neurologic patients.

Many papers extol the virtues of a high-fiber diet to regulate stool consistency and promote peristalsis. However, the evidence for efficacy of this regimen is scant. Cameron et al. added 40 g of wheat bran per day to the diet of SCI patients for 3 weeks and found either no change or an increase in transit time, and no change in stool weight [93]. Use of fiber supplements can result in bloating and flatulence and requires an increased fluid intake, and some types of fiber, such as ispaghula husk, can be allergenic [31].

People with fecal incontinence that is not secondary to severe constipation may find it helpful to keep the stool firm and formed by moderating the fiber content of their diets. Immobile people are often found to have a colon loaded with soft stool, which is more likely to leak than firm stool [29, 94]. Fiber must be used with caution in immobile people, as it has been found to increase the risk of fecal incontinence compared to placebo [95], and a soft impaction can result [94].

Caffeine seems to act as a gut stimulant for some people, and clinically some patients with urgent defecation benefit from caffeine reduction [96].

PRACTICAL TOILETING AIDS FOR PEOPLE WITH DISABILITIES

The practicalities of bowel management can be difficult for anyone with a physical impairment to manage independently. Solutions often need to be imaginative, creative, and tailored to the individual's abilities, lifestyle, physical environment, and the availability of help at appropriate times. White provides a review [97]. Many patients do not feel safe on commode chairs, and transfer from wheelchairs is often difficult. In one study, 37% of 147 SCI patients did not feel safe on commode chairs and 42% felt that the brakes on commodes were ineffective; 35% had falls during transfers, and 23% had needed hospitalization for the resulting injuries [98].

Many adaptations can be made to a toilet to facilitate access and stability in use. Effective bowel evacuation is helped by sitting well supported, with feet slightly raised to enable appropriate use of abdominal effort if needed, and by leaning forward slightly [99]. Horizontal grab rails assist in pushing up; vertical ones can enable pulling up. A raised seat or foot blocks can adjust the height as needed. For lateral transfer from a wheelchair, both seats need to be at the same height.

For cases in which it proves impossible for a person to use the toilet, an alternative, such as a commode or chemical toilet, may be selected containing appropriate features for the individual's needs.

When needs are very particular, REMAP (a voluntary organization of engineers and occupational therapists) can design solutions. The Continence Foundation's *Directory of Continence Products* [100] and the Disabled Living Foundation's *Hamilton Index* [101] provide up-to-date sources of information on products available in the United Kingdom.

Toilet access is often a particular problem when the patient is outside the home, and this factor may be the limiting one in the choice of activities and travel.

People who are at risk of developing pressure sores or who take a long time to evacuate may benefit from the use of an inflatable or gel toilet seat. Some SCI patients take up to 2 hours to complete their bowel routine, and this can create considerable pressure risks [102].

Perineal cleaning can present a problem for someone with limited dexterity, and sometimes minor soiling is simply a result of ineffective wiping after defecation. Use of moist toilet tissue is often more efficient than dry wiping. Toilet tongs or a bottom wiper can extend the reach of someone with limited shoulder or hand flexibility or limited strength. When the toilet is next to the bath, a shower head may be usable. A portable bidet that can be filled with warm water and fits onto any toilet is also available.

MANAGING INTRACTABLE FECAL INCONTINENCE

There are no perfect answers to the problem of coping with leakage from the bowel. Finding anything that reliably disguises bowel leakage and smell is very difficult, and very few products have been designed specifically for fecal leakage.

Pads and Pants

Most of the disposable pads used for urinary incontinence can be used for fecal containment, but some people find them unnecessarily thick and bulky, and not exactly the right shape to contain anal leakage.

The simplest sort of pad for minor leakage is a panty liner, available in supermarkets and drugstores. If the pad is used inside the pants, the area between the buttocks often becomes sore, because stool is on the skin. Some people have found that folding a panty liner between the buttocks and holding it in place with a close-fitting G-string helps to contain soiling and prevents the skin from becoming sore.

More serious incontinence requires larger pads. These come in all shapes and sizes. In the United Kingdom, many are available free of charge from the National Health Service through the district nurse or local continence nurse if a severe or regular problem exists.

Anal Plug

An anal plug has been developed to help people with fecal incontinence. It is designed to be worn inside the rectum to plug the entrance to the anus from the

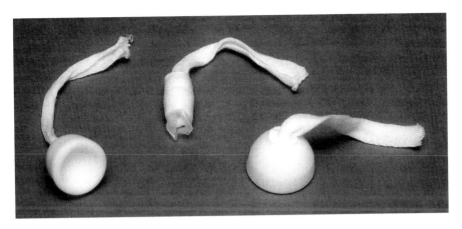

Figure 12.5   Anal plugs.

inside (Figure 12.5). The plug comes wrapped in a water-soluble film, so that it is easy to insert. This film dissolves once the plug is inside the rectum, and the plug opens into a cup shape and has a string for removal.

Some people find that an anal plug is uncomfortable or gives a constant feeling of needing to open the bowels. The plug must be removed before a bowel action, and so is not suitable for someone who needs to open the bowels very frequently. Christiansen and Roed-Peteresen found that 11 of 14 patients (71%) enrolled in a study of the plug withdrew because they experienced discomfort [103]. The problem of discomfort is obviously reduced when anorectal sensation is impaired. The anal plug is certainly worth trying, particularly by patients with passive soiling.

The anal plug is disposable. However, it cannot be flushed down the toilet but must be wrapped in paper or a disposal bag and put in the trash bin.

ODOR CONTROL

Meticulous personal hygiene and prompt disposal of soiled materials do not always ensure good odor control, and this aspect of incontinence can be the most embarrassing for patients. Proprietary deodorants may be helpful. Many other tips that can be tried have been reported [96].

CONCLUSIONS

Knowledge and techniques have not been generalized from one patient group to another. Some techniques have been tried only with SCI patients and others only with spina bifida patients. Cross-fertilization and sharing of techniques is required, and the many methods that have entered the folklore but have never been subjected to a trial need to be rigorously evaluated.

REFERENCES

1. Brittain KR, Peet SM, Castleden CM. Stroke and incontinence. Stroke 1998;29:524–528.
2. Hinds JP, Wald A. Colonic and anorectal dysfunction associated with multiple sclerosis. Am J Gastroenterol 1989;84:587–595.
3. Wald A. Systemic diseases causing disorders of defaecation and continence. Semin Gastrointest Dis 1995;6:194–202.
4. O'Regan S, Yazbeck S, Schick E. Constipation, bladder instability, urinary tract infection syndrome. Clin Nephrol 1985;23:153–154.
5. Banwell JG, Creasey GH, Aggarwal AM, Mortimer JT. Management of the neurogenic bowel in patients with spinal cord injury. Urol Clin North Am 1993;20:517–526.
6. Nelson R, Norton N, Cautley E, Furner S. Community-based prevalence of anal incontinence. JAMA 1995;274:559–561.
7. Drossman DA. Idiopathic Constipation: Definition, Epidemiology and Behavioural Aspects. In MA Kamm, JE Lennard-Jones (eds), Constipation. Petersfield, UK: Wrightson Biomedical Publishing, 1994;11–17.
8. Sultan AH, Kamm MA, Hudson CN, et al. Anal sphincter disruption during vaginal delivery. N Engl J Med 1993;329:1905–1911.
9. Swash M, Snooks SJ, Chalmers DHK. Parity as a factor in incontinence in multiple sclerosis. Arch Neurol 1987;44:504–508.
10. Nakayama H, Jorgensen HS, Pedersen PM, et al. Prevalence and risk factors of incontinence after stroke: The Copenhagen Stroke Study. Stroke 1997;28:58–62.
11. Brocklehurst JC, Andrews K, Richards B, Laycock PJ. Incidence and correlates of incontinence in stroke patients. J Am Geriatr Soc 1985;33:540–542.
12. Glickman S, Kamm MA. Bowel dysfunction in spinal-cord-injury patients. Lancet 1996;347:1651–1653.
13. Levi R, Hultling C, Nash MS, Seiger A. The Stockholm spinal cord injury study: 1. Medical problems in a regional SCI population. Paraplegia 1995;33:308–315.
14. Krogh K, Nielsen J, Djurhuus JC, et al. Colorectal function in patients with spinal cord lesions. Dis Colon Rectum 1997;40:1233–1239.
15. Edwards LL, Quigley EM, Pfeiffer RF. Gastrointestinal dysfunction in Parkinson's disease: frequency and pathophysiology. Neurology 1992;42:726–732.
16. Hinds JP, Eidelman BH, Wald A. Prevalence of bowel dysfunction in multiple sclerosis. Gastroenterology 1990;98:1538–1542.
17. Johanson JF, Lafferty J. Epidemiology of fecal incontinence: the silent affliction. Am J Gastroenterol 1996;91:33–36.
18. Kannisto M, Rintala R. Bowel function in adults who have sustained spinal cord injury in childhood. Paraplegia 1995;33:701–703.
19. Kirshblum SC, Gulati M, O'Connor KC, Voorman SJ. Bowel care practices in chronic spinal cord injury patients. Arch Phys Med Rehabil 1998;79:20–23.
20. Nicholls RJ, Glass R. Coloproctology. Berlin: Springer-Verlag, 1985.
21. Felt-Bersma RJ, Cuesta MA. Faecal incontinence 1994: which test and which treatment? [review]. Neth J Med 1994;44:182–188.
22. Pemberton JH. Anorectal and pelvic floor disorders: putting physiology into practice. J Gastroenterol Hepatol 1990;5(suppl 1):127–143.
23. Chia YW, Gill KP, Jameson JS, et al. Paradoxical puborectalis contraction is a feature of constipation in patients with multiple sclerosis. J Neurol Neurosurg Psychiatry 1996;60:31–35.
24. Edwards LL, Quigley EM, Harned RK, et al. Characterization of swallowing and defecation in Parkinson's disease. Am J Gastroenterol 1994;89:15–25.
25. Law PJ, Bartram CI. Anal endosonography: technique and normal anatomy. Gastrointest Radiol 1989;14:349–353.
26. Bartram CI. The Barium Enema and Evacuation Proctography. In MA Kamm, JE Lennard-Jones (eds), Constipation. Petersfield, UK: Wrightson Biomedical Publishing, 1994;137–143.
27. Lennard-Jones JE. Transit Studies. In MA Kamm, JE Lennard-Jones (eds), Constipation. Petersfield, UK: Wrightson Biomedical Publishing, 1994;125–136.
28. Stiens SA, Bergman SB, Goetz LL. Neurogenic bowel dysfunction after spinal cord injury: clinical evaluation and rehabilitation management. Arch Phys Med Rehabil 1997;78:S86–S104.
29. Barrett JA. Faecal Incontinence and Related Problems in the Older Adult. London: Edward Arnold, 1993.

30. Norton C. Nursing for Continence. Beaconsfield, UK: Beaconsfield Publishers, 1996.
31. Gattuso JM, Kamm MA. Review article: the management of constipation in adults. Aliment Pharmacol Ther 1993;7:487–500.
32. Siegers C-P, von Hertzberg-Lottin E, Otte M, Schneider B. Anthranoid laxative abuse—a risk for colorectal cancer? Gut 1993;34:1099–1101.
33. Passmore AP, Wilson-Davis K, Stoker C, Scott ME. Chronic constipation in long-stay elderly patients: a comparison of lactulose and a senna-fibre combination. BMJ 1993;307:769–771.
34. Culbert P, Gillett H, Ferguson A. Highly effective new oral therapy for faecal impaction. Br J Gen Pract 1998;48:1599–1600.
35. Harari D, Gurwitz JH, Minaker KL. Constipation in the elderly. J Am Geriatr Soc 1993;41:1130–1140.
36. Dunn KL, Galka ML. A comparison of the effectiveness of Therevac SB and bisacodyl suppositories in SCI patients' bowel programs. Rehabil Nurs 1994;19:334–338.
37. Glen House J, Stiens SA. Pharmacologically initiated defaecation for persons with spinal cord injury: effectiveness of three agents. Arch Phys Med Rehabil 1997;78:1062–1065.
38. Stiens SA. Reduction in bowel programme duration with polyethylene glycol based bisacodyl suppositories. Arch Phys Med Rehabil 1995;76:674–677.
39. Graham C, Kunkle C. Do rehabilitation patients continue prescribed bowel medications after discharge? Rehabil Nurs 1996;21:298–302.
40. Abd-El-Maeboud KH, El-Naggar T, El-Hawi EMM. Glycerine suppositories—common sense mode of insertion. Lancet 1991;338:798–800.
41. Binnie NR, Creasey GH, Edmond P, Smith AN. The action of Cisapride on the chronic constipation of paraplegia. Paraplegia 1988;26:151–158.
42. De Both PSM, de Groot GH, Slootman HR. Effects of Cisapride on constipation in paraplegic patients: a placebo-controlled randomised double-blind cross-over study. Eur J Gastroenterol Hepatol 1992;4:1013–1017.
43. Wysowski DK, Bacsanyi J. Cisapride and fatal arrhythmia. N Engl J Med 1996;335:290–291.
44. Edwards LL, Quigley EM, Harned RK, et al. Defecatory function in Parkinson's disease: response to apomorphine. Ann Neurol 1993;33:490–493.
45. Weber J. Constipation in spinal cord lesions, multiple sclerosis and diabetes mellitus. In MA Kamm, JE Lennard-Jones (eds), Constipation. Petersfield, UK: Wrightson Biomedical Publishing, 1994;273–277.
46. Bakke A, Myhr KM, Gronning M, Nyland H. Bladder, bowel and sexual dysfunction in patients with multiple sclerosis—a cohort study. Scand J Urol Nephrol 1996;17(suppl):61–66.
47. Kamm MA. Faecal incontinence: clinical review. BMJ 1998;316:528–532.
48. Read M, Read NW, Barber DC, Duthie HL. Effects of loperamide on anal sphincter function in patients complaining of chronic diarrhoea with faecal incontinence and urgency. Dig Dis Sci 1982;27:807–814.
49. Sun WM, Read NW, Verlinden M. Effects of loperamide oxide in gastrointestinal transit time and anorectal function in patients with chronic diarrhoea and faecal incontinence. Scand J Gastroenterol 1997;32:34–38.
50. Rattan S, Culver PJ. Influence of loperamide on the internal anal sphincter in the opossum. Gastroenterology 1987;93:121–128.
51. Kamm MA. Functional disorders of the colon and anorectum. Curr Opin Gastroenterol 1995;11:9–15.
52. Tobin GW, Brocklehurst JC. Faecal incontinence in residential homes for the elderly: prevalence, aetiology and management. Age Ageing 1986;15:41–46.
53. Whitehead WE, Parker LH, Masek BJ, et al. Biofeedback treatment of faecal incontinence in patients with myelomeningocele. Dev Med Child Neurol 1981;23:313–322.
54. Wald A. Biofeedback therapy for faecal incontinence. Ann Intern Med 1981;95:146–149.
55. Wald A. Biofeedback for neurogenic faecal incontinence: rectal sensation is a determinant of outcome. J Pediatr Gastroenterol Nutr 1983;2:302–306.
56. Killam PE, Jeffries JS, Varni JW. Urodynamic biofeedback treatment of urinary incontinence in children with myelomeningocele. Biofeedback Self-Regul 1985;10:161–171.
57. Loening-Baucke V, Desch L, Wolraich M. Biofeedback training for patients with myelomeningocele and faecal incontinence. Dev Med Child Neurol 1988;30:781–790.
58. Whitehead WE, Parker L, Bosmajian L, et al. Treatment of fecal incontinence in children with spina bifida: comparison of biofeedback and behavior modification. Arch Phys Med Rehabil 1986;67:218–224.

59. Tries J. Biofeedback in the treatment of incontinence. J Head Trauma Rehabil 1990;5:91–100.
60. Sun WM, MacDonagh R, Forster D, et al. Anorectal function in patients with complete spinal transection before and after sacral posterior rhizotomy. Gastroenterology 1995;108:990–998.
61. Jameson JS, Rogers J, Chia YW, et al. Pelvic floor function in multiple sclerosis. Gut 1994;35:388–390.
62. Caruana BJ, Wald A, Hinds JP, Eidelman BH. Anorectal sensory and motor function in neurogenic faecal incontinence. Gastroenterology 1991;100:465–470.
63. Gill KP, Chia YW, Henry MM, Shorvon PJ. Defecography in multiple sclerosis patients with severe constipation. Radiology 1994;191:553–556.
64. Loening-Baucke V. Persistence of chronic constipation in children after biofeedback treatment. Dig Dis Sci 1991;36:153–160.
65. Doughty D. A physiologic approach to bowel training. J Wound Ostomy Continence Nurs 1996;23: 46–56.
66. Younoszai MK. Stooling problems in patients with myelomeningocele. South Med J 1992;85: 718–724.
67. King JC, Currie DM, Wright E. Bowel training in spina bifida: importance of education, patient compliance, age, and anal reflexes. Arch Phys Med Rehabil 1994;75:243–247.
68. Munchiando JF, Kendall K. Comparison of the effectiveness of two bowel programs for CVA patients. Rehabil Nurs 1993;18:168–172.
69. Ouslander JG, Simmons S, Schnelle J, et al. Effects of prompted voiding on fecal continence among nursing home residents. J Am Geriatr Soc 1996;44:424–428.
70. Gattuso JM, Kamm MA, Myers C, et al. Effect of different infusion regimens on colonic motility and efficacy of colostomy irrigation. Br J Surg 1996;83:1459–1462.
71. Shandling B, Gilmour RF. The enema continence catheter in spina bifida: successful bowel management. J Pediatr Surg 1987;22:271–273.
72. Lipak GS, Revell GM. Management of bowel dysfunction in children with spinal cord disease or injury by means of the enema continence catheter. J Pediatr 1992;120:190–194.
73. De Kort LMO, Nesselaar CH, Van Gool JD, De Jong TPVM. The influence of colonic enema irrigation on urodynamic findings in patients with neurogenic bladder dysfunction. Br J Urol 1997;80: 731–733.
74. Scholler-Gyure M, Nesselaar CH, van Wieringen H, Van Gool JD. Treatment of defaecation disorders by colonic enemas in children with spina bifida. Eur J Pediatr Surg 1996;6:32–34.
75. Puet TA, Phen L, Hurst DL. Pulsed irrigation enhanced evacuation: new method for treating faecal impaction. Arch Phys Med Rehabil 1991;72:935–936.
76. Addison R. Digital Rectal Examination and Manual Removal of Faeces. London: Royal College of Nursing, 1995.
77. Engel AF, Kamm MA, Sultan AH, et al. Anterior anal sphincter repair in patients with obstetric trauma. Br J Surg 1994;81:131–134.
78. Parks AG. Anorectal incontinence. J Royal Soc Med 1975;68:21–30.
79. Jameson JS, Speakman CTM, Darzi A, et al. Audit of postanal repair in the treatment of faecal incontinence. Dis Colon Rectum 1994;37:369–372.
80. Malone PS, Ransley PG, Kiely EM. Preliminary report: the antegrade continence enema. Lancet 1990;336:1217–1218.
81. Koyle MA, Kaji DM, Duque M, et al. The Malone antegrade continence enema for neurogenic and structural fecal incontinence and constipation. J Urol 1995;154:759–761.
82. Shandling B, Chait PG, Richards HF. Percutaneous cecostomy: a new technique in the management of faecal incontinence. J Pediatr Surg 1996;31:1–5.
83. MacDonagh R, Sun WM, Smallwood R, Read NW. Control of defaecation in patients with spinal injuries by stimulation of sacral anterior nerve roots. BMJ 1990;300:1494–1497.
84. Baeten CGMI, Geerdes BP, Adang EMM, et al. Anal dynamic graciloplasty in the treatment of intractable faecal incontinence. N Engl J Med 1995;332:1600–1605.
85. Geerdes BP, Heineman E, Konsten J, et al. Dynamic graciloplasty: complications and management. Dis Colon Rectum 1996;39:912–917.
86. Lehur P-A, Michot F, Denis P, et al. Results of artificial sphincter in severe anal incontinence. Dis Colon Rectum 1996;39:1352–1355.
87. Wong WD, Jensen LL, Bartolo DCC, Rothenberger DA. Artificial anal sphincter. Dis Colon Rectum 1996;39:1345–1351.
88. Stone J, Wolfe VA, Nino-Murcia M, Perkash I. Colostomy as treatment for complications of spinal cord injury. Arch Phys Med Rehabil 1990;71:514–518.

89. Markwell S, Sapsford R. Physiotherapy management of obstructed defaecation. Austr J Physiother 1995;41:279–283.
90. Cosman B, Stone J, Perkash I. The gastrointestinal complications of chronic spinal cord injury. J Am Paraplegic Soc 1991;14:175–181.
91. Wald A. Constipation and fecal incontinence in the elderly [review]. Semin Gastrointest Dis 1994;5: 179–188.
92. Resende TL, Brocklehurst JC, O'Neill PA. A pilot study on the effect of exercise and abdominal massage on bowel habit in continuing care patients. Clin Rehabil 1993;7:204–209.
93. Cameron K, Nyulasi I, Collier G, Brown D. Assessment of the effect of increased dietary fibre intake on bowel function in patients with spinal cord injury. Spinal Cord 1996;34:277–283.
94. Barrett JA. Effects of wheat bran on stool size. BMJ 1988;296:1127–1128.
95. Ardron ME, Main ANH. Management of constipation. BMJ 1990;300:1400.
96. Norton C, Kamm MA. Bowel control—information and practical advice. Beaconsfield, UK: Beaconsfield Publishers, 1999.
97. White H. Aids to Continence for People with Physical Disabilities. In C Norton (ed), Nursing for Continence (2nd ed). Beaconsfield, UK: Beaconsfield Publishers, 1996;299–316.
98. Nelson A, Malassigne P, Amerson T, et al. Descriptive study of bowel care practices and equipment in spinal cord injury. Sci Nurs 1993;10:65–67.
99. Chiarelli P, Markwell S. Let's Get Things Moving: Overcoming Constipation. East Dereham, UK: Neen Healthcare, 1992.
100. The Continence Foundation. Continence Products Directory. London: The Continence Foundation, 1998.
101. Disabled Living Foundation. Hamilton Index. London: Disabled Living Foundation, 1995.
102. Nelson A, Malassigne P, Murry J. Comparison of seat pressures on three bowel care/shower chairs in spinal cord injury. Sci Nurs 1994;11:105–107.
103. Christiansen J, Roed-Petersen K. Clinical assessment of the anal continence plug. Dis Colon Rectum 1993;36:740–742.

13
Treatment of Sexual Dysfunction and Infertility in Patients with Neurologic Diseases

Dimitrios G. Hatzichristou

Since 1983, a revolution has occurred in the field of sexual dysfunction and infertility. The introduction of intracavernosal injections of vasoactive agents shed light not only on the diagnosis and treatment of male erectile dysfunction but also on the basic mechanisms of erection. As a result, new treatment options were added to the armamentarium of physicians, and more will be available for physicians and patients in the near future [1]. Regarding infertility, the newly developed methods for assisted reproduction have made it feasible for many men and women with neurologic diseases to become parents [2, 3]. Unfortunately, female sexual dysfunction has not yet received a great deal of attention, and current knowledge does not provide the necessary information for the development of specific treatment modalities [3–5]. This chapter focuses mainly on the treatment of erectile dysfunction and infertility problems, with only a brief overview of empirical treatments available for female sexual dysfunction.

TREATMENT OF MALE ERECTILE DYSFUNCTION

Since the mid-1980s, intracavernosal pharmacotherapy has been the cornerstone for the medical treatment of male erectile dysfunction. New treatment possibilities have been introduced, and current research has focused on pharmacologic treatment. Among these new possibilities, the oral and intraurethral treatment methods are the most significant developments. Vacuum devices and penile prosthesis implantation, however, remain as possible alternatives.

Intracavernosal Pharmacotherapy

Theoretically, intracavernosal injections work best in patients with neurogenic impotence who have a normal arterial inflow and a normal corporal veno-occlusion

209

mechanism [6]. Patients with diabetic vasculopathy or older patients with atherosclerosis are the least likely to respond to this form of therapy [7]. In general, intracavernosal pharmacotherapy may be offered to most patients with neurogenic impotence [6–10]. The pioneering work in this area involved the use of papaverine hydrochloride, a direct smooth muscle relaxant, alone or in combination with phentolamine mesylate, a nonselective α-blocking agent [1]. Several substances are available in the current market and are briefly described here.

Alprostadil

The most widely used agent for intracavernosal injection therapy is the synthetic prostanoid prostaglandin E_1 (PGE_1, alprostadil), a direct smooth muscle relaxant [11–13]. Two types of alprostadil powder (Viridal DUO, available in three packages—5, 10, and 20 μg alprostadil; and Caverject, available in two packages—10 and 20 μg alprostadil) have been approved worldwide for the treatment of erectile dysfunction. Information on PGE_1's efficacy, safety profile, and long-term patient compliance and satisfaction are available from international multicenter clinical trials [11–13]. The recommended dose of alprostadil has ranged from 5 to 60 μg in various studies [11]. Patients with neurogenic impotence respond well to alprostadil therapy, whereas men with coexisting vasculogenic impotence require the largest maintenance dosage [7, 9].

The response rate to PGE_1 is approximately 70% [11]. With both patients and their partners reporting sexual activity and satisfaction after more than 90% of injections, alprostadil represents the most efficacious monotherapy and also improves several aspects of patients' quality of life [14, 15]. The main side effect of alprostadil is penile pain, which occurs in approximately half of patients [11, 12]. Prolonged erection or priapism is a rare complication but occurs in 1% of patients [11, 12]. The incidence of both pain and prolonged erections decreases with time [13]. The only significant systemic side effect is hypotension; however, it is extremely rare in patients with neurogenic impotence because it is associated with the use of large doses [11]. The main late complication is the appearance of fibrotic nodules or scarring within the corpora, which has an incidence of approximately 10% [12, 13, 16]. In most cases, fibrotic alterations disappear after temporary discontinuation of the treatment, usually for 1 month. Due to its efficacy and safety profile, alprostadil has been suggested as the initial choice when intracavernosal pharmacotherapy is considered [17].

Moxisylyte Hydrochloride

Multicenter clinical trials have shown that the α-adrenergic blocking agent moxisylyte hydrochloride (Erecnos by Fournier), when administered intracavernously in doses of 10 mg, can produce rigid erections in patients with neurogenic impotence. The incidence of local or systemic adverse effects is very low [18, 19]. Although PGE_1 has proved to be significantly more efficacious than moxisylyte hydrochloride (71% versus 50%), PGE_1 has a higher incidence of prolonged erections and pain. Therefore, moxisylyte hydrochloride may be an alternative, specifically in those neurogenically impotent patients with supersensitivity to the injections and in those with significant pain after PGE_1 [19]. Moxisylyte hydrochloride has been given official approval for the treatment of erectile dysfunction in some countries.

Drug Combinations

The rationale for the use of drug combinations is their different mechanisms of action and the synergistic effect of the vasoactive agents. Historically, the first vasoactive agent combination included papaverine hydrochloride and phentolamine mesylate [1]. This combination is equally effective with PGE_1; it has a lower incidence of pain but a considerably higher risk of priapism and local fibrotic complications [20]. The combination of PGE_1 with phentolamine mesylate also seems to be effective [21]. In cases in which vasculopathy is also present, the combination of papaverine hydrochloride, phentolamine mesylate, and PGE_1 (tri-mix) may be used; it is the most effective intracavernosal treatment available today, and it features a low incidence of pain [22, 23]. The combination of vasoactive intestinal peptide with phentolamine mesylate (Invicorp by Senetec) also has been shown to induce an erection of sufficient rigidity for intercourse in most patients with psychogenic, neurogenic, or arteriogenic impotence [24]. Penile pain and transient facial flushing are rare side effects; no cases of priapism have been reported. The drug combination is available in some European markets in a user-friendly autoinjector system.

In general, intracavernosal pharmacotherapy is a highly effective treatment with tolerable side effects but limited patient compliance; consequently, there is a high dropout rate during the early phases of treatment [25–27]. The reasons for such high attrition include fear of the needle, artificiality of the therapy, and practical problems in solution preparation and administration [27]. To overcome these problems, several self-injection devices have been manufactured (Figures 13.1 and 13.2) [28]. Such devices may offer benefits to certain groups of patients with neurogenic impotence, reduced manual dexterity, or poor visual acuity. In such patients, drugs may also administered by their partners. For those in whom a transient hypotensive episode could have a deleterious effect (e.g., patients with

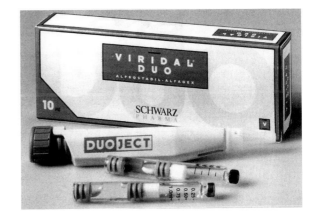

Figure 13.1 The DUO system uses an injector for user-friendly preparation and administration of intracavernosal alprostadil. The injector is for multiple uses. The kit includes everything the patient needs for an injection. (Photograph courtesy of Schwarz Pharma Inc., Milwaukee, WI.)

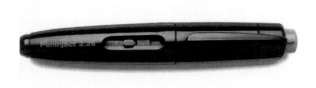

Figure 13.2   PenInject 2.25 is a patient-friendly, fully automatic device designed to facilitate self-injection. At a push of the button, the autoinjector advances the needle to a preset depth of penetration and delivers the drug properly. (Photograph courtesy of Pharmacia & Upjohn Company, Kalamazoo, MI.)

unstable cardiovascular disease and transient ischemic attacks), careful assessment should be made before offering this treatment. Patients with significant psychiatric disease or the potential for misuse or abuse of this therapy should not be supplied. Patients should also be told that this form of therapy does not affect orgasm or ejaculation and is used only for restoration of erectile capabilities. The usual therapeutic goal is to be able to create an erection that is rigid enough for vaginal penetration and lasts between 20 and 60 minutes [9].

The most common complication of intracavernosal pharmacotherapy is priapism, an erection that persists for 4–6 hours or longer. No general agreement exists on the time limits at which treatment of prolonged erection is necessary. Irreversible histologic changes of the erectile tissue have been identified after 12 hours of priapism [9]. An initial intracavernosal injection of 500 μg of phenylephrine hydrochloride is usually successful in producing detumescence and may be repeated once or twice at 20-minute intervals. Blood aspiration from the corpora through a 23-gauge butterfly needle and irrigation of the corpora with 20–100 ml of an α-adrenergic agonist solution (1 mg phenylephrine hydrochloride to 1,000 ml normal saline) has been an effective alternative in cases of persistent priapism [9].

The main problem with intracavernosal pharmacotherapy is the simplistic approach often taken to this treatment modality; clinicians usually prescribe the drugs without the appropriate dose titration, patient education, counseling, or regular follow-up. Practical clinical guidelines are briefly described here to offer the necessary information for the development of an efficient pharmacologic erection program [9].

Pharmacologic Erection Program

Patients who enter a pharmacologic erection program should be well-informed and should sign a detailed consent form that states the known complications of this treatment and discusses the possibility of long-term side effects.

The training program consists of three phases [9]: the dose-determination phase, the self-injection phase, and the at-home self-injection phase. After the introductory period, regular follow-up visits may take place.

- During the dose-determination phase, the patient is simply instructed to observe the techniques involved in self-injection. A basic principle for safe intracavernosal pharmacotherapy is to use low drug doses to reduce the potential complications and to minimize the therapy cost. Patients with neurogenic impotence should initially receive an extremely low dose (for example, 5 μg of PGE_1). Instructing the patient to compress the site of the injection firmly after each and every intracavernosal injection to reduce the possibility of a local hematoma is also important.

- The self-injection phase begins with instructions in sterile injection techniques and review of the results of the first injection in terms of erection duration and quality. If only tumescence or poor erection of short duration is achieved with the first dose, the second dose of vasoactive agents is increased (for example, 10 μg of PGE_1). In cases in which erectile response continues to be inadequate, further testing with increasing doses or a combination of vasoactive agents is indicated. In cases in which the erectile response to the initial injection was overly prolonged, the dose should be lowered. If full tumescence but not rigid erection occurs with the second injection, then a prescription of the appropriate medication is provided to the patient for home use on a trial basis. In cases in which a drug combination must be used, prefilled syringes with the appropriate dose of the mixture (usually up to 1 ml of the tri-mix solution: 300 mg papaverine hydrochloride, 10 mg phentolamine mesylate, and 100 μg PGE_1) should be used. The use of a 27- to 30-gauge needle minimizes discomfort.

- In the at-home self-injection phase, the patient is asked to describe his experience from the initial at-home use of injections. Technical points, the quality of the erection, patient satisfaction, and partner's acceptance are also discussed. If this initial trial is satisfactory, medication is prescribed. Patients are told not to inject more than once per day. Medication vials usually should be kept in a refrigerator at home, and syringes must be stored in a secure place.

Physician follow-up should occur once per month for the first 3 months and then at regular intervals, usually once every 3 months. Follow-up visits may include physical examination of the penis. If fibrotic nodules develop, discontinuation of the treatment for 1 month is recommended. A small group of patients may also need dose readjustment.

Intraurethral Pharmacotherapy

Several formulations of vasoactive agents, such as nitroglycerin plasters or paste, have been tested for topical application with limited efficacy, as drug absorption through the skin is poor. However, studies have indicated that the urethra is an effective route for vasoactive drug administration, with absorption through the venous drainage channels of the glans, corpus spongiosum, and corpora cavernosa [29]. A new formulation of alprostadil has been approved for intraurethral administration (MUSE). A medicated pellet is inserted into the urethra through a specially developed delivery system (Figure 13.3). When 125–1,000 μg of intraurethral alprostadil was used in a clinical setting, 65.9% of the patients tested achieved erectile responses sufficient for intercourse [30]. Of these men,

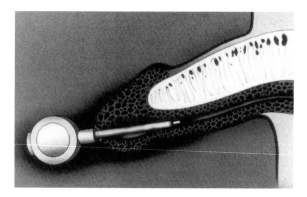

Figure 13.3   MUSE is administered by inserting the applicator stem into the urethra after urination. While keeping the penis stretched, the patient slowly inserts the applicator stem into the urethra up to the collar of the applicator. The pellet containing alprostadil is delivered by depressing the applicator button. A penile massage helps the medication become absorbed. (Diagram courtesy of Vivus Inc., Menlo Park, CA.)

961 were entered in a randomized, placebo-controlled trial at home, and 64.9% of those treated with alprostadil reported successful intercourse at least once, as compared with 18.6% of those who received placebo. In multicenter clinical trials that involved 2,595 patients and included a follow-up between 6 and 24 months, penile pain was reported by 29% of patients, urethral bleeding by 5%, dizziness by 2%, fibrosis by 1%, and priapism by fewer than 0.1% [31]. Such a profile shows that, compared to intracavernosal injection of alprostadil, intraurethral application of alprostadil has much higher dose requirements and a lower efficacy rate, but the incidence of adverse effects is lower. Overall, the efficacy and safety profile of intraurethral alprostadil makes the new formulation a suitable alternative for patients with neurogenic impotence. Long-term follow-up studies will determine patient compliance and attrition rates.

Oral Medication

Orally administered drugs have not been available in the past for the successful treatment of male erectile dysfunction [32]. However, numerous publications have shown that sildenafil citrate (Viagra), a highly selective and potent inhibitor of type 5 cGMP phosphodiesterase (PDE_5), enhances erection by the augmentation of nitric oxide–mediated relaxation pathways, through increased cGMP accumulation in the corpus cavernosum [33, 34]. Its pharmacokinetic and pharmacodynamic properties (rapid absorption with maximal plasma concentration occurring within 1 hour after oral administration and a mean terminal half-life of 3–5 hours) suggested that sildenafil citrate is the first effective oral agent for use on demand, before sexual activity [33, 34]. In a placebo-controlled pilot clinical study in 12 men, sildenafil citrate significantly improved the erectile response during video sexual stimulation [34].

In a 24-week, double-blind, placebo-controlled, fixed-dose study, 532 patients with organic, psychogenic, or mixed erectile dysfunction were treated with 25, 50, or 100 mg of oral sildenafil citrate (316 patients) or with placebo (216 patients) [35]. The dropout rate was 10% and 17% for the sildenafil citrate and placebo groups, respectively. Increasing doses of sildenafil citrate were associated with improved frequency of penetration and maintenance of erection after sexual penetration, independently of the cause of erectile dysfunction. At the end of the study, improved erections were reported by 56%, 77%, and 84% of the men taking 25-, 50-, and 100-mg doses of sildenafil citrate, respectively, as compared with 25% of those taking placebo [35].

In a 12-week flexible dose-escalation study, 329 men were treated with placebo or 50 mg of sildenafil citrate approximately 1 hour before sexual activity [35]. At each follow-up visit, the dose was adjusted (25–100 mg) according to the therapeutic response and the adverse effects. At the end of the study, the proportions of men taking 25, 50, and 100 mg of sildenafil citrate were 2%, 23%, and 74% respectively, whereas for the men taking placebo, the corresponding proportions were 0%, 5%, and 95%. The mean scores in the domains of erectile function, orgasmic function, intercourse satisfaction, and overall satisfaction, as assessed by the International Index of Erectile Function, were higher in the sildenafil citrate group than in the placebo group. Sexual desire was comparable, as expected in men seeking treatment for erectile dysfunction. In the last 4 weeks of treatment, 69% of all attempts at sexual intercourse were successful in the sildenafil citrate group, compared with 22% in the placebo group. At the end of the study, improved erections were reported by 74% of the men taking sildenafil citrate and 19% of those taking the placebo. The dropout rate in this study was 2% for the sildenafil citrate group and 5% for the placebo group.

Side effects noted in these two studies included transient headache (14–30%), flushing (13.27%), dyspepsia (3–16%), rhinitis (1–11%), and visual disturbances, such as changes in the perception of color or brightness (2–9%). The incidence of side effects was dose-related. Two hundred and twenty-five of the men who completed the dose-escalation study without reporting any serious side effect were enrolled in a 32-week open-label extension study. Ninety-two percent completed the study; 4 patients (2%) withdrew because of treatment-related adverse effects [35]. The safety and tolerability of sildenafil citrate have been studied in large-scale clinical trials involving more than 4,000 patients worldwide [36]. Sildenafil may have lethal effects in patients using nitrates, and co-commitant use of nitrates is an absolute contraindication. There have been 130 "spontaneous" reports to the U.S. Food and Drug Administration of death, and although no death directly related to the drug has been documented, a proper medical workup of any patient with erectile dysfunction is mandatory before prescribing the drug, as erectile dysfunction is a symptom often occurring in conjunction with more than one disorder.

Some studies in subpopulations have shown that sildenafil citrate is efficacious in patients with diabetes mellitus, spinal cord injury patients, patients with neurogenic impotence after radical prostatectomy, and patients with depression [37–40]. Data are emerging of its high efficacy in men with multiple sclerosis.

In a multicenter, randomized, double-blind, placebo-controlled study, 268 men (mean age, 57 years) with erectile dysfunction (mean duration, 5.6 years) and diabetes (mean duration, 12 years), were randomized to receive sildenafil or placebo for 12 weeks [37]. Improved erections were reported by 56% of the patients in the sildenafil group compared with 10% in the placebo group, while the proportion of men with at least one successful attempt at sexual intercourse was 61% for the sildenafil group versus 22% for the placebo group ($P < .001$). Adverse events related to treatment were reported for 16% of those taking sildenafil versus 1% of those receiving placebo.

The efficacy and safety of sildenafil in spinal cord injury patients was also evaluated in a double-blind, placebo-controlled study. All patients had spinal cord injury between T6–L5 level and reflexogenic erectile response to penile vibratory stimulation [38]. A total of 27 patients were randomized to receive 50 mg of sildenafil or placebo. After 28 days of treatment, 75% of patients on sildenafil and 7% on placebo reported that treatment had improved their erections ($P = .0043$). An analysis of diary data showed no difference between the groups with respect to the frequency of erections hard enough for sexual intercourse or that lasted as long as the subject would have liked. Furthermore, the mean proportion of attempts at sexual intercourse that were successful was 30% and 15% for the sildenafil and placebo groups, respectively ($P = .21$). However, 67% of patients on sildenafil and 15% on placebo indicated that they wished to continue treatment ($P = .018$), and a significant improvement in satisfaction with their sex life was reported by patients taking sildenafil ($P = .012$). No patients discontinued treatment because of adverse events.

The efficacy of sildenafil citrate was also evaluated in patients with erectile dysfunction after radical prostatectomy, without any preoperative neoadjuvant/adjuvant hormonal or adjuvant radiation therapy [39]. Twenty-eight health patients presenting with erectile dysfunction after radical prostatectomy reported what their erectile status was before surgery, before sildenafil therapy, and after using a minimum of four doses of sildenafil. Of the 15 patients who had bilateral nerve-sparing procedures, 80% had a positive response to sildenafil, with a mean duration of 6.92 minutes of vaginal intercourse and a spousal satisfaction rate of 80%. None of the three patients who had undergone a unilateral nerve-sparing procedure responded, nor did any of the 10 patients who had undergone a non–nerve-sparing procedure. The two most common side effects of the drug were transient headaches (39%) and abnormal color vision (11%), although no patients discontinued the medication because of side effects. Such findings support the role of nerve-sparing surgery, as the ability to restore potency with an oral medication after radical prostatectomy minimizes surgical morbidity of radical prostatectomy.

Finally, one study evaluated the efficacy of sildenafil citrate in nine men and five women with depression under treatment [40]. Twelve of the 14 patients were treated with a serotonin reuptake inhibitor and 2 with mirtazepine. Statistically significant improvements in all domains of sexual functioning, including libido, arousal, orgasm, sexual satisfaction, and (in men) erectile function, with a 69% rate of patients reporting themselves as much or very much improved, were reported. Only one patient reported side effects (hot flushes). Such findings indicate that sildenafil may be useful in both men and women with antidepressant-induced sexual dysfunction. Large-scale, placebo-controlled studies, however, are necessary before the final conclusions are reached; specifically, for the use of the drug in women with sexual dysfunction.

Based on the described efficacy and safety profile, sildenafil citrate may be considered as the first-line treatment for patients with erectile dysfunction; for patients with neurogenic impotence, sildenafil is efficacious when patients experience reflexogenic erections or at least penile tumescence during sexual stimulation.

Figure 13.4 ErecAid system for external vacuum therapy. The diameter of the cylinder should match the diameter of the engorged penis as closely as possible. After the cylinder is properly positioned, the operation of the pump removes air from the cylinder, creating a negative-pressure environment. At the end of the procedure, a restrictive ring is applied at the base of the penis to impede venous outflow from the penis. (Diagram courtesy of Osbon Medical Systems, Augusta, GA.)

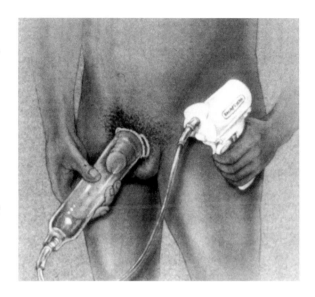

Vacuum Constrictor Devices

Vacuum therapy is an alternative long-term treatment option with an overall clinical success rate, in those prepared to use it, as high as 90%. The therapy has limited side effects (e.g., difficulty with ejaculation, numbness, penile pain, ecchymoses, hematomas, petechiae, and penile congestion from the tourniquet effect) and contraindications (e.g., bleeding disorders, significant intracavernosal scarring, and Peyronie's disease) [41].

A variety of external penile appliances are currently available. The majority have three common components: a vacuum chamber, a vacuum pump that creates negative pressure within the chamber, and a constrictor or tension band that is applied to the base of the penis after the erection is achieved (Figure 13.4). Vacuum-induced erection is significantly different from physiologically induced erection because rigidity occurs only distal to the constricting band, allowing for the penis to pivot at its base [41].

In a study in which vacuum induction of erection was compared to intracavernosal pharmacotherapy, both patients and their partners reported a superior quality of erection, greater ability to attain orgasm, and greater overall sexual satisfaction with intracavernosal injection therapy [42]. Patient acceptance of vacuum devices is therefore low, particularly among younger men. Vacuum constrictor devices, however, have shown significant success rates in patients with spinal cord injury. In one study, 41% of spinal cord–injured men with erectile dysfunction and 45% of their partners were satisfied with the use of vacuum constrictor devices, and 60% of men and 42% of women reported improvement of their sexual relationships [43]. Such findings indicate that nearly every patient showing erec-

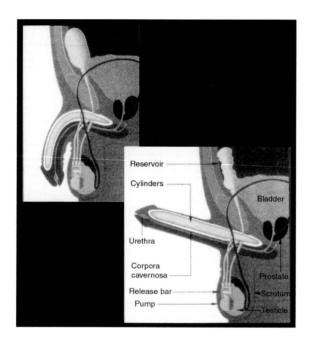

Figure 13.5   Diagram showing the Mentor Alpha-1 three-piece hydraulic device in position, with the penis in the flaccid and erect state. (Diagram courtesy of Mentor Corporation, Santa Barbara, CA.)

tile dysfunction of any degree or duration, as well as patients who have failed other therapeutic choices, are candidates for vacuum therapy. Moreover, vacuum constrictor devices may be useful in enhancing the final results of other treatment modalities (intracavernosal and intraurethral pharmacotherapy) [44].

Penile Prosthesis Implantation

Penile prosthesis implantation represents one of the oldest treatment options for erectile dysfunction. Significant improvements have been made in both the available devices and surgical practices [45].

Two types of penile prostheses are available: the semirigid and the multicomponent inflatable prosthesis (two-piece and three-piece inflatable devices). The semirigid devices are relatively low in cost, have a low postoperative complication rate, and are relatively easy to implant, but have an aesthetically less desirable detumescent phase. By contrast, the inflatable devices are based on hydraulic principles, so that the patient can inflate and deflate his device (Figure 13.5). Although more than 80% of patients report satisfaction after prosthetic surgery, implantation of a penile prosthesis has become the last treatment option to be considered for impotence because of the advent of intracavernosal pharmacotherapy [17, 45].

The modern multicomponent inflatable prostheses seem to be superior to self-contained devices in terms of mechanical reliability and patient satisfaction, with no differences in rate of complications [46]. In a multi-institutional, large-scale retrospective study with a mean follow-up of 22.2 months, no morbidity of any type was found in 90.8% of the 434 patients who underwent implantation of a three-piece prosthesis; 80% reported satisfaction with regard to intercourse ability and confidence, device rigidity and function, and fulfillment of expectations. Factors adversely affecting satisfaction included partner feelings of dissatisfaction and need for explantation or revision surgery [47].

Overall, penile prosthesis implantation, although not a first-line treatment option, is associated with a high long-term satisfaction rate. Multicomponent devices may be implanted in an outpatient setting [48], whereas the risk of infection is significantly greater when penile reconstruction is required [49]. Patients should be fully informed about possible surgical morbidity and the possibility of reoperation due to component failure, postoperative infection, or device erosion (10% of cases). The actual postoperative penile length is also a critical factor for paraplegic patients using condoms for bladder emptying; in patients with insufficient penile length, surgical procedures that allow patients to gain additional functional length for satisfactory intercourse are recommended [50, 51].

Psychological Counseling and Rehabilitation

Sexual and psychological counseling are important during the evaluation period, as well as in selection of the appropriate treatment. Restoration of erectile function should not be the only treatment objective; it is also essential to address personal and emotional factors in the patient, conflicts in his relationship with his partner, and sexual problems in his partner, all of which may be instrumental in causing or maintaining the negative feelings for sexual activity [52, 53]. Furthermore, autonomic dysreflexia, bladder emptying, coital positioning, and alternate sexual activities are important topics that should be discussed and require skilled professional guidance [5].

In conclusion, neurogenic erectile dysfunction requires minimal investigation because no reliable diagnostic test is available today [54], the underlying pathophysiology is usually known, and the dysfunction may be easily treated in most cases with low doses of alprostadil administered either intraurethrally or intracavernosally. In cases of supersensitivity to alprostadil (not uncommon in younger men), the use of agents such as moxisylyte hydrochloride is recommended to avoid prolonged erections. Patients with upper motor neuron lesions and preserved reflexogenic erections may also respond to oral medications such as sildenafil citrate. Therefore, factors including the level of the injury, upper extremity function, partner availability, and motivation may determine the appropriate treatment for each patient.

MALE INFERTILITY

Infertility may be a significant problem for male patients with neurologic diseases [55–57]. In rare instances (1.1% of cases), male infertility may lead to identification of significant neurologic pathology, mainly brain and spinal cord tumors [58]. Ejaculatory failure and impaired sperm quality are the major causes of infertility in these patients.

Although anejaculation is relatively uncommon in the general population, more than 12,000 new cases are reported annually in the United States in patients with neurologic diseases [59]. Anejaculation may result from spinal cord injury, retroperitoneal lymph node dissection, diabetes mellitus, transverse myelitis, multiple sclerosis, or other neurologic disorders. Ejaculations are reported to occur in only 5% of men with spinal cord injury who have complete upper motor lesions, in 18% of those who have complete lower motor lesions, and in up to 70% of men with incomplete lesions [57]. According to the available data, at least 30% of these patients are or will be married, and many will seek help to remedy their infertile states [59].

Several methods have been used to induce ejaculation, including intrathecal injection of neostigmine, subcutaneous injection of physostigmine salicylate, direct aspiration of sperm from the vas deferens, vibratory stimulation, electroejaculation, and direct stimulation of the hypogastric nerve [5, 60, 61]. The most commonly used methods today are vibratory stimulation and electroejaculation.

Vibratory stimulation, applied to the frenular undersurface of the glans penis, was first introduced to induce normal antegrade ejaculation [5]. Vibratory tactile stimuli from the penile area result in a rapid sequence of sympathetic outflow from T10–L3 and induction of emission followed by the precisely timed efferent outflow from S2–S4 to stimulate contractions of the perineal musculature and create antegrade semen flow. The method is applicable only in patients with an intact and functional lower thoracolumbosacral cord segment [60, 61]. In ideal circumstances, the patient and his spouse are able to use vibratory stimulation coupled with self-insemination of the resultant semen to achieve pregnancy. Successful induction of ejaculation with the technique is possible in 60–75% of patients with injury above T12 [61–63]. Particular care needs to be given to monitoring men undergoing these procedures who are prone to autonomic dysreflexia. Supportive measures and administration of sublingual nifedipine (10 mg) to counteract hypertension may be necessary.

Rectal probe electroejaculation has also been used widely to induce ejaculation in patients with spinal cord injuries [59–61]. The basic concept involves direct electrical stimulation with resultant contraction and discharge of the structures responsible for elaboration of the constituents of semen (seminal vesicles, vasal ampullae, and prostate) and deposition of the seminal fluid into the posterior urethra [5]. As no true antegrade ejaculation occurs, the bulbous and pendulous portions of the urethra need to be milked and the posterior urethra and bladder catheterized after stimulation to recover all the seminal fluid delivered into the posterior urethra. The collected semen is washed and the motile sperm fraction isolated and prepared for intrauterine insemination or other advanced reproductive techniques such as in vitro fertilization. Rectal probe electroejaculation elicits seminal emissions in 60–90% of spinal cord patients [59–61, 64]. Impregnations using electroejaculates have been documented since 1975 in case reports and small series; the pregnancy rate is as high as 40% [64]. In general, however, electroejaculates exhibit high sperm counts but low motility and poor sperm function [65–70].

Little is known about the effects of neurologic diseases on male reproductive function. Factors contributing to poor semen quality include long anejaculatory status, stasis of prostatic fluid, testicular hyperthermia, recurrent urinary tract infections, abnormal testicular histology, possible changes in the hypothalamic-pituitary-testicular axis, possible sperm antibodies, long-term use of various medications, and type of bladder management [65–72].

When evaluated by strict criteria, electroejaculates exhibit specific defects in sperm morphologic profile. A pervasive pattern of teratozoospermia exists that may reflect underlying defects contributing to decreased fertility in men with spinal cord injury [65]. Numerous studies have also documented asthenospermia (low sperm motility) despite the presence of normal sperm concentrations in most men undergoing these procedures. Low sperm motility may also be related to high levels of reactive oxygen species in their sperm, as human spermatozoa exhibit a capacity to generate reactive oxygen species and initiate peroxidation of the unsaturated fatty acids in the sperm plasma membrane, which plays a key role in the etiology of male infertility [69, 70]. Autoimmunity should also be considered as among the important causes underlying seminal dysfunction, because a high incidence of antisperm antibodies has been observed in men with neurogenic infertility [68].

The matter of potential functional obstruction of the epididymis as an underlying cause for infertility in such patients has also been discussed. Preliminary data support the hypothesis that functional obstruction of the epididymis in patients with neurogenic infertility exerts a spermatic insult similar to that of typical postinflammatory anatomic obstruction. In such cases, the putative cause for neurogenic infertility is more likely to be at the post-testicular level [67]. Such data clearly show the multifactorial etiology of reproductive dysfunction in such patients.

The role of genitourinary tract infections is also clear. In one study of patients with spinal cord injury, a high incidence of infected urine and infected semen (41% and 56%, respectively) was found in comparison to patients with normal bladder function (0% and 11%) [71]. Urinary infection was associated with slightly lower sperm quality and lower pregnancy rates (10% versus 30% in the presence of sterile urine). Semen infection, on the other hand, had no effect on sperm counts or pregnancy rates. Antibiotics did not reduce the incidence of urine or semen infection but did improve sperm counts slightly. Continuous prophylaxis was associated with bacterial resistance to many oral antibiotics and had no advantage over a short course of antibiotics before procedures for assisted reproduction.

Bladder management also seems to be critical. Individuals managing their neuropathic bladder by catheter (intermittent self-catheterization, indwelling urethral or suprapubic catheter) have significantly enhanced semen quality compared to those voiding by reflex or straining [72]. Differences have also been noted within the group of patients using catheters; those practicing intermittent self-catheterization show a higher percentage of motile sperm present. In cases in which intermittent self-catheterization was used to empty the neurogenic bladder, slightly better sperm quality was reported, and the total infertility rate was less than in cases in which patients used an alternative bladder management strategy. Better pregnancy rates were also obtained (44% for those using intermittent self-catheterization versus 7% for those using other methods) [72].

The evolution in the 1990s of assisted reproductive techniques, such as zygote intrafallopian transfer, gamete intrafallopian transfer, in vitro fertilization, and intracytoplasmic sperm injection, has provided men with spinal cord injury a means of producing their own biological offspring [2, 73–75]. Before the introduction of intracytoplasmic sperm injection, the fertilization rate was approximately 30%; intracytoplasmic sperm injection increased the fertilization rate to

88%. No association was found between the pregnancy rate and the sperm count, level of injury, or fertilization technique [2]. Although fertilization rates are encouraging, pregnancy rates cannot be accurately estimated because of the lack of reports of large series in the literature.

FEMALE SEXUAL DYSFUNCTION AND INFERTILITY

Sexual dysfunction in women includes decrease in libido, arousal, lubrication, and vaginal and clitoral sensation, as well as dyspareunia and anorgasmia [3–5]. Data are lacking with respect to female sexual dysfunction, especially dysfunction that is neurogenic in origin. The few available studies, most of them epidemiologic, relate to the sexual function of women with diabetes, multiple sclerosis, and spinal cord injury [3, 5, 76–78]. Unfortunately, treatment options remain empirical—for example, management of decreased vaginal lubrication with use of water-soluble lubricants [76].

The only currently available information on the pathophysiology of female sexual dysfunction comes from studies of women with spinal cord injuries [3]. Patients with complete upper motor neuron lesions lack autonomic input to the pelvic area and therefore suffer from a lack of vaginal lubrication during sexual excitation. However, manifestations of this excitement stage mediated by fibers above the lesion still occur. These include a change in respiration, pulse, and blood pressure, breast changes, and a "sexual flush." Sensation around the breast area is still intact, making this area valuable as an erogenous zone. Incomplete upper motor neuron lesions allow more of the normal sexual cycle components to occur. With lower motor neuron lesions, psychogenic vaginal lubrication may be evident. Factors such as the inability to move in response to a partner, inability to initiate physical activity, and inability to experience orgasm are often psychologically discouraging [4, 76, 77]. A lack of bladder control, use of incontinence pads or an indwelling catheter, concerns about flaccid musculature, and a lack of abdominal control can seriously detract from the woman's feelings of adequacy [76, 77].

The preinjury menstrual pattern is regained in nearly all patients of childbearing age within 6 months of spinal cord injury, and approximately 50% do not miss a single period [3, 76]. Irrespective of the injury level, these women clearly have the potential to become pregnant. Level or completeness of injury does not seem to play a role in the postinjury fertility status [3, 78]. Autonomic dysreflexia may complicate labor if the injury is above the T6 level. Premature labor is common but may be successfully treated with bedrest or terbutaline sulfate. Most of these women are able to deliver vaginally [3, 5]. Ovulation induction in combination with intrauterine insemination may be necessary in cases of severe male-factor infertility.

CONCLUSIONS

Patients with neurologic diseases generally have a predictable erectile, ejaculatory, and orgasmic dysfunctional pattern. Currently, several treatment options are available, making a return of some sexual function and fertility feasible in many patients. Several treatment options are available or will be available in the near future to help men with neurogenic erectile dysfunction.

The major obstacle to success in treatment of fertility is the poor quality of the sperm samples obtained. Assisted reproductive technology has been used in conjunction with electroejaculation with promising results. Achieving conception requires a team approach involving a neurologist, urologist/andrologist, gynecologist/reproductive endocrinologist, and sperm-processing laboratory.

Female sexual function may be assisted exclusively by empirical therapies. The research focus should be on the physiology and pathophysiology in women to allow an etiologic approach to female sexual dysfunction in the future.

REFERENCES

1. Hatzichristou DG. Current treatment and future perspectives for erectile dysfunction. Int J Impotence Res 1998;10(suppl):3–13.
2. Hultling C, Rosenlund B, Levi R, et al. Assisted ejaculation and in-vitro fertilization in the treatment of infertile spinal cord–injured men: the role of intracytoplasmic sperm injection. Hum Reprod 1997;12:499–502.
3. Nygaard I, Bartscht KD, Cole S. Sexuality and reproduction in spinal cord injured women. Obstet Gynecol Surv 1990;45:727–732.
4. Heiman JR. Female Sexual Dysfunction: Definitions, History Taking Techniques, and Work-Up. In C Singer, WJ Weiner (eds), Sexual Dysfunction. A Neuro-Medical Approach. New York: Futura Publishing, 1994;61–76.
5. Hatzichristou DG, Seftel AD, Saenz de Tejada I. Sexual Dysfunction in Diabetes and Other Autonomic Neuropathies. In C Singer, WJ Weiner (eds), Sexual Dysfunction. A Neuro-Medical Approach. New York: Futura Publishing, 1994;167–198.
6. Beck RO, Fowler CJ. Neurogenic impotence. Cur Opin Urol 1994;4:333–335.
7. Basile G, Goldstein I. Medical treatment of neurogenic impotence. Sex Dis 1994;12:81–94.
8. Betts CD, Jones SJ, Fowler CG, Fowler CJ. Erectile dysfunction in multiple sclerosis: associated neurological and neurophysiological deficits and treatment of the condition. Brain 1994;117:1303–1310.
9. Hatzichristou DG, Payton T, Goldstein I. Intracavernous Injection Therapy for Impotence. In HM Nagler, ED Whitehead (eds), Management of Impotence and Infertility. Philadelphia: Lippincott, 1994;12–26.
10. Seftel AD, Oates RD, Krane RJ. Disturbed sexual function in patients with spinal cord disease. Neurol Clin 1991;9:757–778.
11. Porst H. The rationale for prostaglandin E_1 in erectile failure: a survey of worldwide experience. J Urol 1996;155:802–815.
12. Hatzichristou DG, Bertero E, Goldstein I. Decision making in the evaluation of impotence: the patient profile–oriented algorithm. Sex Dis 1994;12:81–95.
13. Bennet CJ, Seager SW, Vasher EA, McGuire EJ. Sexual dysfunction and electroejaculation in men with spinal cord injury: review. J Urol 1988;139:453–457.
14. Frith JA, McLeod JG. Pregnancy and multiple sclerosis. J Neurol Neurosurg Psychiatry 1988;51: 495–498.
15. Linsenmeyer TA, Perkash I. Infertility in men with spinal cord injury. Arch Phys Med Rehabil 1991;72:747–754.
16. Honig SC, Lipshultz LI, Jarow J. Significant medical pathology uncovered by a comprehensive male infertility evaluation. Fertil Steril 1994;62:1028–1034.
17. Witt MA, Grantmyre JE. Ejaculatory failure. World J Urol 1993;11:89–95.
18. Lipschultz LI, McConnell J, Benson GS. Current concepts of the mechanisms of ejaculation: normal and abnormal states. J Reprod Med 1981;26:499–504.
19. Linsenmeyer TA. Male infertility following spinal cord injury. J Am Paraplegia Soc 1991;14:116–121.
20. Dahlberg A, Ruutu M, Hovatta O. Pregnancy results from a vibrator application, electroejaculation, and a vas aspiration program in spinal-cord injured men. Hum Reprod 1995;10:2305–2307.
21. Sonksen J, Biering-Sorensen F, Kristensen JK. Ejaculation induced by penile vibratory stimulation in men with spinal cord injuries: the importance of the vibratory amplitude. Paraplegia 1994;32:651–660.

22. Chung PH, Yeko TR, Mayer JC, et al. Assisted fertility using electroejaculation in men with spinal cord injury—a review of literature. Fertil Steril 1995;64:1–9.
23. Sedor JF, Hirsch IH. Evaluation of sperm morphology of electroejaculates of spinal cord–injured men by strict criteria. Fertil Steril 1995;63:1125–1127.
24. Brackett NL, Santa-Cruz C, Lynne CM. Sperm from spinal cord injured men lose motility faster than sperm from normal men: the effect is exacerbated at body compared to room temperature. J Urol 1997;157:2150–2153.
25. Hirsch IH, Sedor J, Kulp D, et al. Objective assessment of spermatogenesis in men with functional and anatomic obstruction of the genital tract. Int J Androl 1994;17:29–34.
26. Hirsch IH, Sedor J, Callahan HJ, Staas WE. Antisperm antibodies in seminal plasma of spinal cord–injured men. Urology 1992;39:243–247.
27. Sharma RK, Agarwal A. Role of reactive oxygen species in male infertility. Urology 1996;48: 835–850.
28. De Lamirande E, Leduc BE, Iwasaki A, et al. Increased reactive oxygen species formation in semen of patients with spinal cord injury. Fertil Steril 1995;63:637–642.
29. Ohl DA, Denil J, Fitzgerald-Shelton K, et al. Fertility of spinal cord injured males: effect of genitourinary infection and bladder management on results of electroejaculation. J Am Paraplegia Soc 1992;15:53–59.
30. Rutkowski SB, Middleton JW, Truman G, et al. The influence of bladder management on fertility in spinal cord injured males. Paraplegia 1995;33:263–266.
31. Brackett NL, Abae M, Padron OF, Lynne CM. Treatment by assisted conception of severe male factor infertility due to spinal cord injury or other neurologic impairment. J Assist Reprod Genet 1995;12: 210–216.
32. Watkins W, Lim T, Bourne H, et al. Testicular aspiration of sperm for intracytoplasmic sperm injection: an alternative treatment to electro-emission: case report. Spinal Cord 1996;34:696–698.
33. Yamamoto M, Momose H, Yamada K. Fathering of a child with the assistance of electroejaculation in conjunction with intracytoplasmic sperm injection: case report. Spinal Cord 1997;35:179–180.
34. Lundberg PO, Hutler B. Female sexual dysfunction in multiple sclerosis: a review. Sex Dis 1996;14: 65–72.
35. Lemon MA. Sexual counseling and spinal cord injury. Sex Dis 1993;11:73–98.
36. Frith JA, McLeod JG. Pregnancy and multiple sclerosis. J Neurol Neurosurg Psychiatry 1988;51: 495–498.
37. Rendell MS, Rajfer J, Wicker PA, Smith MD. Sildenafil for treatment of erectile dysfunction in men with diabetes: a randomized controlled trial. Sildenafil Diabetes Study Group. JAMA 1999;281: 421–426.
38. Maytom MC, Derry FA, Dinsmore WW, et al. A two-part pilot study of sildenafil (VIAGRA) in men with erectile dysfunction caused by spinal cord injury. Spinal Cord 1999;37:110–116.
39. Zippe CD, Kedia AW, Kedia K, et al. Treatment of erectile dysfunction after radical prostatectomy with sildenafil citrate (Viagra). Urology 1998;52:963–966.
40. Fava M, Rankin MA, Alpert JE, et al. An open trial of oral sildenafil antidepressant-induced sexual dysfunction. Psychother Psychosom 1998;67:328–331.
41. Lewis RW, Witherington R. External vacuum therapy for erectile dysfunction: use and results. World J Urol 1997;15:78–82.
42. Soderdahl DW, Thrasher JB, Hansberry KL. Intracavernosal drug-induced erection therapy versus external vacuum devices in the treatment of erectile dysfunction. Br J Urol 1997;79:952–957.
43. Denil J, Ohl DA, Smythe C. Vacuum erection device in spinal cord injured men: patient and partner satisfaction. Arch Phys Med Rehabil 1996;77:750–753.
44. John H, Lehmann K, Hauri D. Intraurethral prostaglandin improves quality of vacuum erection therapy. Eur Urol 1996;29:224–226.
45. Lewis R. Long-term results of penile prosthetic implants. Urol Clin North Am 1995;22:847–856.
46. Wilson SK, Cleves M, Delk JR 2nd. Long-term results with Hydroflex and Dynaflex penile prostheses: device survival comparison to multicomponent inflatables. J Urol 1996;155:1621–1623.
47. Goldstein I, Newman L, Baum N, et al. Safety and efficacy outcome of Mentor alpha-1 inflatable penile prosthesis implantation for impotence treatment. J Urol 1997;157:833–839.
48. Garber BB. Outpatient inflatable penile prosthesis insertion. Urology 1997;49:600–603.
49. Jarow JP. Risk factors for penile prosthetic infection. J Urol 1996;156:402–404.
50. Knoll LD, Fisher J, Benson RC, et al. Treatment of penile fibrosis with prosthetic implantation and flap advancement with tissue debulking. J Urol 1996;156:394–397.
51. Gross AJ, Sauerwein DH, Kutzenberger J, et al. Penile prostheses in paraplegic men. Br J Urol 1996;78:262–264.

52. Riley AJ, Athanasiadis L. Impotence and its non-surgical management. Br J Clin Pract 1997;51: 99–103.

53. Hartmann U. Psychological subtypes of erectile dysfunction: results of statistical analyses and clinical practice. World J Urol 1997;15:56–64.

54. Hatzichristou DG, Bertero E, Goldstein I. Decision making in the evaluation of impotence: the patient profile-oriented algorithm. Sex Dis 1994;12:81–95.

55. Bennet CJ, Seager SW, Vasher EA, McGuire EJ. Sexual dysfunction and electroejaculation in men with spinal cord injury: review. J Urol 1988;139:453–457.

56. Frith JA, McLeod JG. Pregnancy and multiple sclerosis. J Neurol Neurosurg Psychiatry 1988;51: 495–498.

57. Linsenmeyer TA, Perkash I. Infertility in men with spinal cord injury. Arch Phys Med Rehabil 1991; 72:747–754.

58. Honig SC, Lipshultz LI, Jarow J. Significant medical pathology uncovered by a comprehensive male infertility evaluation. Fertil Steril 1994;62:1028–1034.

59. Witt MA, Grantmyre JE. Ejaculatory failure. World J Urol 1993;11:89–95.

60. Lipschultz LI, McConnell J, Benson GS. Current concepts of the mechanisms of ejaculation: normal and abnormal states. J Reprod Med 1981;26:499–504.

61. Linsenmeyer TA. Male infertility following spinal cord injury. J Am Paraplegia Soc 1991;14: 116–191.

62. Dahlberg A, Ruutu M, Hovatta O. Pregnancy results from a vibrator application, electroejaculation, and a vas aspiration program in spinal-cord injured men. Hum Reprod 1995;10:2305–2307.

63. Sonksen J, Biering-Sorensen F, Kristensen JK. Ejaculation induced by penile vibratory stimulation in men with spinal cord injuries. The importance of the vibratory amplitude. Paraplegia 1994;32:651–660.

64. Chung PH, Yeko TR, Mayer JC, et al. Assisted fertility using electroejaculation in men with spinal cord injury—a review of literature. Fertil Steril 1995;64:1–9.

65. Sedor JF, Hirsch IH. Evaluation of sperm morphology of electroejaculates of spinal cord injured men by strict criteria. Fertil Steril 1995;63:1125–1127.

66. Brackett NL, Santa-Cruz C, Lynne CM. Sperm from spinal cord injured men lose motility faster than sperm from normal men: the effect is exacerbated at body compared to room temperature. J Urol 1997;157:2150–2153.

67. Hirsch IH, Sedor J, Kulp D, et al. Objective assessment of spermatogenesis in men with functional and anatomic obstruction of the genital tract. Int J Androl 1994;17:29–34.

68. Hirsch IH, Sedor J, Callahan HJ, Staas WE. Antisperm antibodies in seminal plasma of spinal cord-injured men. Urology 1992;39:243–247.

69. Sharma RK, Agarwal A. Role of reactive oxygen species in male infertility. Urology 1996;48: 835–850.

70. de Lamirande E, Leduc BE, Iwasaki A, et al. Increased reactive oxygen species formation in semen of patients with spinal cord injury. Fertil Steril 1995;63:637–642.

71. Ohl DA, Denil J, Fitzgerald-Shelton K, et al. Fertility of spinal cord injured males: effect of genitourinary infection and bladder management on results of electroejaculation. J Am Paraplegia Soc 1992;15:53–59.

72. Rutkowski SB, Middleton JW, Truman G, et al. The influence of bladder management on fertility in spinal cord injured males. Paraplegia 1995;33:263–266.

73. Brackett NL, Abae M, Padron OF, Lynne CM. Treatment by assisted conception of severe male factor infertility due to spinal cord injury or other neurologic impairment. J Assist Reprod Genet 1995;12:210–216.

74. Watkins W, Lim T, Bourne H, et al. Testicular aspiration of sperm for intracytoplasmic sperm injection: an alternative treatment to electro-emission: case report. Spinal Cord 1996;34:696–698.

75. Yamamoto M, Momose H, Yamada K. Fathering of a child with the assistance of electroejaculation in conjunction with intracytoplasmic sperm injection: case report. Spinal Cord 1997;35:179–180.

76. Lundberg PO, Hutler B. Female sexual dysfunction in multiple sclerosis: a review. Sex Dis 1996;14:65–72.

77. Lemon MA. Sexual counseling and spinal cord injury. Sex Dis 1993;11:73–98.

78. Frith JA, McLeod JG. Pregnancy and multiple sclerosis. J Neurol Neurosurg Psychiatry 1988;51: 495–498.

IV
SPECIFIC CONDITIONS

14

Cerebral Control of Bladder, Bowel, and Sexual Function and Effects of Brain Disease

Ryuji Sakakibara and Clare J. Fowler

Although the nerve supplies to the pelvic organs converge at the same sacral roots and the organs have some commonality of peripheral innervation, no single cortical region exists that, if involved in disease, causes bladder, bowel, and sexual dysfunction. That little overlap of cortical representation exists for pelvic functions is not surprising—control of each organ is critically dependent on cortical influences for inhibition and initiation of its activity in a way that determines and is determined by human social interaction.

Only in the last few years have the techniques for investigating cortical control been applied to examine bladder function, and the initial results using functional imaging techniques to explore cortical control of the bladder have produced interesting results. As yet, little has been done to investigate cortical control of sexual function, and work to look at the mechanism of perception of bowel sensation is only preliminary. Future studies are awaited with interest and will contribute greatly to our understanding of various pelvic dysfunctions in patients with brain disease—an area of neurology that remains largely unexplored.

CORTICAL CONTROL OF BLADDER FUNCTION

Observations with Functional Brain-Imaging Techniques

The first full report on functional imaging of cortical control of the bladder was published in Japan and described the use of single photon emission computed tomography (SPECT) during micturition [1]. Ten healthy male volunteers were instructed to void while standing and, immediately after the initiation of urine flow, were injected with a radioactive blood flow tracer. Scanning was performed 15 minutes later and continued for 30 minutes. Preliminary studies revealed no difference in cerebral blood flow between lying and standing in healthy subjects, so a second radioactive tracer injection was given, and the subjects were scanned

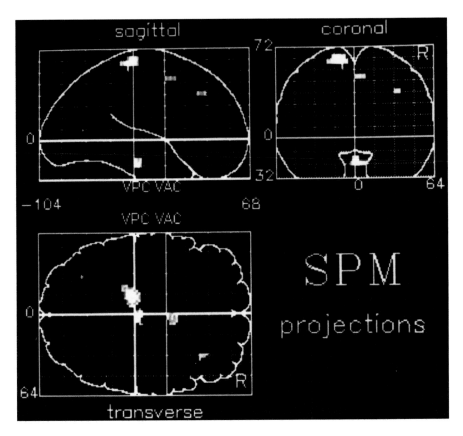

Figure 14.1 Three-dimensional projection of the areas activated during micturition using single photon emission computed tomographic scanning. (R = right; SPM= Statistical Parametric Mapping [Hammersmith Hospital, London]; VAC, VPC = vertical lines through anterior and posterior commissure, respectively.) (Reprinted with permission from H Fukuyama, S Matsuzaki, Y Ouchi, et al. Neural control of micturition in man examined with single photon emission computed tomography using mTc-HMPAO. Neuroreport 1996;7:3009–3012.)

while lying supine at rest over 15 minutes. The two scans were subtracted from one another to remove the resting effects. The image obtained showed the areas activated during micturition (Figure 14.1).

As judged from increased cerebral blood flow during voiding versus during the resting state, small areas in the midpons extending into the midbrain, the left sensorimotor cortex, the right lateral frontal cortex, and bilateral supplementary motor areas were shown to have been activated by voiding. The pontomidbrain area that enhanced was thought to be the periaqueductal gray matter, a region that had been shown to act as a sensory-integration relay center for micturition in animals [2].

The first reports using positron emission tomographic (PET) scanning to look at micturition in humans came from the Netherlands. Holstege's group had previously carried out experiments looking at control of micturition in cats; extending what was already known about brain stem mechanisms from the early work of Barrington [3]

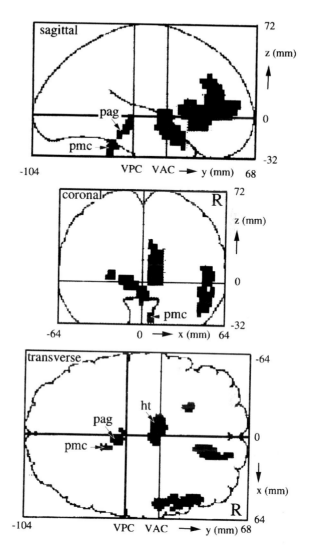

Figure 14.2 Differences in regional cerebral blood flow, comparing successful micturition with voluntary withholding of urine. (ht = hypothalamus; pag = periaqueductal gray; pmc = pontine micturition center; R = right; VAC, VPC = vertical lines through anterior and posterior commissure, respectively.) (Adapted with permission from B Blok, T Willemsen, G Holstege. A PET study of brain control of micturition in humans. Brain 1997;129:111–121.)

(see later) and others [4, 5], they defined in detail the brain stem sites involved in bladder storage and voiding [6, 7]. Because of this previous work, when the Dutch workers started PET imaging studies, they focused on the brain stem and diencephalon.

Seventeen right-handed male volunteers were trained to void while supine. One bolus injection of radioactively labeled water was given 15 minutes before micturition when the bladder was full, another just after the command to start micturition, and a third and fourth 15 and 30 minutes after voiding. Scans were performed after each injection. Ten subjects were able to void within 30 seconds of the command to do so and within 30 seconds of scan 2, whereas the other seven could not switch on micturition. In the successful micturition group, scan 1 showed increased activity in the periaqueductal gray and hypothalamus and the dorsomedial pons compared with scan 2 (Figure 14.2). In the cortex, significant activity was

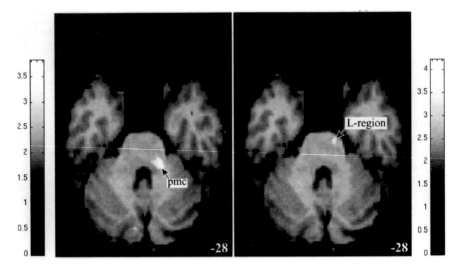

Figure 14.3   Left: Significant differences in regional cerebral blood flow (rCBF) in the right dorsomedial tegmentum (indicated by pmc [pontine micturition center]) during successful micturition compared with an empty bladder. Right: Significant differences in rCBF in the right ventral tegmentum (indicated by L-region) during unsuccessful micturition compared with an empty bladder. (L = left; R = right.) (Reprinted with permission from B Blok, L Sturms, G Holstege. Brain activation during micturition in women. Brain 1998;121:2033–2042.)

seen in the right inferior frontal gyrus and the right anterior cingulate gyrus during voiding that was not present during the withholding phase. In the unsuccessful micturition group, activation was found in the right ventral pons. A significant difference was also seen in the right cingulate gyrus; more activity was seen in the posterior and superior region during withholding.

The differences noted in activity in the dorsomedial tegmentum between the successful and unsuccessful voiding group (Figure 14.3) were of great interest. In the group who voided, activity was seen in a medioposterior region, and this was suggested to be the human homologue of Barrington's nucleus or the M-region [2]. In animals, stimulation of this region results in an immediate decrease in urethral pressure and silence of pelvic floor electromyographic signals, followed by a rise in detrusor pressure. In the unsuccessful voiders, a region in the ventrolateral pontine tegmentum was seen to be active on the PET scans. This was proposed to be the homologue of the cat L-region that, when stimulated, results in powerful contraction of the urethral sphincter [6]. Direct projections between the L-region and Onuf's nucleus, the nucleus containing the anterior horns that innervate the sphincters, have been demonstrated in the cat [7]. A study of similar design using 18 female volunteers has confirmed the same specific nuclei to be involved, although in women activation of the periaqueductal gray matter could not be demonstrated [8]. These PET scanning studies therefore show that a brain stem controlling mechanism similar to that known to exist in the cat is also found in humans.

The differences between the results of the SPECT study [1] and the results of the PET study [9] (see Figure 14.1 compared with Figure 14.2) may be due in part to the different techniques used, but they may also reflect the difference in timing during the micturition cycle on which each study had focused: The SPECT study looked at sustaining micturition, whereas the PET study looked at initiation of micturition. The cerebral contribution to these different neurologic processes is likely to be different. Future studies examining the mechanism of bladder storage are awaited with interest.

The authors of the PET study drew attention to the lateralization of micturition control on the right in their right-handed subjects, both men [9] and women [8]. The same group has also used PET scanning to study cortical activation in response to pelvic floor muscle contraction [10]. In this study, six female volunteers were scanned under four conditions: at rest and during repetitive pelvic floor contraction, sustained pelvic floor contraction, and sustained abdominal straining. Activity was demonstrated in the most medial portion of the motor cortex during pelvic floor contraction and somewhat more laterally during abdominal contraction. Activation was also seen in the cerebellum, supplementary motor cortex, and thalamus during these procedures but not in subcortical structures—the "emotional motor system" [11]—possibly because the activities occurred voluntarily rather than as part of complex reflex mechanisms.

Studies of Patients with Brain Lesions

Before the findings of these functional brain-imaging experiments, what was known about the cortical control of the bladder came from clinical studies of patients with brain lesions. The most authoritative work in this area was the 1964 study by Andrew and Nathan [12], in which the authors described 38 patients with disturbances of micturition as a result of lesions in the anterior frontal lobe. Ten patients had intracranial tumors, 2 had anterior frontal lobe damage after rupture of an aneurysm, 4 had penetrating brain wounds, and 22 had undergone leukotomy. The leukotomy cases were the most useful in terms of localization of important brain structures, and the authors concluded that lesions in the plane of the genu of the corpus callosum involving some of the white matter anterior to the anterior horns of the lateral ventricle cause a permanent disorder of control of micturition.

A typical case of frontal lobe incontinence described by Andrew and Nathan [12] was that of a patient with severe urgency and frequency of micturition and urge incontinence without dementia who was socially aware and embarrassed by the incontinence. Micturition was normally coordinated, indicating that the disturbance was in the higher control of this process. The infrequency with which such patients are encountered is stressed by the authors, who explain that they had each been collecting cases separately over a period of 24 years and only just before writing did they learn of each other's interest and combine to present a joint paper.

Two years later, Andrew et al. [13] described six cases with disturbances of micturition due to aneurysms of anterior communicating or anterior cerebral arteries. In this paper, they reviewed the animal experimentation literature on neurologic bladder control and hypothesized that it was the disconnection of the frontal or anterior cingulate regions from the septal and hypothalamic areas that allowed micturition to proceed automatically and involuntarily after brain damage.

Although the paper of Andrew and Nathan [12] has been the most influential in the study of frontal lobe control of the bladder, it was not in fact the first.

In 1960, Ueki [14], a neurosurgeon from Japan, published a report (of which Andrew and Nathan were unaware at the time they were writing) that analyzed the urinary symptoms of 462 patients who had come to surgery for brain tumors, 34 patients who had undergone frontal lobectomy, and 16 patients who had undergone bilateral anterior cingulectomy. He illustrated his conclusions with a diagram of the brain showing a strong positive influence on micturition of an area in the pons and an inhibitory input from the frontal lobe, the left more than the right and bilateral paracentral lobules.

In 1901, Czyhlarz and Marburg [15] had published on this subject in German. They described two cases identified by them and others taken from the literature. One of the inevitable defects of such a study was that at that time, tumors could be localized only on clinical grounds, and by the time a postmortem examination was performed, the lesions responsible for the clinical condition were considerably larger and inevitably poorly localized. However, from the clinical evidence available, the authors concluded that the cortical field of the bladder was in the motor zone, in a region between the arm and the leg, and that the clinical manifestation of a disturbance of this region was difficulty initiating micturition and thus urinary retention. The authors reported cases of lesions in other parts of the central nervous system in which micturition was affected—in particular, the pons. Nathan concludes his translation of the study with the comment, "this paper was written because people did not believe that there was such a thing as a cerebral disturbance of the bladder" (written communication, July 1997).

After the paper by Andrews and Nathan [12], Maurice-Williams [16] reported on a series of 50 consecutive cases of frontal lobe tumor and found seven patients exhibiting the syndrome previously described. The syndrome was not found in 100 consecutive cases of nonfrontal intracranial tumor, indicating the localizing value of the syndrome. The author [16; p. 434] also observed that "it is odd that the syndrome may be relieved by excision of both the causative lesions and the area of brain it involves" because, in five of the reported cases, resection of a tumor relieved the micturition symptoms for up to 2 years. It was concluded that the phenomenon was a positive rather than a negative one, with the lesion activating some system rather than releasing one from control. This author also noted an apparent preponderance of right-sided tumors, which accounted for six out of seven cases in the series he reported.

Mochizuki and Saito [17] reported their findings on 26 patients with lesions involving the medial frontal lobes. Fifteen patients had had cerebral infarctions of the anterior cerebral artery region; two, cerebral hemorrhages; six, subarachnoid hemorrhages due to anterior communicating artery aneurysms; two, traumatic frontal lobe damage; and one, a frontal brain tumor for which surgery had been performed. Common clinical features included hemiparesis predominantly involving the lower extremity, verbal adynamia, and emotional disturbance characterized by depressed motivation, dementia, and memory disturbance. More extensive injury produced akinetic mutism, or motor neglect and dressing apraxia. Ten of the patients had urinary incontinence; in eight of them, it was persistent, and these eight suffered from bilateral superior prefrontal damage. Transitory urinary incontinence occurred after unilateral right superior prefrontal damage.

Urinary retention has also been described with brain lesions. In the series by Andrew and Nathan [12], two of their patients were in urinary retention at some stage. Yamamoto et al. [18] described a 70-year-old woman who was demonstrated to have urinary retention and detrusor hyporeflexia on cystometry. Her high fever and worsening cognitive state prompted brain imaging, and she was found to have a right frontal lobe abscess. Both her general condition and her bladder function were improved by antibiotic administration that successfully treated the abscess. Lang et al. [19] reported on two patients with voiding difficulty and retention. One was an 87-year-old woman who had a diffuse subdural hematoma with a marked inter-hemispheric component and presented with disorientation, nuchal rigidity, and bilat-eral extensor plantar responses. She then developed urinary retention, and a general worsening of her neurologic condition necessitated burr-hole evacuation of the hematoma. Postoperatively, her ability to void recovered. The other patient, a 63-year-old woman, presented with a complaint of difficulty initiating micturition and only mild hyperreflexia of her limbs. Cystometry showed detrusor hypocontractil-ity, and a magnetic resonance imaging (MRI) scan revealed left frontal convexity meningioma. She refused surgery and used a suprapubic urinary catheter for blad-der management; she died several years later from raised intracranial pressure.

Perhaps with the increasing availability and decreasing cost of brain imaging, case histories such as these will not be uncommon, and one can make an argu-ment for requesting such tests for more patients with nonurologic, unexplained bladder dysfunction.

Changes in Bladder Control after Cerebrovascular Accidents

Studies of patients' bladder function after cerebrovascular accidents (CVAs) have examined the relationship in two different and interesting ways: Some studies have examined urodynamic changes after CVAs in small groups of patients and have correlated the site of the lesion with the urodynamic findings, but a more sub-stantial body of work has looked at incontinence after stroke. Because the empha-sis of these two approaches is quite different, the findings are reviewed separately.

Urodynamic Studies of Patients after Cerebrovascular Accidents

A study by Khan et al. [20] examined 20 patients who had presented to a urol-ogy department with urinary incontinence 3 or 4 months after a CVA. Computed tomographic (CT) scanning was performed to localize the area of brain injury. In four patients, the basal ganglia had been affected; in eight, the frontoparietal region; in one, the frontal region; and in one, the parietal region. In four patients, diffuse bilateral ischemic damage was present, and CT scans were normal in two. The most common cystometric finding in this disparate group of patients was detrusor hyperreflexia, which was found in all but one. In this single patient, inability to communicate due to aphasia and poor mobility appeared to be the cause of incontinence, because stable bladder filling occurred.

A similar finding was reported by Tsuchida et al. [21], who looked at 39 hemi-plegic patients. The patients were evaluated by urodynamic studies and CT scanning. Again, the most common finding was urinary urge incontinence, although 13 patients complained of difficulty with micturition. Ten of the 11 patients who had frontal and internal capsular lesions showed bladder hyperreflexia, as did 9 of the 10 patients who had putaminal lesions. Normal sphincter relaxation was coordinated in all these patients. In the remaining patients, no correlation was found between urodynamic dysfunction and type of brain injury. Another study of similar design—that is, of patients who had had a stroke presenting with incontinence—showed that, of 134 patients with chronic hemiplegia, complaints of urinary frequency were more common in those with left than with right hemiplegia [22].

It is not clear how these observations might fit with those of a study showing that, of 85 patients admitted to a rehabilitation center, incomplete bladder emptying occurred initially in 48 and was persistent in 28 [23]. Twenty-two of this group were able to void voluntarily and 15 were continent, but the authors emphasized that urinary retention in stroke patients with apparently normal bladder function was a frequent problem that should be assessed as part of routine rehabilitation management.

Khan et al. [24] followed up their first report with another study of a similar design. Thirty-three patients with voiding problems after a CVA were assessed, and again the predominant finding was of involuntary contractions of the bladder. This condition was present in 26, all of whom had normal coordinated voiding. The majority of patients with cerebral cortex or internal capsular lesions had uninhibited relaxation of the sphincter during involuntary bladder contractions, whereas all of the patients with lesions only in the basal ganglia or thalamus had normal sphincter function. The conclusion of the investigators was that bladder dysfunction could not be correlated with the area of brain injury.

Sakakibara et al. [25] reported on the bladder symptoms of 72 patients who had been admitted to the hospital with an acute hemispheric stroke. When assessed at 3 months, 53% were found to have significant urinary complaints. The most common problem was nocturnal urinary frequency, which affected 36%; urge incontinence affected 29%, and difficulty in voiding affected 25%. Urinary retention was seen in the acute phase of illness in 6%. A significant correlation was found between the occurrence of a urinary disturbance and hemiparesis (P <.05) and a negative correlation between urinary disturbance and hemianopia (P <.05); brain-imaging techniques confirmed a more anterior location of brain lesions in the former group (Figure 14.4). Urodynamic studies of 22 symptomatic patients showed detrusor hyperreflexia in 68%, detrusor-sphincter dyssynergia in 14%, and uninhibited sphincter relaxation in 36%. Patients with urinary retention had detrusor areflexia and a nonrelaxing sphincter. No statistically significant correlation could be demonstrated between any particular lesion site and urodynamic findings.

In this study, no preponderance of right-sided lesions was found in the group of patients with urinary symptoms. There was some indication that lesion size was related to the occurrence of urinary symptoms. These findings further supported the idea that lesions of the anteromedial frontal lobe and its descending pathway and of the basal ganglia are mainly responsible for micturitional dysfunction in stroke patients.

Table 14.1 summarizes the possible causes of incontinence due to cortical lesions.

Epidemiologic Studies of Incontinence after Cerebrovascular Accident

Epidemiologic studies of urinary incontinence after CVA lead to the almost unanimous and somewhat surprising conclusion that urinary incontinence occurring within 7 days after a stroke is a specific indicator of poor prognosis.

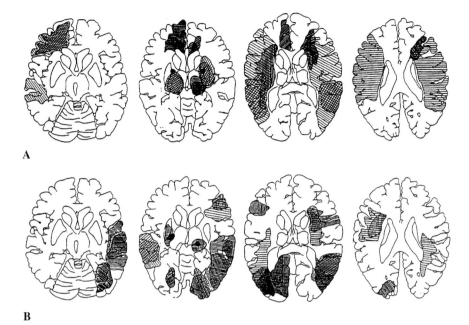

Figure 14.4 (**A**) Lesions on brain computed tomography (CT) or magnetic resonance imaging (MRI) in patients with micturitional disturbance. (**B**) Lesions on brain CT or MRI in patients without micturitional disturbance. (Reprinted with permission from R Sakakibara, T Hattori, K Yasuda, T Yamanishi. Micturitional disturbance after acute hemispheric stroke: analysis of the lesion site by CT and MRI. J Neurol Sci 1996;137:47–56.)

Wade and Langton-Hewer [26] analyzed the symptoms of 532 patients seen within 7 days of their stroke and found that the presence of urinary incontinence was a more powerful prognostic indicator for poor survival and eventual functional dependence than was a depressed level of consciousness. The authors stress that they did not attempt to investigate the cause of incontinence in these patients and pointed out that many patients were immobile or aphasic. In discussing the possible significance of their finding, they argued that disturbed cognitive function is associated with poor recovery, independent of its close association with other indices of severity of stroke, and demented patients are often incontinent. They offered two alternative proposals: Either incontinence

Table 14.1   Possible causes of incontinence due to cortical lesions

Pathophysiology	Effect
Neurogenic bladder dysfunction	True incontinence
Immobility and/or dementia	Functional incontinence
A combination of both of the above	

was the result of a severe general rather than specific loss of function, or those who were incontinent may have been less motivated to remain continent and to recover loss of function.

Barer and Mitchell [27] studied a similar large number of patients after CVA and concluded that single variables, such as power in the affected arm and continence, were as good as the more complex discriminate functions in predicting discharge within the first month or first 6 months. Barer [28] took this matter further and looked at the prevalence and time course of recovery of urinary incontinence; associations with other variables; and the relationship between bladder control and the neurologic, functional, and overall outcome. Outcome was so much better in those who remained or became dry that possibly recovery of continence may promote morale and self-esteem, which can actually hasten overall recovery.

Brocklehurst et al. [29] concluded that incontinence after a CVA was commonly a by-product of immobility and dependency and was mostly a transient phenomenon.

Incontinence probably is a strong predicting factor for poor prognosis for a number of reasons: The same lesion might cause neurogenic bladder dysfunction and motor or cognitive impairment; urinary incontinence may cause psychological problems; or urinary continence may be an important factor in rehabilitation, independence, and quality of life.

The role of diffuse brain disease in causing incontinence is not clear, although this problem has immense socioeconomic importance because of the cost of caring for demented incontinent patients. The onset of incontinence has been shown to bear a close relationship to the duration and stage of illness in patients with Alzheimer's disease [30]. Other causes of urinary incontinence in the elderly are discussed in Chapter 17.

Brain Stem Control of Micturition

Since the studies of Barrington [3], the mechanisms for coordinating bladder and sphincter activity have been known to reside in brain stem centers. Kuru and Yamamoto suggested that the area in the rostral pons, which when electrically stimulated in the cat results in a marked contraction of the detrusor muscle, be named the *pontine detrusor nucleus of Barrington* [31]. Subsequent studies by the groups of de Groat [4, 5] and then Holstege [6, 7] defined in great detail the brain stem activity involved in bladder storage and voiding in animals and culminated in the PET imaging studies in humans [9], reviewed earlier in this chapter.

In 1926, Holman [32] noted that voiding difficulty could be a sign of posterior fossa tumors. In a series studying patients with brain tumors reported by Ueki [14], voiding difficulty occurred in 46 (30%) of 152 patients with posterior fossa tumors, and urinary incontinence in 3 (1.9%). Analysis in greater detail revealed that voiding difficulty occurred in 77.3% with lesions of the pons, 66.7% with fourth-ventricle lesions, 40.9% with lesions in the midline of the cerebellum, 24.2% with lesions of the cerebellar hemisphere, and 9.1% with lesions of the cerebellopontine angle in posterior fossa tumors. Renier and Gabreels [33] found urinary retention in 71% of 17 children with pontine glioma.

Betts et al. [34] reported voiding dysfunction and diplopia as the presenting symptoms in a young man with a probable dermoid involving the upper pons.

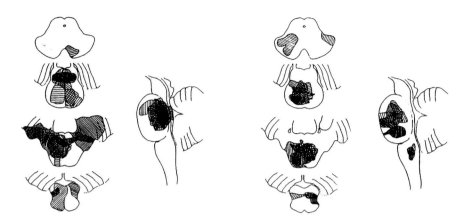

Figure 14.5 Lesions on brain magnetic resonance imaging in patients with micturitional disturbance (left) and those without (right). (Reprinted with permission from R Sakakibara, T Hattori, K Yasuda, T Yamanishi. Micturitional disturbance and the pontine tegmental lesion: urodynamic and MRI analyses of vascular cases. J Neurol Sci 1996;141:105–110.)

Manenete et al. [35] described the MRI appearances of a low-grade pontine glioma in a woman complaining of weakness of her lower limbs and difficulty in micturition. Sakakibara et al. [36] reported on a patient with herpetic brain stem encephalitis who, on recovering consciousness, had urinary retention and abnormalities of eye movements.

An analysis of urinary symptoms of 39 patients who had had brain stem strokes produced evidence that dorsally situated lesions (Figure 14.5) were those that resulted in disturbance of micturition [37]. Forty-nine percent of all patients had urinary symptoms; nocturnal urinary frequency and voiding difficulty were seen in 28%, urinary retention in 21%, and urinary incontinence in 8%. The problems were more common in those with hemorrhage, possibly because the damage was usually bilateral. MRI showed that the responsible lesions were in the pontine reticular nucleus and the reticular formation, adjacent to the medial parabrachial nucleus and the locus ceruleus. A correlation was found between urinary symptoms with sensory disturbance, abnormal eye movement, and lack of coordination. Urodynamics in 11 symptomatic patients showed detrusor hyperreflexia in 8 (73%), low bladder compliance in 1 (9%), detrusor areflexia in 3 (27%) (at 3 months, 6 months, and 3 years after the occurrence), nonrelaxing sphincter on voiding in 5 (45%), and uninhibited sphincter relaxation in 3 (27%). Three asymptomatic patients had normal findings.

The authors of these various papers all draw attention to the fact that such patients confirm that the neurophysiology of micturition control in humans appears to be very similar to that described in experimental animals. The proximity of the medial longitudinal fasciculus in the dorsal pons to the presumed pontine micturition center means that a disorder of eye movements, such as an internuclear ophthalmoplegia, is highly likely in patients with pontine pathology, causing a voiding disorder.

CORTICAL CONTROL OF DEFECATION

Very much less has been written about cortical control of the bowel than about cortical control of the bladder. Andrew and Nathan mentioned bowel control in the patients they described and reported that, in general, defecation was affected much less often than micturition [12]. Three of the 10 patients with brain tumors they studied had fecal frequency, fecal incontinence, and constipation. After aneurysm surgery, one of two patients had fecal incontinence, occasionally with diarrhea. Two of four brain-injured patients had fecal incontinence without warning. One reported not to feel feces passing, whereas the other had fecal incontinence only when asleep. Rectal examination showed that these patients had full voluntary control of their levator ani muscles and of the external anal sphincter. After leukotomy, some patients were incontinent of feces, and in such cases this incontinence was always accompanied by urinary dysfunction. Most of the other papers reviewed previously that described disorders of bladder function in frontal lobe disease do not mention the patients' bowel symptoms.

One paper concentrated primarily on the anorectal abnormalities experienced by six out of seven patients with frontal lobe damage of various types [38]. Anorectal manometric recordings and urodynamic investigations were carried out in seven patients who had either right, left, or bilateral frontal lobe injury. Two patients lacked sensation of bladder filling; two other patients had increased perception threshold for rectal distention; five had uninhibited detrusor hyperreflexia or spontaneous rectal contractions; and one patient had lost reflex micturition and the rectoanal inhibitory reflex. The authors concluded that the frontal lobe was involved in neurologic control of anorectal motility as it is for bladder function, but the lack of correlation between urinary and anorectal abnormality in individual cases suggests that these functions depend on distinct areas of the frontal lobes.

The site of lesions responsible for problems with bowel control seems to be similar to that involved in cases with disturbances of bladder control—that is, the medial prefrontal area and the anterior cingulate gyrus. The hypothesis was that, as a result of such a lesion, the patient experienced lack of awareness of visceral events and an inability to inhibit a reflex process of elimination once it had begun [13].

One study used PET to examine the areas of brain activation after rectal distention. The emphasis of the study was to compare responses in healthy control subjects with responses in a group of patients with irritable bowel syndrome in whom a hyperalgesia of visceral events is hypothesized to occur. A balloon catheter was inserted into the rectum, and different degrees of distention were produced at timed intervals. The subjects were asked to rate any discomfort. Differences in response were found between the control subjects and patients both on maximal filling and in anticipation of filling, but in healthy subjects activation of the anterior cingulate cortex could be demonstrated on filling only to pressures that were perceived as painful [39].

CORTICAL CONTROL OF SEXUAL FUNCTION

Little is known about the contribution of the cortex to sexual function, although cerebral processing is thought to determine libido and desire; the ability to effect a sexual response is determined by spinal, autonomic reflexes [40]. Libido is hormone-dependent, with a major hypothalamic component. Loss of libido commonly affects patients with a pituitary disorder, and this may be the earliest symptom of a pituitary tumor [41, 42].

In experimental animals, the deep anterior midline structures that form the limbic system have been shown to be important in determining sexual responses, and the medial preoptic–anterior hypothalamic area has been shown to be an integrating area [43]. Electrical stimulation of the hypothalamic and limbic pathways in experimental animals results in erection. Brain stimulation in awake humans has been carried out as part of various forms of stereotaxic neurosurgery, but Brindley, who reviewed reports of brain stimulation in humans, stated categorically that no reliable reports exist of erection occurring during such surgery [44].

A study using the technique of SPECT scanning showed an increase in activity in the right frontal lobe region during ejaculation in healthy male subjects [45], but no focal activation was found in the medial anterior parietal lobe corresponding to somatosensory cortex of the genital projection area. This finding was interpreted as implying that the right prefrontal cortex is important for the emotional responses of male sexuality.

Otherwise, most of what is known about human cerebral regions involved in sexuality comes from observations of patients with brain lesions. The frontotemporal regions are important in sexual activity [46], and these regions of the brain can be involved by pathology that causes epilepsy or by trauma, tumors, cerebrovascular disease, or encephalitis. Sexual dysfunction has long been observed to be more common in both men and women with epilepsy. Although various types of abnormal sexual behavior and, occasionally, hypersexuality have been described in patients with temporal lobe epilepsy, the picture most commonly seen is that of sexual apathy [47]. Studies comparing sexual dysfunction in groups of patients with generalized epilepsy to that in groups with focal temporal lobe epilepsy [47, 48] provide sufficient evidence that the deficit is a function of the specific area of brain involvement rather than a consequence of epilepsy, psychosocial factors, or antiepileptic medication. The problem is usually a low or even absent libido, of which patients rarely complain. The role of hormonal dysfunction has yet to be fully determined, but based on measurements of sex hormone level and pituitary function, some have suggested that the hyposexuality of temporal lobe epilepsy is due to a subclinical hypogonadotrophic hypogonadism [49] and that dysfunction of medial temporal lobe structures may dysmodulate hypothalamic-pituitary secretion.

However, erectile dysfunction with preserved libido and of which a patient therefore complains can also occur in men with temporal lobe damage and epilepsy [50] and may be characterized by loss of nocturnal penile tumescence [51]. Surgery for epilepsy rarely restores function [48], although a survey of operated patients showed a higher level of satisfaction with sexual function among those who were seizure-free [52].

Sexual problems are not uncommon after head injury, particularly if cognitive damage or a personality change has occurred [53] and appears to contribute significantly to the long-term failure of relationships that predated the injury. A study of people who had been admitted to the hospital for a minimum of 24 hours after a closed head injury found significant sexual dysfunction in 50% over a 15-year period. The most common complaint was of infrequency [54], and some evidence exists that hypogonadotrophic hypogonadism may be a significant factor

[55]. Sexually demanding behavior combined with a loss of empathic sensitivity can also occur after head injury [56].

REFERENCES

1. Fukuyama H, Matsuzaki S, Ouchi Y, et al. Neural control of micturition in man examined with single photon emission computed tomography using mTc-HMPAO. Neuroreport 1996;7:3009–3012.
2. Blok B, Holstege G. Direct projections from the periaqueductal gray to the pontine micturition centre (M-region): an anterograde and retrograde tracing study in the cat. Neurosci Lett 1994;166:93–96.
3. Barrington RJF. The effect of lesions of the hind and midbrain on micturition in the cat. Q J Exp Physiol Cogn Med 1925;15:81–102.
4. De Groat W. Nervous control of the urinary bladder of the cat. Brain Res 1975;87:201–211.
5. Noto H, Roppolo J, Steers W, de Groat W. Electrophysiological analysis of the ascending and descending components of the micturition reflex pathway in the rat. Brain Res 1991;549:95–105.
6. Holstege G, Griffiths D, de Wall H, Dalm E. Anatomical and physiological observations on supraspinal control of bladder and urethral sphincter muscles in the cat. J Comp Neurol 1986;250:449–461.
7. Griffiths D, Holstege G, de Wall H, Dalm E. Control and coordination of bladder and urethral function in the brain stem of the cat. Neurourol Urodyn 1990;9:63–82.
8. Blok B, Sturms L, Holstege G. Brain activation during micturition in women. Brain 1998;121:2033–2042.
9. Blok B, Willemsen T, Holstege G. A PET study of brain control of micturition in humans. Brain 1997;129:111–121.
10. Blok B, Sturms L, Holstege G. A PET study on cortical and subcortical control of pelvic floor musculature in women. J Comp Neurol 1997;389:535–544.
11. Blok B, Holstege G. Neuronal control of micturition and its relation to the emotional system. Prog Brain Res 1996;107:113–126.
12. Andrew J, Nathan PW. Lesions of the anterior frontal lobes and disturbances of micturition and defaecation. Brain 1964;87:233–262.
13. Andrew J, Nathan P, Spanos N. Disturbances of micturition and defaecation due to aneurysms of anterior communication or anterior cerebral arteries. J Neurosurg 1966;24:1–10.
14. Ueki K. Disturbances of micturition observed in some patients with brain tumour. Neurol Med Chir (Tokyo) 1960;2:25–33.
15. Czyhlarz E, Marlburg O. Über cerebrale Blasenstorungen. Jahrb Psychiatry Neurol 1901;20:134–174.
16. Maurice-Williams RS. Micturition symptoms in frontal tumours. J Neurol Neurosurg Psychiatry 1974;37:431–436.
17. Mochizuki H, Saito H. Mesial frontal lobe syndromes: correlations between neurological deficits and radiological localizations. J Exp Med 1990;161:231–239.
18. Yamamoto S, Soma T, Hatayama T, et al. Neurogenic bladder induced by brain abscess. Br J Urol 1995;76:272.
19. Lang E, Chesnut R, Hennerici M. Urinary retention and space-occupying lesions of the frontal cortex. Eur Neurol 1996;36:43–47.
20. Khan Z, Hertanu J, Yang W, et al. Predictive correlation of urodynamic dysfunction and brain injury after cerebrovascular accident. J Urol 1981;126:86–88.
21. Tsuchida S, Noto H, Yamaguchi O, Itoh M. Urodynamic studies on hemiplegic patients after cerebrovascular accident. Urology 1983;21:315–318.
22. Kuroiwa Y, Tohgi H, Itoh M. Frequency and urgency of micturition in hemiplegic patients: relationship to hemisphere laterality of lesions. J Neurol 1987;234:100–102.
23. Garrett V, Scott J, Costich J, et al. Bladder emptying assessment in stroke patients. Arch Phys Med Rehabil 1989;70:41–43.
24. Khan Z, Starer P, Yang W, Bhola A. Analysis of voiding disorders in patients with cerebrovascular accidents. Urology 1990;35:263–270.
25. Sakakibara R, Hattori T, Yasuda K, Yamanishi T. Micturitional disturbance after acute hemispheric stroke: analysis of the lesion site by CT and MRI. J Neurol Sci 1996;137:47–56.
26. Wade D, Langton-Hewer R. Outlook after an acute stroke: urinary incontinence and loss of consciousness compared in 532 patients. QJM 1985;56:601–608.
27. Barer D, Mitchell J. Predicting the outcome of acute stroke: do multivariate models help? QJM 1989;70:27–39.

28. Barer D. Continence after stroke: useful predictor or goal therapy. Age Ageing 1989;18:183–191.
29. Brocklehurst J, Andrews K, Richards B, Laycock P. Incidence and correlates of incontinence in stroke patients. J Am Geriatr Soc 1985;33:540–542.
30. Del-Ser T, Munoz D, Hachinski V. Temporal pattern of cognitive decline and incontinence is different in Alzheimer's disease and diffuse Lewy body disease. Neurology 1996;46:682–686.
31. Kuru M, Yamamoto H. Fiber connections of the pontine detrusor nucleus (Barrington). J Comp Neurol 1964;123:161–185.
32. Holman E. Difficult urination associated with intracranial tumours of the posterior fossa: a physiologic and clinical study. Arch Neurol Psychiatry 1926;15:371–380.
33. Renier WO, Gabreels FJM. Evaluation of diagnosis and non-surgical therapy in 24 children with a pontine tumour. Neuropaediatrie 1980;11:262–273.
34. Betts CD, Kapoor R, Fowler CJ. Pontine pathology and micturition dysfunction. Br J Urol 1992;70:100–102.
35. Manente G, Melchionda D, Uncini A. Urinary retention in bilateral pontine tumour: evidence for a pontine micturition centre in humans. J Neurol Neurosurg Psychiatry 1996;61:528–536.
36. Sakakibara R, Hattori T, Fukutake T, et al. Micturitional disturbance in herpetic brainstem encephalitis; contribution of the pontine micturition center (PMC). J Neurol Neurosurg Psychiatry 1998;64:269–272.
37. Sakakibara R, Hattori T, Yasuda K, Yamanishi T. Micturitional disturbance and the pontine tegmental lesion: urodynamic and MRI analyses of vascular cases. J Neurol Sci 1996;141:105–110.
38. Weber J, Delanger T, Hannequin D, et al. Anorectal manometric anomalies in seven patients with frontal lobe brain damage. Dig Dis Sci 1990;35:225–230.
39. Silverman D, Munakata J, Ennes H, et al. Regional cerebral activity in normal and pathological perception of visceral pain. Gastroenterology 1997;112:64–72.
40. Lundberg P, Brattberg A. Impotence—the neurological risk factor. Int J Impot Res 1993;5:241–243.
41. Hutling A-L, Muhr C, Lundberg P, Werner S. Prolactinomas in men: clinical characteristics and the effect of bromocriptine treatment. Acta Med Scand 1985;217:101–109.
42. Lundberg P, Hulter B. Sexual dysfunction in patients with hypothalamo-pituitary disorders. Exp Clin Endocrinol 1991;98:81–88.
43. De Groat W. Neural Control of the Urinary Bladder and Sexual Organs. In R Bannister, C Mathias (eds), Autonomic Failure (3rd ed). Oxford, UK: Oxford University Press, 1992;129–159.
44. Brindley G. Neurophysiology. In R Kirby, C Carson, G Webster (eds). Impotence: Diagnosis and Management of Male Erectile Dysfunction. Oxford, UK: Butterworth–Heinemann, 1991;27–31.
45. Tiihonen J, Kikka J, Kuplia J, et al. Increase in cerebral blood flow of right prefrontal cortex in man during orgasm. Neurosci Lett 1994;170:241–243.
46. Miller B, Cummings J, McIntyre H. Hypersexuality or altered sexual preference following brain injury. J Neurol Neurosurg Psychiatry 1986;49:867–873.
47. Shukla G, Srivastava O, Katiyar B. Sexual disturbance in temporal lobe epilepsy: a controlled study. Br J Psychiatry 1979;134:288–292.
48. Blumer D, Walker A. Sexual behavior in temporal lobe epilepsy. Arch Neurol 1967;16:37–43.
49. Murialdo G, Galimberti C, Fonzi S, et al. Sex hormones and pituitary function in male epileptic patients with altered or normal sexuality. Epilepsia 1995;36:360–365.
50. Hierons R, Saunders M. Impotence in patients with temporal lobe lesions. Lancet 1966;2:761.
51. Guldner G, Morrell M. Nocturnal penile tumescence and rigidity evaluation in men with epilepsy. Epilepsia 1996;37:1211–1214.
52. Christianson S, Silfvenius H, Saisa J, Nilsson M. Life satisfaction and sexuality in patients operated for epilepsy. Acta Neurol Scand 1995;92:1–6.
53. Elliott M, Biever L. Head injury and sexual dysfunction. Brain Inj 1996;10:703–717.
54. O'Carroll R, Woodrow J, Maroun F. Psychosexual and psychosocial sequelae of closed head injury. Brain Inj 1991;5:303–313.
55. Clark J, Raggatt P, Edwards O. Hypothalamic hypogonadism following major head injury. Clin Endocrinol 1988;29:153–165.
56. Lezak M. Living with the characterologically altered brain injured patient. J Clin Psychiatry 1978;39:592–598.

15
Urogenital Disorders in Parkinson's Disease and Multiple System Atrophy

Vijay A. Chandiramani and Clare J. Fowler

The distinction between idiopathic Parkinson's disease (PD) and multiple system atrophy (MSA) may not always be clear, even to specialists, but certain features suggest the latter diagnosis. Poor response to administration of L-dopa, rapid progression, early postural instability, cerebellar features, and respiratory stridor are all red flags that raise the alert for a diagnosis of MSA; so too, however, are early and severe urogenital symptoms [1, 2]. In a patient with bladder symptoms and parkinsonism, knowing if the patient has MSA is important both to ensure accuracy of neurologic diagnosis and because the urinary symptoms may be severe enough that surgical intervention is considered, and patients with MSA do not have a good outcome from urologic surgery [3].

BLADDER DYSFUNCTION IN MULTIPLE SYSTEM ATROPHY AND IDIOPATHIC PARKINSON'S DISEASE

Bladder and Multiple System Atrophy

Neuronal atrophy in MSA affects the central nervous system at many different sites, and the neurologic features reflect the diffuse nature of cell loss that can occur in the striatum, olives, pons, cerebellum, intermediolateral cell columns, and Onuf's nucleus in the spinal cord [1]. Because many of these structures are concerned with the neurologic control of micturition, premonitive urinary symptoms are not unusual.

Detrusor hyperreflexia is thought to be due to cell loss in the midbrain, whereas incomplete bladder emptying and poor flow are due to loss of parasympathetic drive on the detrusor after atrophy of preganglionic cells in the intermediolateral cell columns [4]. The balance of pathophysiology may change during the course of the disease [5]. Whereas early on, symptoms due to detrusor hyperreflexia pre-

Table 15.1   Possible pathophysiologic causes of various urinary symptoms
in multiple system atrophy

Symptom	Cause
Degeneration of cells in midbrain	Detrusor hyperreflexia (frequency, urgency, urge incontinence)
Degeneration in dorsal pons	Hesitancy
Cell loss in intermediolateral cell column	Detrusor failure (incomplete emptying and poor flow)
Atrophy of anterior horn cells (Onuf's nucleus)	Sphincter weakness
Postural hypotension	Nocturnal polyuria/nocturia

dominate, as the disease progresses, symptoms may change to those due to incomplete bladder emptying.

Of particular importance is the group of anterior horn cells in the sacral spinal cord that innervate the striated muscles of the urethral and anal sphincters. They were first described by Onufrowicz in 1900 and hence became known as *Onuf's nucleus*. Postmortem studies of patients who died with Shy-Drager syndrome demonstrated a selective loss of anterior horn cells in Onuf's nucleus [6], which are spared in amyotrophic lateral sclerosis [7]. The resulting denervation of the urethral sphincter, together with detrusor hyperreflexia, is a further reason why urge incontinence is such a pronounced and early feature of MSA.

Postural hypotension, a disorder characterized by nocturnal polyuria, affects a proportion of patients with MSA [8]. It is probably due to a combination of factors, including compensatory supine hypertension at night leading to increased glomerular filtration and alterations in the production of atrial natriuretic peptide [9].

Table 15.1 summarizes the possible pathophysiologic causes of urinary dysfunction in MSA.

Clinical Consequences of Changes in Bladder Behavior in Multiple System Atrophy

Onset of Urinary Symptoms in Relation to the Diagnosis of Parkinsonism

Two retrospective studies [3, 10] confirmed that approximately 60% of patients with MSA develop urinary symptoms either preceding or at the time of presentation with parkinsonism. Many of these patients sought urologic advice early in the course of their disease.

Nature of the Urinary Symptoms

Although urinary symptoms may also be a feature of PD, the incontinence that occurs in patients with MSA is more severe. Incomplete bladder emptying may be a factor that contributes significantly to the incontinence in MSA, and a raised postmicturitional residual volume is much more likely in MSA than in PD. Worsening urinary control after urologic surgery (transurethral resection of the prostate in men or anti-incontinence procedures in women) is common in patients with

Table 15.2   Urogenital criteria suggesting a diagnosis of multiple system atrophy

Urinary symptoms preceding or presenting with parkinsonism

Male erectile dysfunction preceding or presenting with parkinsonism
Urinary incontinence
Significant postmicturition residue (>100 ml)
Worsening bladder control after urologic surgery

MSA: In one study, all patients who underwent prostatic surgery were incontinent either immediately after or within 1 year after surgery [3].

Suggested Clinical Urogenital Criteria for a Diagnosis of Multiple System Atrophy

As described in the section Sexual Dysfunction in Idiopathic Parkinson's Disease and Multiple System Atrophy, male erectile dysfunction (MED) is often the first symptom of MSA. The clinical criteria relating to the urogenital symptoms suggesting a diagnosis of MSA are shown in Table 15.2. The urologist confronted with a patient showing these features should be cautious of embarking on an operative approach [10]. The neurologist encountering a patient with marked urinary symptoms might consider future investigation by sphincter electromyography (EMG) if available.

Sphincter Electromyography

Selective atrophy of the anterior horn cells (Onuf's nucleus) is a characteristic feature of MSA. The changes of chronic reinnervation that occur in the motor units of the anal sphincter [11] and the urethral sphincter [4] have been demonstrated by EMG. Because in PD the anterior horn cells of Onuf's nucleus are not affected, sphincter EMG was proposed as a means of distinguishing between PD and MSA [12].

The mean prolongation of the duration of response of sphincter motor units is the most important indicator by which changes of chronic reinnervation are identified. The reference range of values for duration of motor unit response is wide [3, 5, 13–15], but a mean duration of greater than 10 milliseconds is higher than the upper limit of all normal studies [16]. In a retrospective analysis of sphincter EMG in 126 patients with parkinsonism, Palace et al. [17] found that 82% of patients who were subsequently diagnosed as having MSA had had an abnormal sphincter EMG (i.e., mean duration greater than 10 milliseconds).

The neurophysiologic details of sphincter EMG are discussed in Chapter 9. Both the anal and urethral sphincters are innervated by the anterior horn cells in Onuf's nucleus, and similar changes of chronic reinnervation—that is, prolongation of the mean duration of motor unit responses—have been demonstrated in both sphincters in patients with MSA [3]. As the anal sphincter is more superficial and needle EMG of this sphincter causes less discomfort, testing this sphincter is preferable. By varying the position of the needle electrode, 10 different motor

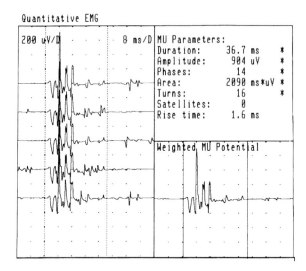

Figure 15.1   A motor unit recorded from the anal sphincter of a patient with multiple system atrophy shows an abnormally prolonged duration (upper range of normal is less than 10 milliseconds) and stable low-amplitude late components. See Chapter 9. (D = division; EMG = electromyography; MU = motor unit.)

units can be identified and the overall mean duration calculated. The highly stable but low-amplitude late components, which may be separated from the initial part of the complex by an isoelectric period of several milliseconds (Figure 15.1), should be included in the measurement of duration of individual units [17].

Bladder and Idiopathic Parkinson's Disease

Urodynamics studies of several series of patients with PD have found that the most common abnormality is detrusor hyperreflexia [18–24]; the reported incidence varies between 45% and 93%. Several possible causes have been postulated for detrusor hyperreflexia in PD. The hypothesis that has been most widely proposed is that the basal ganglia have an inhibitory effect on the micturition reflex in health, and, with cell loss in the substantia nigra, detrusor hyperreflexia emerges. Experimental evidence of an inhibitory role for the basal ganglia comes from animal data: In cats, electrical stimulation of the areas in and around the nucleus ruber, substantia nigra, and subthalamus inhibited the rhythmic contractions of the bladder that had been induced by distension [25, 26]. These rhythmic contractions were also inhibited by intracerebroventricular administration of a D1-receptor agonist but were not affected by a D2-receptor agonist [25]. Marmosets with parkinsonism induced by MPTP (1-methyl-4-phenyl-1,2,3,6-tetrahydropyridine) were found to have detrusor hyperreflexia [27], and evidence that D1 receptors are the main inhibitory influence on the micturition reflex was also established for the primate model [28].

Clinical studies examining the effect of L-dopa or apomorphine hydrochloride on bladder behavior in patients with PD have produced conflicting results. In patients showing "on-off" phenomena, cystometry performed in both states showed a lessening of hyperreflexia with L-dopa administration in some patients and a worsening in others [24]. In one study [29], a similar unpredictable effect was found on detrusor hyperreflexia when subcutaneous apomorphine hydrochloride was given, although in another, all those with detrusor hyperreflexia improved [30].

Some authors have suggested that an impaired relaxation, or *bradykinesia*, of the urethral sphincter can result in voiding dysfunction due to bladder outflow obstruction [21, 29, 31], whereas an earlier study suggested that the effect of L-dopa was to increase bladder neck obstruction [32]. A study in which subcutaneous apomorphine hydrochloride was given to patients with PD and urinary symptoms showed that administration of apomorphine hydrochloride reduced bladder outflow resistance and improved voiding in all 10 patients [29]. The authors proposed that this intervention be used to demonstrate the reversibility of outflow obstruction in men with PD before prostatic surgery is undertaken.

Clinical Consequences of Change in Bladder Behavior in Parkinson's Disease

In patients with true PD and bladder symptoms, establishing the pathophysiologic basis of symptoms may be fairly difficult, and treatment is often problematic. Typically, patients present with advanced disease, with the bladder symptoms appearing some years after initiation of treatment for PD [10]. Patients complain of urgency and frequency that may be severe, as well as of urge incontinence, particularly if poor mobility compounds their bladder disorder so that they may not reach the toilet in time. Due to a combination of detrusor overactivity and unimpaired detrusor contractions during voiding, these patients usually have a relatively small postmicturition residue [10, 33].

Many male patients with PD may be in the age group in which bladder outflow obstruction due to benign prostatic hyperplasia is a common coexisting disorder. Those with outflow obstruction complain of voiding symptoms, such as a hesitancy and a poor flow, and may also have urgency, because obstruction itself can cause detrusor overactivity [34]. Thus, urinary symptoms in a patient with PD can be similar to those associated with benign prostatic enlargement. A flow rate test and cystometry with pressure-flow measurements is recommended, although sometimes the bladder overactivity (due either to detrusor hyperreflexia caused by PD or to detrusor instability as a consequence of benign prostatic hyperplasia) is so severe that the bladder capacity is inadequate to allow assessment of flow rate with a reasonable volume (Figure 15.2).

Treatment of Urinary Symptoms

Inappropriate urologic surgery should be avoided in patients with MSA; a conservative approach with medical measures to manage incontinence can be highly effective. Detrusor hyperreflexia is treated with anticholinergic medication, such as oxybutynin chloride, propantheline bromide, or tolterodine tartrate, which diminishes the parasympathetic effect on bladder smooth muscle. This therapy is usually tried in patients with urgency and frequency, but side effects due to the anticholinergics—a dry mouth, in particular—may be exacerbated because of the anticholinergic medication given to treat parkinsonian tremor.

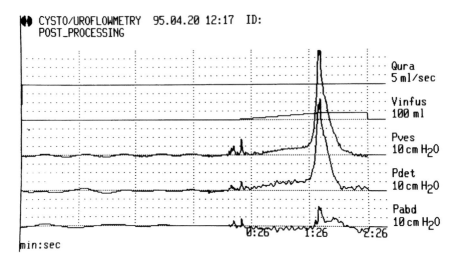

Figure 15.2   Bladder capacity at which an overactive bladder contraction is recorded is much reduced at 50 ml. A medium rate of filling (50 ml/minute) was used. The high pressure of the detrusor contraction (Pdet 100 cm H_2O) resulted in urge incontinence. Filling such bladders to a reasonable volume to obtain a reliable voiding study may prove difficult. (cysto = cystometrogram; Pabd = abdominal [rectal] pressure; Pves = intravesical pressure; Qura = flow of urine; Vinfus = volume infused.)

Pergolide mesylate, which acts on both D1 and D2 receptors, has been tried in a small number of patients with Parkinson's disease and bladder symptoms, and treatment with 100–250 µg was reported to produce a significant improvement both symptomatically and urodynamically in a limited trial [35].

Many patients with MSA progress to develop incomplete bladder emptying. Estimation of the postvoid residual urine volume is a simple and useful test in such patients, as they may be unaware that their bladders do not empty completely. If the patient has a significant postmicturition residue and is symptomatic, this aspect of the problem should be managed by intermittent catheterization if possible. In patients with advanced disease and severe neurologic disability, however, a permanent indwelling catheter or urosheath drainage may be required.

Nocturnal polyuria can be estimated by a frequency volume chart and controlled by desmopressin acetate, which may also be beneficial for stabilizing the blood pressure in those with autonomic failure [7].

A number of the earlier studies examining "Parkinson's disease" and the bladder probably included patients with MSA, and the notion that patients with PD have a poor outcome after prostatic surgery may well have been due to the inadvertent inclusion of some men with MSA in these studies [22, 36]. However, more recent research studies have recognized the potential problem and have provided information regarding the certainty of neurologic diagnosis. Urologic intervention is not contraindicated in men with PD, but treating

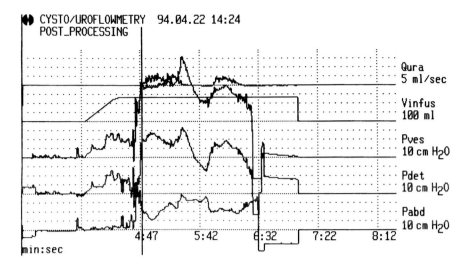

```
CYSTO/UROFLOWMETRY  94.04.22 14:24
POST_PROCESSING
```

Qura
5 ml/sec

Vinfus
100 ml

Pves
10 cm H₂0

Pdet
10 cm H₂0

Pabd
10 cm H₂0

4:47   5:42   6:32   7:22   8:12

min:sec

Figure 15.3 Voiding cystometrogram was recorded from a man aged 65 with Parkinson's disease. The top trace (Qura) shows the urine flow rate, which is measured in milliliters per second. This study shows some evidence of detrusor hyperreflexia during the filling phase; the bladder capacity was 280 ml. The voiding pressure is high and the flow rate poor, indicating bladder outflow obstruction. The patient had a transurethral resection of the prostate and was maintained on anticholinergic therapy for his detrusor overactivity with a good therapeutic result. (cysto = cystometrogram; Pabd = abdominal [rectal] pressure; Pdet = detrusor pressure; Pves = intravesical pressure; Vinfus = volume infused.)

these patients with anticholinergic medication first is reasonable if storage symptoms are prominent. If conservative measures fail, then a voiding cystometrogram to demonstrate obstructed voiding should be performed before urologic intervention is considered. If convincing evidence of prostatic obstruction is found, a prostatectomy should be considered, as some men with PD do benefit from a transurethral resection of the prostate [10, 36]. Patients who do undergo outflow surgery often need to continue their anticholinergic medication postoperatively to suppress detrusor overactivity (Figure 15.3). Obviously, in patients with troublesome frequency and urgency and advanced neurologic disease, any urologic intervention will not have the expected benefits, and conservative management must be considered. With advances in medical therapy for benign prostatic hyperplasia [37–39], trial of any of the uroselective α-blockers, such as tamsulosin hydrochloride, alfuzosin hydrochloride, or doxazocin mesylate, or of the 5-α reductase inhibitor finasteride should be given. Such an approach is certainly the appropriate one for a patient with a combination of detrusor hyperreflexia, obstructed voiding, and a small capacity bladder (Figure 15.4), for whom prostatic surgery should be avoided if possible.

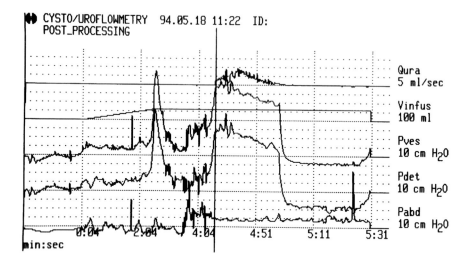

Figure 15.4   Urodynamic tracing recorded from a 70-year-old man shows high-amplitude detrusor hyperreflexia during the filling phase, a small functional bladder capacity, and some evidence of bladder outflow obstruction (poor peak flow rate with high voiding pressure). The combination of these findings is difficult to manage, and medical measures should be tried as outlined in the text. (cysto = cystometrogram; Pabd = abdominal [rectal] pressure; Pdet = detrusor pressure; Pves = intravesical pressure; Qura = flow of urine; Vinfus = volume infused.)

SEXUAL DYSFUNCTION IN PARKINSON'S DISEASE AND MULTIPLE SYSTEM ATROPHY

Both animal experiments and human studies provide evidence that dopaminergic mechanisms are involved in determining libido and causing penile erection. In animals, the medial preoptic area of the hypothalamus has been shown to regulate sexual drive, and selective stimulation of D2 dopaminergic receptors in this region of the brain increases sexual activity in rats [40]. An increase in libido in some patients with Parkinson's disease treated with L-dopa is a well-observed problem [41], although the extent to which this problem occurs is not known.

Estimates of the prevalence of MED in men with PD show that it is a significant problem, affecting 60% of a group of men in one study; by comparison, the prevalence in an age-matched healthy nonparkinsonian group was 37.5% [42]. The cause of MED in PD is unclear, but it usually affects men only some years after the neurologic disease has been established [10]. A survey of young patients with Parkinson's disease (mean age, 49.6 years) and their partners revealed a high level of dysfunction; the most severely affected couples were those in which the patient was male. MED and premature ejaculation were complaints in a significant proportion, although in general terms sexual dysfunction appeared to be multifactorial with no simple single cause identified [43].

Dopaminergic agonists induce erection in rats and monkeys, and spontaneous erections have been reported in patients treated with L-dopa. Administration of apomorphine hydrochloride induced a "durable erection" in 7 of 10 selected men with psychogenic impotence; the side effect of nausea was diminished by using a sublingual preparation [44]. Subcutaneous injections of apomorphine hydrochloride used to treat complicated motor fluctuations have also been found to benefit sexual function [45].

A striking feature of MSA is that the first symptom in men is often MED. Appearance of this symptom usually predates the onset of any other neurologic symptoms by several years [3]. The disorder appears chronologically to be quite separate from the development of postural hypotension [46], and the reason for the apparent early selective development of MED is not known. Preserved erectile function is a clinical feature that argues strongly against a diagnosis of MSA. Nothing is known about the sexual dysfunction of women with MSA.

REFERENCES

1. Quinn N. Parkinsonism—recognition and differential diagnosis. BMJ 1995;310:447–452.
2. Wenning GK, Ben Shlomo Y, Magalhaes M, et al. Clinical features and natural history of multiple system atrophy—an analysis of 100 cases. Brain 1994;117:835–845.
3. Beck RO, Betts CD, Fowler CJ. Genito-urinary dysfunction in multiple system atrophy: clinical features and treatment in 62 cases. J Urol 1994;151:1336–1341.
4. Kirby RS, Fowler CJ, Gosling J, Bannister R. Urethro-vesical dysfunction in progressive autonomic failure with multiple system atrophy. J Neurol Neurosurg Psychiatry 1986;49:554–562.
5. Sakakibara R, Hattori T, Tojo M, et al. Micturitional disturbance in multiple system atrophy. Jpn J Psychiatry Neurol 1993;47:591–598.
6. Sung JH, Mastri AR, Segal E. Pathology of the Shy-Drager syndrome. J Neuropathol Exp Neurol 1978;38:253–268.
7. Mannen T, Iwata M, Toyokura Y, Nagashima K. Preservation of a certain motor neurone group in amyotrophic lateral sclerosis: its clinical significance. J Neurol Neurosurg Psychiatry 1977;4:464–469.
8. Wilcox CS, Aminoff MJ, Penn W. Basis of nocturnal polyuria in patients with autonomic failure. J Neurol Neurosurg Psychiatry 1974;37:677–684.
9. Mathias CJ, Fosbraey P, da Costa DF, et al. The effect of desmopressin on nocturnal polyuria, overnight weight loss and morning postural hypotension in patients with autonomic failure. BMJ 1986;293:353–354.
10. Chandiramani VA, Palace J, Fowler CJ. How to recognize patients with parkinsonism who should not have urological surgery. Br J Urol 1997;80:100–104.
11. Sakuta M, Nakanishi T, Toyokura Y. Anal muscle electromyograms differ in amyotrophic lateral sclerosis and Shy-Drager syndrome. Neurology 1978;28:1289–1293.
12. Eardley I, Quinn NP, Fowler CJ. The value of urethral sphincter electromyography in the differential diagnosis of parkinsonism. Br J Urol 1989;64:360–362.
13. Stocchi F, Carbone A, Inghilleri M, et al. Instrumental diagnosis of multiple system atrophy. Adv Neurol 1996;69:421–424.
14. Valldeoriola F, Valls-Sole J, Tolosa E, Marti M. Striated anal sphincter denervation in patients with progressive supranuclear palsy. Mov Disord 1995;10:550–555.
15. Fowler CJ, Kirby RS, Harrison MJG, et al. Individual motor unit analysis in the diagnosis of disorders of urethral sphincter innervation. J Neurol Neurosurg Psychiatry 1984;47:637–641.
16. Fowler CJ. Pelvic Floor Neurophysiology. In C Binnie (ed), Clinical Neurophysiology (vol 1). Oxford, UK: Butterworth–Heinemann, 1995;233–250.
17. Palace J, Chandiramani VA, Fowler CJ. Value of sphincter electromyography in the diagnosis of multiple system atrophy. Muscle Nerve 1997;20:1396–1403.
18. Andersen JT, Hebjorn S, Frimodt-Moller C, et al. Disturbances of micturition in Parkinson's disease. Acta Neurol Scand 1976;53:161–170.
19. Murnaghan GF. Neurogenic disorders of the bladder in parkinsonism. Br J Urol 1961;33:403–409.
20. Raz S. Parkinsonism and neurogenic bladder: experimental and clinical observations. Urol Res 1976;4:133–138.

21. Pavlakis AJ, Siroky MB, Goldstein I, Krane RJ. Neurourologic findings in Parkinson's disease. J Urol 1983;129:80–83.
22. Berger Y, Blaivas JG, DeLaRocha ER, Salinas JM. Urodynamic findings in Parkinson's disease. J Urol 1987;138:836–838.
23. Berger Y, Salinas JN, Blaivas JG. Urodynamic differentiation of Parkinson disease and the Shy Drager syndrome. Neurol Urodyn 1990;9:117–121.
24. Fitzmaurice H, Fowler CJ, Rickards D, et al. Micturition disturbance in Parkinson's disease. Br J Urol 1985;57:652–656.
25. Lewin RJ, Dillard GV, Porter RW. Extrapyramidal inhibition of the urinary bladder. Brain Res 1967;4:301–307.
26. Yoshimura N, Sas M, Yoshida O, Takaori S. Dopamine D1 receptor–mediated inhibition of micturition reflex by central dopamine from the substantia nigra. Neurourol Urodyn 1992;11:535–545.
27. Albanese A, Jenner P, Marsden C, Stephenson J. Bladder hyperreflexia induced in marmosets by 1-methyl-4-phenyl-1,2,3,6-tetrahydropyridine. Neurosci Lett 1988;87:46–50.
28. Yoshimura N, Mizuta E, Kuno S, et al. The dopamine D1 receptor agonist SKF 38393 suppresses detrusor hyperreflexia in the monkey with parkinsonism induced by MPTP. Neuropharmacology 1993;32:315–321.
29. Christmas TJ, Chapple CR, Lees AJ, et al. Role of subcutaneous apomorphine in parkinsonian voiding dysfunction. Lancet 1988;2:1451–1453.
30. Aranda B, Cramer P. Effect of apomorphine and L-dopa on parkinsonian bladder. Neurourol Urodyn 1993;12:203–209.
31. Galloway NTM. Urethral sphincter abnormalities in parkinsonism. Br J Urol 1983;55:691–693.
32. Murdock M, Olsson C, Sax D, Krane R. Effects of levodopa on the bladder outlet. J Urol 1975;113:803.
33. Hattori T, Yasuda K, Kita K, Hirayama K. Voiding dysfunction in Parkinson's disease. Jpn J Psychiatry Neurol 1992;46:181–186.
34. Abrams PH, Farrar DJ, Turner-Warwick R, et al. The results of prostatectomy: a symptomatic and urodynamic analysis of 152 patients. J Urol 1979;121:640–642.
35. Yamamoto M. Pergolide improves neurogenic bladder in patients with Parkinson's disease. Mov Disord 1997;12(suppl 1):P328.
36. Staskin DS, Vardi Y, Siroky MB. Post-prostatectomy continence in the parkinsonian patient: the significance of poor voluntary sphincter control. J Urol 1988;140:117–118.
37. Boyle P, Gould A, Roehrborn C. Prostate volume predicts outcome of treatment of benign prostatic hyperplasia with finasteride: meta-analysis of randomised clinical trials. Urology 1996;48:398–405.
38. Kirby R, Pool J. Alpha adrenoreceptor blockade in the treatment of benign prostatic hyperplasia: past, present and future. Br J Urol 1997;80:521–533.
39. Lepor H, Williford W, Barry M, et al. The efficacy of terazosin, finasteride, or both in benign prostatic hyperplasia. N Engl J Med 1996;335:533–539.
40. Argiolas A, Melis M, Mauri A, Gessa G. Paraventricular nucleus lesion prevents yawning and penile erection induced by apomorphine and oxytocin but not ACTH in rats. Brain Res 1987;421:349–352.
41. Uitti R, Tanner C, Rajput A et al. Hypersexuality with antiparkinsonism therapy. Clin Neuropharmacol 1989;5:375–383.
42. Singer C, Weiner WJ, Sanchez-Ramos JR, Ackerman M. Sexual dysfunction in men with Parkinson's disease. J Neurol Rehabil 1989;3:199–204.
43. Brown RG, Jahanshahi M, Quinn N, Marsden CD. Sexual function in patients with Parkinson's disease and their partners. J Neurol Neurosurg Psychiatry 1990;53:480–486.
44. Heaton J, Morales A, Adams M, et al. Recovery of erectile function by the oral administration of apomorphine. Urology 1995;45:200–206.
45. O'Sullivan J, Hughes A. Apomorphine-induced penile erections in Parkinson's disease. Mov Disord 1998;13:536–539.
46. Kirchhof K, Mathias CJ, Fowler CJ. The relationship of uro-genital dysfunction to other features of autonomic failure in MSA. Clin Auton Res 1999: in press.

16
Disorders of Bowel Function in Parkinsonism

Fabrizio Stocchi

In his classic 1817 monograph, James Parkinson described the gastrointestinal dysfunction of patients with the shaking palsy: "food is with difficulty retained in the mouth until masticated; and then as difficultly swallowed. . . . the saliva fails of being directed to the back part of the fauces, and hence is continually draining from the mouth. . . . the bowels which all along had been torpid, now in most cases, demand stimulating medicines of very considerable power: the expulsion of the feces from the rectum sometimes requiring mechanical aid" [1].

At this point, interest in the intestinal dysfunction associated with Parkinson's disease (PD) and other parkinsonian syndromes has been renewed [2–4], because not only does this dysfunction interfere with effective treatment of the condition, but it also causes distressing symptoms. The majority of patients with parkinsonism depend for their mobility on the blood level of L-dopa, which is a large neutral amino acid absorbed only from the small bowel. L-Dopa has a short half-life, and any factor that limits or delays its absorption results in the reappearance of parkinsonian symptoms. This chapter reviews the intestinal dysfunction of PD patients.

SWALLOWING ABNORMALITIES AND ESOPHAGEAL ALTERATIONS

Dysphagia and a variety of swallowing abnormalities are well-recognized complications of PD (Table 16.1). Logemann et al. reported abnormal lingual control of swallowing [5]. Blonsky et al. described lingual "festination," in which elevation of the tongue prevented passage of the bolus into the pharynx [6]. Robbins et al. [7] described delay of the swallowing reflex and noted a tendency to aspiration. Bushmann et al. reported a repetitive and involuntary reflux from the vallecula and piriform sinuses into the oral cavity and observed that some patients have great difficulty swallowing pills, with prolonged retention in the vallecula [8].

Table 16.1   Swallowing abnormalities associated with Parkinson's disease

Disturbed lingual peristalsis
Piecemeal swallowing
Vallecular and piriform sinus residue
Coating of pharyngeal walls
Decreased relaxation of pharynx after swallow
Increased oral transit time
Bolus falling over base of tongue
Vestibular aspiration
Decreased laryngeal elevation
Decreased oral mobility
Drooling of saliva

Dopaminergic drugs improve swallowing in some patients [9], whereas anticholinergics may inhibit the process.

The main esophageal alterations in patients with parkinsonism are nonperistaltic swallowing, belching, segmental spasms, esophageal dilatation, and gastroesophageal reflux [10]. Belching can be related to "on-off" fluctuations [11] and may disappear when the patient is "on." Bramble et al. suggested that cholinergic rather than dopaminergic mechanisms are more important in the control of esophageal motility in patients with parkinsonism and showed that intravenous administration of atropine sulfate produced marked disruption of coordination in response to swallows in patients with PD compared with control subjects [12].

Patients with swallowing or esophageal problems may benefit from the use of a liquid formulation of L-dopa (L-dopa methyl ester), dispersible Madopar [13], or from the subcutaneous injection of the dopamine receptor agonist apomorphine hydrochloride [14]. Anticholinergic drugs should be withdrawn, but in some patients with severe drooling of saliva, peripheral anticholinergic belladonna folium may be useful. Drooling is not related to salivary hypersecretion, however, but rather to pooling of saliva within the mouth as a consequence of impaired deglutition [15]. Some patients suffer from achalasia, which can be treated with injection of botulinum toxin into the cardia.

STOMACH

Gastroparesis or delayed gastric emptying can occur in PD [16, 17] and other causes of parkinsonism and can produce a variety of symptoms, such as early satiety, abnormal discomfort with bloating, nausea, vomiting, weight loss, and even malnutrition.

L-Dopa is not absorbed from the stomach, and delayed gastric emptying may delay and blunt the achievement of peak plasma L-dopa levels, adversely affecting the clinical response to the dose [18]. When L-dopa is taken after meals, it may be poorly absorbed because of delayed gastric emptying due to the bulk, tonicity, and composition of the food [19, 20]. Lipids and carbohydrates, as well as some drugs, such as dopamine agonists or anticholinergics, may delay gastric emptying as well. Excessive gastric acidity also delays gastric emptying, but excessive neutralization of stomach contents may lead to incomplete dissolution of the L-dopa tablets and thus incomplete absorption [21]. Gastric emptying may also be delayed by PD itself or by constipation because of the gastrocolic reflex. Research has demonstrated that in patients with parkinsonism, tablets may remain in the stomach for a long time, delaying L-dopa from reaching intestinal absorptive sites. Moreover, the enzyme dopa-decarboxylase is present in the gastric mucosa and may convert L-dopa trapped in the stomach due to gastroparesis into dopamine, making it unavailable for central nervous system delivery and use [22]. Furthermore, dopamine formed in the stomach may stimulate gastric dopamine receptors, promote stomach relaxation, and inhibit gastric motility, potentially worsening the gastroparesis [23, 24].

Many authors have shown that the direct infusion of liquid L-dopa into the duodenum ensures a more reliable and predictable response to the drug [25]. Moreover, the L-dopa plasma levels are more stable after intraduodenal infusion than after intragastric infusion [26]. These studies indicate the relevant role of the stomach in the pathophysiology of motor fluctuations in patients with parkinsonism. L-Dopa is absorbed only from the small bowel, mostly the duodenum, although some absorption occurs in the jejunum and ileum. Despite the high capacity of the large neutral amino acid transporters, there may be competition between L-dopa and other dietary large neutral amino acids, such as valine, leucine, and isolucine [27].

Liquid L-dopa may improve symptoms in patients with motor fluctuations, ensuring better absorption. L-Dopa methyl ester and dispersible Madopar are absorbed more quickly than are standard L-dopa preparations (Figure 16.1), especially when the drug is taken after meals [13]. Subcutaneous infusion of dopamine agonists (apomorphine hydrochloride and lisuride maleate) [28] are effective in controlling motor fluctuations, bypassing the gastrointestinal tract. Patients with parkinsonism should be told to eat small meals, to avoid protein during the day, and to take the drugs when fasting. Use of domperidone and cisapride sometimes may help. Other common gastric symptoms in patients with parkinsonism are epigastric fullness and bloating, and vomiting.

SMALL BOWEL

The literature contains references both to symptoms and to radiologic signs suggestive of small intestine motor dysfunction in patients with PD, but the frequency and functional significance of these findings remain uncertain.

Weight loss is a frequent finding in elderly patients with Parkinson's disease [29, 30], although the reasons for this have not been fully explained. An increase in energy expenditure has been shown in two studies [29,31]; other possible contributing factors include dietary deficiency [32] and malabsorption due to small bowel bacterial overgrowth. Davies et al. [33] showed a reduced absorption of mannitol with an increase in the lactulose-to-mannitol ratio; these findings suggest a reduction in the absorptive surface area of the small intestine in patients with parkinsonism, possibly a specific alteration in the enterocyte brushborder membrane. These authors did not find any evidence of small bowel bacterial contamination, whereas other studies have suggested small bowel bacterial

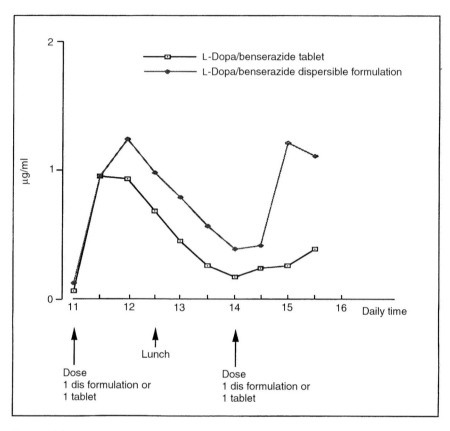

Figure 16.1   L-Dopa plasma levels after administration of L-dopa/benserazide hydrochloride tablet (125 mg) and L-dopa/benserazide hydrochloride dispersible (dis) formulation (125 mg) before and after lunch. Note the better absorption of the liquid formulation.

overgrowth as a cause of malabsorption, even when the small bowel is anatomically normal [34, 35].

Davies et al. also found a significantly prolonged orocecal transit time in patients with Parkinson's disease compared with healthy elderly subjects. This prolongation was not related to disease severity or duration and may be due to disordered gastrointestinal autonomic function. Lewy bodies have been found in the sympathetic vertebral chain and in the ganglionic coeliacus of patients with Parkinson's disease [36, 37], resulting in an autonomic or enteric nervous system dysfunction.

LARGE BOWEL

With regard to the large bowel, the symptoms are clearer and their frequency is known to be high in the PD population [38, 39]. Constipation is by far the most common bowel complaint, and in one survey 50% of patients had a defecation frequency of less than once daily, compared with 12% in age-matched control subjects [40]. In a questionnaire study we conducted of a group of PD patients, 76.5% of the patients reported a bowel frequency of less than three evacuations per week; 94% reported hard stools and straining difficulty of defecation; and 88% reported continuous use of laxatives or enemas, or both. In our series of a group of severe PD patients [41], 41% of the patients were referred for fecal incontinence, 35% for liquid stools, and 5% for solid feces. Seventy-six percent of the patients reported that the onset or worsening of these bowel dysfunctions followed the onset of neurologic symptoms.

Constipation is defined as a decrease in frequency of bowel movements to less than three bowel movements per week [42]. The stools may be hard and pelletlike or large and difficult to pass. In general, constipation may be caused by one or several mechanisms: (1) functional obstruction due to increased segmental contractions, (2) poor colonic contractions (colonic inertia or pseudo-obstruction), or (3) functional outlet obstruction [43]. Particular symptoms may suggest the likely underlying cause of constipation. All patients usually have abdominal discomfort, but patients with increased segmental contractions are more likely to have lower abdominal cramps associated with irritable bowel syndrome. Patients with nausea and vomiting are more likely to have an absence of postprandial colonic contractions [44]. Straining at stool and incomplete evacuation suggest outlet obstruction.

In PD, constipation may be the result of several malfunctions. For stool expulsion to occur, fecal material must first be propelled by colonic muscle contraction and then expelled through the coordinated action of the rectum, anal sphincters, and pelvic floor muscles, as well as the musculature of the abdominal wall and diaphragm [45]. In parkinsonism, constipation may be due to outlet-type dysfunction, but colonic inertia may also be present [46–48]. In colonic inertia, the problem seems to be in the musculature of the colon, which causes a slow transit of feces through the colon [48, 49]. Several authors showed that the mean colon transit time is considerably prolonged in PD patients [50–52]. Although the role of dopamine in colonic motility has not been defined, constipation may be related to a direct involvement of the colonic myenteric plexus by the PD process. Singaram et al. [53] compared colonic tissue from 11 patients with advanced PD, 17 with adenocarcinoma (nonmalignant tissue was studied), and 5 who underwent colectomy for severe constipation. Immunohistochemical techniques were used to stain myenteric and submucosal neurons for dopamine, tyrosine hydroxylase, and vasoactive intestinal polypeptide (VIP). Each class of neuron was quantified as a percentage of the total neuronal population stained for the neuronal marker protein gene product (PGP) 9.5. Nine of the 11 Parkinson's disease patients had substantially fewer dopaminergic myenteric neurons than the other subjects. Little difference was found between the groups in numbers of tyrosine hydroxylase and VIP neurons. High-performance liquid chromatography showed lower levels of dopamine in the muscularis externa (but not mucosa) in four PD patients compared with controls, but levels of dopamine metabolites were similar in two groups. The authors also confirmed the findings of others [54, 55] who showed that most Lewy bodies in the gut were in VIP-immunoreactive neurons, whereas in the sympathetic ganglia all Lewy-body-containing neurons were immunoreactive for tyrosine hydroxylase. These findings suggest that slow colonic transit may be related to direct involvement of the colonic myenteric plexus by the PD process.

Outlet-type dysfunction in patients with PD is due mainly to an inability to relax the pelvic floor and so reduce the anorectal angle [45, 56]. Normal defecation occurs at a socially convenient time, after rectal distension by fecal material is perceived. Defecation is achieved by inhibition of the tonic resting activity in the striated sphincter musculature and relaxation of the puborectalis muscle sling, which permits straightening of the rectoanal angle, allowing the contents of the rectum into the anal canal. Simultaneously, relaxation occurs in the external anal sphincter muscle. When the individual strains to defecate, co-contraction of glottic, diaphragm, and abdominal wall muscles occurs. Rectal evacuation is achieved by a combination of raised intra-abdominal pressure and relaxation of the anal sphincter muscles, often aided by colonic pressure waves. Previous descriptions of electromyographic (EMG) activity during simulated defecation have confirmed that, in normal subjects, inhibition of the external anal sphincter and puborectalis muscles occurs [57]. In subjects with normal EMG sphincter muscle relaxation, activity in the adjacent gluteal muscles does not change when recorded under laboratory conditions [56]. Mathers et al. [45] showed that the selective pattern of muscle contraction and inhibition that accompanies defecation is disturbed in some patients with parkinsonism who suffer from constipation. Paradoxical activation of the puborectalis and external anal sphincter muscles occurred, and some patients also showed a tendency to recruit gluteal muscles during simulated defecation straining.

When the puborectalis fails to relax or even contracts during defecation, the forward passage of stool is impaired, and defecation is obstructed. Paradoxical anal sphincter muscle contraction resembling anismus-type pelvic outlet obstruction may occur as well [56].

Anorectal manometry has revealed several abnormalities in patients with parkinsonism, including low basal and impaired squeeze pressures, prominent phasic fluctuations during squeeze, and a hypercontractile response to rectosphincteric reflex [52].

We studied anorectal function in 17 patients, 8 men and 9 women; the mean age was 62 years [41]. The mean duration of disease was 10.5 years (standard deviation, 5 years); the Hoehn and Yahr stage ranged from 2 to 5. Four hours after the patient received a cleansing enema, anorectal manometry was performed with a multilumen catheter (outer diameter of 4 mm) with distal side openings spaced 5 mm apart.

Three lumens were continuously perfused (0.5 ml/minute) with bubble-free distilled water by means of a low-compliance pneumohydraulic capillary infusion system and were connected through an external transducer to a multichannel polygraph. A latex balloon was attached to the tip of the catheter, 5 cm from the nearest recording side hole. When suspended in air and inflated with 50 ml of air, the balloon was 6.5 cm long and 4 cm wide. Intraluminal balloon pressures were recorded and transmitted to the polygraph via a fourth lumen. With the subject lying on the left side, the manometric probe was introduced into the rectum so that all recording holes were positioned within the ampulla. The manometric catheter was then withdrawn through the anal canal using a station pull-through technique. The probe was then reintroduced into the rectum and withdrawn into the anal canal, with the recording sensors at 10, 15, and 20 mm from the anal verge. The operator kept the manometric probe firmly in place throughout the study period. The protocol included three maneuvers: anal sphincter squeezing, progressive intermittent distension of the intrarectal balloon, and straining. In the PD patients, we found a mean resting anal pressure of 49 ± 19 mm Hg and a maximal contraction pressure of 99 ± 40 mm Hg lasting 15.6 ± 6.8 seconds; all these results were lower than normal. Three patients were unable to contract the anal sphincter. Resting and squeezing anal pressures were inversely related to disease duration. Maximal anal contraction pressure was higher in patients with a lower degree of disability (Hoehn and Yahr stage 2–3). The threshold of the inhibitory anal reflex and rectal compliance was within the normal range; the mean threshold of rectal sensitivity (70 ± 58 ml air) was in the upper range of the normal values. Manometric recordings during straining showed a lack of anal inhibition in 11 patients (65%).

Altered voluntary anal contraction and paradoxical anal contraction during straining have been reported in PD patients before [52]. Our study confirmed the presence of inadequate relaxation of the sphincter canal during straining. One possible explanation is manometric expression of abdominopelvic dyssynergia, as recorded by EMG in other studies [58].

In PD and in multiple system atrophy (MSA), the manometric finding of a paradoxical contraction or insufficient inhibition of the anal canal during straining could be considered part of the generalized extrapyramidal motor disorder and so could be unrelated to degeneration of the sacral nuclei. Its frequent occurrence in patients with idiopathic constipation [59] and in children with functional megarectum [60] indicates that the abnormality is not strictly related to the specific neurologic alterations of idiopathic PD or MSA but rather is related to a focal dystonia [56] of the abdominopelvic muscles.

The finding of a low resting anal tone has not been consistently reported in PD patients; the investigation described earlier confirms that, although resting anal pressure may be within the normal range in PD, some patients have marked hypotonia. Because the resting anal pressure is essentially due to the contractile activity of the internal anal sphincter—a function mainly regulated by the sympathetic nervous system—this abnormality may reflect a degenerative lesion of the spinal cord intermediolateral columns or autonomic ganglia [36].

Alternative explanations for the reduced anal pressure during rest and voluntary contraction can be found in the possible presence of anatomic changes in the internal and external anal sphincter due to age-related degeneration or continuous straining efforts or both; in the attempt to overcome the defecation difficulty, these changes may possibly lead to traction neuropathy involving the distal fibers of the pudendal nerves.

Irrespective of its pathophysiology, the reduced anal tone during resting conditions and voluntary contraction could explain the relatively high frequency of episodes of fecal incontinence with liquid stools frequently reported by PD patients, especially after laxative treatment. The inefficient voluntary anal contraction found in PD patients may be due to their inability to recruit the external anal sphincter muscles.

Although many therapies have been advocated for the treatment of constipation in PD, few have been subjected to clinical trial. Jost and Schimrigk reported both symptomatic improvement and an acceleration of colon transit in PD patients with constipation after treatment with the prokinetic agent cisapride (an agent that increases the release of acetylcholine in the myenteric plexus) [61]. Ashraf et al. reported that use of psyllium increased stool frequency and weight but did not alter colonic transit or anorectal function in PD patients with confirmed constipation [62]. Astarloa et al. reported that following a diet rich in insoluble fiber produced a significant improvement in constipation, as indicated by an increase in stool frequency and an improvement in stool consistency [63]. A fascinating observation of this study was a parallel improvement in extrapyramidal function, which in turn appeared to relate to an increase in the bioavailability of orally administered L-dopa. The authors suggested that this increase in L-dopa absorption and resultant improvement in clinical status was related to an augmentation of gastrointestinal motility and thereby of drug delivery. Suppression of defecation could result in delayed gastric emptying, possibly via a gastrocolic reflex [64, 65], which could explain why treatments that improve constipation may improve the extrapyramidal disorder.

Difficulty in relaxing the pelvic floor and paradoxical puborectalis contraction generally respond well to dopaminergic drugs. Paradoxical EMG activity of the pelvic floor and sphincter tend to persist even in the "on" phase. However, a definite improvement in pelvic outlet obstruction was demonstrated with proctography after administration of apomorphine hydrochloride [45].

The practical outcome of this is that patients should try to defecate when in the "on" phase or should take a quick-acting drug, such as L-dopa methyl esther [13] or apomorphine hydrochloride injection, to quickly turn the patient "on." Unfortunately, some patients still experience difficulty, even when motor disability has otherwise been reversed by dopaminergic drugs. In these patients, the injection of botulinum toxin in the puborectalis muscle or in the external anal sphincter may be useful. Botulinum toxin injection may also be helpful in patients with painful anismus.

Laxatives may help patients with normal pelvic floor relaxation. On the other hand, encouraging laxative use in patients who cannot defecate effectively due to pelvic floor dystonia only produces adverse effects and adds further to their difficulties.

REFERENCES

1. Parkinson J. An essay on the shaking palsy. London: Whittingham and Rowland, 1817.
2. Edwards LL, Quigley EMM, Pfeiffer RF. Gastrointestinal dysfunction in Parkinson's disease: frequency and pathophysiology. Neurology 1992;42:726–732.
3. Edwards LL, Pfeiffer RF, Quigley EMM, et al. Gastrointestinal symptoms in Parkinson's disease. Mov Disord 1991;6:151–156.
4. Edwards LL, Quigley EMM, Hofman R, et al. Gastrointestinal symptoms in Parkinson's disease: 18-month follow-up study. Mov Disord 1993;8:83–86.
5. Logemann JA, Blonsky ER, Boshes B. Lingual control in Parkinson's disease. Trans Am Neurol Assoc 1973;98:276–278.
6. Blonsky ER, Logemann JA, Boshes B, et al. Comparison of speech and swallowing function in patients with tremor disorders and in normal geriatric patients: a cinefluorographic study. J Gerontol 1975;30:299–303.
7. Robbins JA, Logemann JA, Kirschner HS. Swallowing and speech production in Parkinson's disease. Ann Neurol 1986;19:283–287.
8. Bushmann M, Dobmeyer SM, Leeker L, et al. Swallowing abnormalities and their response to treatment in Parkinson's disease. Neurology 1989;39:1309–1314.
9. Calne DB, Shaw DG, Spiers ASD, et al. Swallowing in parkinsonism. Br J Radiol 1970;43:456–457.
10. Gibberd FB, Gleeson JA, Gossage AAR, et al. Oesophageal dilatation in Parkinson's disease. J Neurol Neurosurg Psychiatry 1974;37:938–940.
11. Kempster PA, Lees AJ, Crichton P, et al. Off-period belching due to a reversible disturbance of oesophageal motility in Parkinson's disease and its treatment with apomorphine. Mov Disord 1989;4:47–52.

12. Bramble MG, Cunliffe J, Dellipiani W. Evidence for a change in neurotransmitter affecting oesophageal motility in Parkinson's disease. J Neurol Neurosurg Psychiatry 1978;41:709–712.
13. Steiger MJ, Stocchi F, Bramante L, et al. The clinical efficacy of single morning doses of levodopa methyl esther, dispersible madopar and sinemet plus in Parkinson's disease. Clin Neuropharmacol 1992;15:501–504.
14. Muguet D, Broussolle E, Chazot G. Apomorphine in patients with Parkinson's disease. Biomed Pharmacother 1995;49:197–209.
15. Eadie MJ, Tyrer JH. Alimentary disorders in parkinsonism. Aust Ann Med 1965;114:3–22.
16. Sulla M, Hardoff R, Gilardi N, et al. Gastric emptying time and gastric motility in patients with untreated Parkinson's disease [abstract]. Mov Disord 1996;11(suppl 1):167.
17. Djaletti R, Baron J, Ziv I, et al. Gastric emptying in Parkinson's disease: patients with and without response fluctuations. Neurology 1996;46:1051–1054.
18. Baruzzi A, Contin M, Riva R, et al. Influence of meal ingestion time on pharmacokinetics of orally administered levodopa in parkinsonian patients. Clin Neuropharmacol 1987;10:527–537.
19. Dubois A. Diet and gastric digestion. Am J Clin Nutr 1985;42:1002–1005.
20. Kelly KA. Motility of the Stomach and Gastroduodenal Junction. In LR Johnson (ed), Physiology of the Gastrointestinal Tract. New York: Raven Press, 1981.
21. Leon AS, Speigel H. The effect of antacid administration on the absorption and metabolism of levodopa. J Clin Pharmacol 1972;12:263–267.
22. Evans MA, Broe GA, Triggs EJ, et al. Gastric emptying rate and the systemic availability of levodopa in the elderly parkinsonian patient. Neurology 1981;31:1288–1294.
23. Valenzuala JE. Dopamine as a possible neurotransmitter in gastric relaxation. Gastroenterology 1976;71:1019–1022.
24. Berkowitz DM, McCallum RW. Interaction of levodopa and metoclopramide on gastric emptying. Clin Pharmacol Ther 1980;27:414–420.
25. Ruggieri S, Stocchi F, Carta A, et al. Jejunal delivery of levodopa methyl ester [letter]. Lancet 1989;2:8653:45–46.
26. Kurlan R, Rothfield KP, Woodward WR, et al. Erratic gastric emptying of levodopa may cause "random" fluctuations of parkinsonian mobility. Neurology 1988;38:419–421.
27. Wade DN, Mearrik PT, Birkett DJ, et al. Active transport of L-dopa in the intestine. Nature 1973;242:463–465.
28. Stocchi F, Ruggieri S, Viselli F, et al. Subcutaneous Lisuride Infusion. In JPWF Lakke, EM Delhaas, AWF Rutgers (eds), New Trends in Clinical Neurology: Parenteral Drug Therapy in Spasticity and Parkinson's Disease. Carnforth, UK: Parthenon Publishing Group, 1992.
29. Levi S, Cox M, Lugon M, et al. Increased energy expenditure in Parkinson's disease. BMJ 1990;301:1256–1257.
30. Yapa RSS, Playfer JR, Lye M. Anthropometric and nutritional assessment of elderly patients with Parkinson's disease. J Clin Exp Geront 1989;11:155–164.
31. Markus HS, Cox M, Tomkins AM. Raised energy expenditure in Parkinson's disease and its relationship to muscular rigidity. Clin Sci 1992;83:199–204.
32. Davies KN, King D, Davies H. A study of the nutritional status of elderly patients with Parkinson's disease. Age Ageing 1994;23:142–145.
33. Davies KN, King D, Billington D, Barrett JA. Intestinal permeability and orocaecal transit time in elderly patients with Parkinson's disease. Postgrad Med J 1996;72:164–167.
34. McEvoy A, Dutton J, James OFW. Bacterial contamination of the small intestine is an important cause of malabsorption in the elderly. BMJ 1983;287:789–793.
35. Montgomery RD, Haboubi NY, Mike NH, et al. Cause of malabsorption in the elderly. Age Ageing 1986;15:235–240.
36. Den Hartog Jager WA, Bethlem J. The distribution of Lewy bodies in the central and autonomic nervous system in idiopathic paralysis agitans. J Neurol Neurosurg Psychiatry 1960;23:283–290.
37. Ohama E, Ikuta F. Parkinson's disease: distribution of Lewy bodies and monoamine neuron system. Acta Neuropathol 1976;34:311–319.
38. Kupsky WJ, Grimes MM, Sweeting J, et al. Parkinson's disease and megacolon: concentric hyaline inclusions (Lewy bodies) in enteric ganglionic cells. Neurology 1987;37:1253–1255.
39. Lewitan A, Nathanson L, Slade WR. Megacolon and dilatation of the small bowel in parkinsonism. Gastroenterology 1952;17:367–374.
40. Pallis CA. Parkinsonism: natural history and clinical features. BMJ 1971;3:683–690.
41. Stocchi F, Badiali D, Vacca L, et al. Anorectal function in multiple system atrophy and Parkinson's disease. Mov Disord 1999 (in press).
42. Thompson WG, Dotevall G, Drossman DA, et al. Irritable bowel syndrome: guidelines for the diagnosis. Gastroenterol Int 1989;2:92–95.

43. Reynolds JC, Ouyang A, Lee C, et al. Chronic severe constipation. Gastroenterology 1987;92:414–420.
44. Bazzocchi G, Ellis J, Villanueva-Meyer J, et al. Postprandial colonic transit and motor activity in chronic constipation. Gastroenterology 1990;98:686–693.
45. Mathers SE, Kempster PA, Law PJ, et al. Anal sphincter dysfunction in Parkinson's disease. Arch Neurol 1989;46:1061–1064.
46. Lubowski DZ, Swash M, Henry M. Neural mechanisms in disorders of defecation. Baillieres Clin Gastroenterol 1988;2:210–223.
47. Martelli H, Devroede G, Arhan P, et al. Mechanisms of idiopathic constipation: outlet obstruction. Gastroenterology 1978;75:623–631.
48. Arhtan P, Devroede G, Jehannin B, et al. Segmental colon transit time. Dis Colon Rectum 1981;24:625–629.
49. McLean RG, Smart RC, Gaston-Perry D, et al. Colon transit scintigraphy in health and constipation using oral I-131-cellulose. J Nucl Med 1990;31:985–989.
50. Metcalf AM, Phillips SF, Zinsmeister AR, et al. Simplified assessment of segmental colonic transit. Gastroenterology 1987;92:40–47.
51. Jost WH, Schimrigk K. Constipation in Parkinson's disease. Wien Klin Wochenschr 1991;69:906–909.
52. Edwards LL, Quigley EMM, Harned RK, et al. Characterisation of swallowing and defecation in Parkinson's disease. Am J Gastroenterol 1994;89:15–25.
53. Singaram C, Ashraf W, Gaumnitz EA, et al. Dopaminergic defect of enteric nervous system in Parkinson's disease patients with chronic constipation. Lancet 1995;346:861–864.
54. Wakabayashi K, Takahachi H, Ohama E, Ikuta F. Tyrosine hydroxylase-immunoreactive intrinsic neurons in the Auerbach's and Meissner's plexuses of humans. Neurosci Lett 1989;96:259–263.
55. Wakabayashi K, Takahachi H, Ohama E, Ikuta F. Parkinson's disease: an immunohistochemical study of Lewy body–containing neurons in the enteric nervous system. Acta Neuropathol 1990;79:581–583.
56. Mathers SE, Kempster PA, Swash M, et al. Constipation and paradoxical puborectalis contraction in anismus and Parkinson's disease: a dystonic phenomenon? J Neurol Neurosurg Psychiatry 1988;51:1503–1507.
57. Floyd WF, Walls EW. Electromyography of the sphincter ani externus in man. J Physiol 1953;122:599–609.
58. Ger G-C, Wexner SD, Jorge JMN, Salanga VD. Anorectal manometry in the diagnosis of paradoxical puborectalis syndrome. Dis Colon Rectum 1993;36:816–825.
59. Whitehead WE, Devroede G, Habib FI, et al. Functional disorders of the anorectum. Gastroenterol Int 1992;5:92–108.
60. Loening-Baucke VA, Cruikshank BM. Abnormal defecation dynamics in chronic constipated children with encopresis. J Pediatr 1986;108:562–566.
61. Jost WH, Schimrigk K. Cisapride treatment of constipation in Parkinson's disease. Mov Disord 1993;8:339–343.
62. Ashraf W, Pfeiffer RP, Park F, et al. Constipation in Parkinson's disease: objective assessment and response to psyllium. Mov Disord 1997;6:946–951.
63. Astarloa R, Mena MA, Sanchez V, et al. Clinical and pharmacological effects of a diet rich in insoluble fiber on Parkinson's disease. Clin Neuropharmacol 1992;15:375–380.
64. Kellow JE, Gill RC, Wingate DL. Modulation of human upper gastrointestinal motility by rectal distension. Gut 1987;28:864–868.
65. Tjeerdsma HC, Smout AJPM, Akkermans LMA. Voluntary suppression of defecation delays gastric emptying. Dig Dis Sci 1993;38:832–836.

17
Urinary Incontinence in the Elderly

Derek J. Griffiths

Bladder problems are common among the elderly. Although the number of possible symptoms is quite limited (e.g., incontinence, voiding difficulty, frequency, urgency), the possible causes are varied. They include changes in the bladder itself, the pelvic floor, or the urethra, or changes in the control of these organs. Good control requires an intact nervous system, from the cerebral cortex to the peripheral level, and dysfunction at any level may affect it.

Characteristic changes in the lower urinary tract occur in middle age. Urinary incontinence, which is involuntary loss of urine that constitutes a medical or hygienic problem [1], is one possible consequence. Its overall prevalence is at least 5%; the incidence is higher in women than in men [2]. Among middle-aged women, especially after multiple births, the muscles of the pelvic floor may weaken, allowing the bladder base to descend or become more mobile. These changes are associated with loss of urine during mechanical stress, such as coughing or sneezing (see the following section, Types of Urinary Incontinence). Descent of the bladder base (cystocele) is sometimes also associated with poor bladder emptying—that is, a low urinary flow rate and substantial residual urine after voiding. Among men aged 50–60 years, the prostate may become enlarged. Enlargement may lead to urethral obstruction, so that during voiding the rate of flow of urine is reduced and the bladder (detrusor) pressure becomes abnormally elevated. Incomplete bladder emptying and symptoms of frequency and urgency often accompany prostatic enlargement or urethral obstruction. As men and women become elderly, new problems may develop: For example, the prevalence of urinary incontinence rises to approximately 15% among elderly men and women living in the community and to more than 50% among those living in institutions [2].

Urodynamic measurements show that the strength of voiding detrusor contractions tends to decline with age [3]. Correspondingly, the volume of postvoid residual urine becomes noticeably larger among elderly patients. This decline in contractility appears to be associated with degenerative changes in the bladder, particularly in muscle cells and nerve axons [4]. Among older men, elevated postvoid residual urine levels are often ascribed to prostatic obstruction. However, the volume of residual urine tends to become larger with age in women also.

265

In some cases, urinary incontinence may develop in later life because of acute causes, such as a urinary infection, a recent stroke, or acute confusion, and is potentially transient—that is, it is reversible either spontaneously or by appropriate treatment. In other cases, the incontinence may become established and may present a more serious clinical problem. This chapter is concerned with established incontinence.

TYPES OF URINARY INCONTINENCE

The International Continence Society has defined four types of urinary incontinence—urge, stress, reflex, and overflow [1]—on the basis of symptoms and urodynamic characteristics. Reflex incontinence occurs almost exclusively in patients with suprasacral spinal cord lesions. The bladder and urethra operate automatically and involuntarily, often in an uncoordinated (dyssynergic) manner. Overflow incontinence is defined as leakage of urine from an overdistended bladder. It occurs in association with a few specific conditions, such as end-stage prostatic obstruction, late-stage diabetes, and sacral cord lesion. Reflex and overflow incontinence are not considered further in this chapter.

The defining urodynamic characteristic of stress incontinence is the leakage of urine during a period of raised abdominal pressure, in the absence of a detrusor contraction. The term *genuine stress incontinence* is used to describe this urodynamically diagnosed condition [1]. Although it is the predominant type of incontinence among middle-aged women, stress incontinence is relatively less common among the female geriatric population. Surveys suggest that the prevalence of stress incontinence stabilizes or decreases in older women [5].

Urge incontinence is defined as leakage of urine accompanied by an urgent desire to void. The characteristic symptom is "not being able to make it to the bathroom in time." It is often accompanied by the symptoms of urinary frequency and nocturia. Urodynamically, urge incontinence is associated with involuntary contraction of the detrusor, which is a manifestation of overactive bladder function, considered in more detail later. It represents a failure of voluntary control of the voiding reflex. Objective urodynamic demonstration of urge incontinence requires observation of leakage of urine during an involuntary detrusor contraction, accompanied by the sensation of urgency, and in the absence of elevated abdominal pressure.

Urinary incontinence that first appears in later life appears to be mainly urge incontinence. Among geriatric patients, for example, urinary incontinence is most frequently of this type [6]. As pointed out earlier, elderly people often fail to empty the bladder completely when they void. The combination of involuntary detrusor contraction, leading to urge incontinence, and incomplete bladder emptying has been termed *detrusor hyperactivity with impaired contractile function* [7]. The condition is particularly difficult to treat, because interventions aimed at reducing involuntary detrusor contractions usually impair detrusor contractility further.

Overactive bladder function is a topic with a number of controversial aspects, and the following is a personal view. Involuntary detrusor contractions may be responsible for urine loss both in patients with spinal cord injuries or neurologic diseases, and in some patients without overt neurologic abnormality. In the early years of urodynamics, it was agreed to refer to involuntary contractions as *detrusor hyperreflexia* if they appeared to be due to a neurologic lesion and as *detru-*

sor instability if no obvious neurologic lesion was present [8]. The term *overactive bladder function* was introduced to cover both of these possibilities. Detrusor hyperreflexia is clearly abnormal, but involuntary detrusor contractions are frequently observed in symptom-free volunteers [8], especially if observations are continued for long periods [9]. Therefore, involuntary detrusor contractions probably should not be considered abnormal unless they are associated with symptoms. Consequently, neither detrusor instability nor overactive bladder function is necessarily abnormal, although they may be so. During urodynamic investigations, merely demonstrating involuntary detrusor contractions is not sufficient; they must also be shown to cause relevant symptoms, such as urge incontinence.

A further complication is that correct use of the terms *detrusor instability* and *detrusor hyperreflexia* depends on whether a relevant neurologic lesion can be recognized, and this may change over time. Until recently, urge incontinence in an elderly patient probably would have been ascribed to detrusor hyperreflexia if it followed a clearly defined cerebrovascular accident, but to detrusor instability in many other situations. Now, partly as a result of the research described in this chapter, nearly all detrusor overactivity leading to urge incontinence in the frail elderly would probably be classified as detrusor hyperreflexia.

In an attempt to resolve this unsatisfactory situation, a different classification of overactive bladder function has been introduced [10]. It is based mainly on urodynamic observations rather than presumed etiology. With some simplification, if phasic involuntary contractions of the detrusor are observed during bladder filling, the condition is called *phasic detrusor instability*. If just one involuntary contraction occurs that terminates bladder filling and causes urine leakage, the condition is called *uninhibited overactive bladder*; bladder sensation is often reduced as well. The authors of this scheme have shown that uninhibited overactive bladder is particularly common among the elderly and appears to be associated with cortical dysfunction [10]. Phasic detrusor instability is more common in younger patients who have symptoms of frequency, urgency, or urge incontinence but do not show overt neurologic disease. The reflex detrusor contractions observed in patients with suprasacral spinal cord injury are termed *spinal detrusor hyperreflexia*.

For many years, researchers have known that voluntary voiding is controlled in the brain and that the regions involved include the medial surface of the frontal lobe (the superior frontal gyrus and anterior cingulate gyrus) [11]. Therefore, when incontinence develops in later life, a satisfying chain of hypotheses would be that it is related to lesions in these areas of the cortex, that these impair voluntary control of the bladder and cause urge incontinence, and that the underlying type of overactive bladder function is the uninhibited overactive bladder. Results bearing on the hypothesis are discussed in this chapter.

RESEARCH FINDINGS

Urodynamic Findings in the Frail Elderly with Established Incontinence

One study was concerned with 128 elderly patients (76 women and 52 men) referred for established incontinence from a tertiary geriatric rehabilitation program [6, 12]. Any who were bedridden or who had an indwelling catheter, mul-

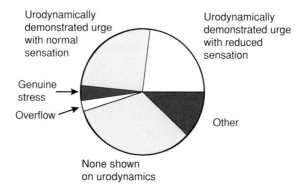

Figure 17.1   Relative frequency of different types of incontinence among 128 incontinent geriatric patients as assessed by videourodynamics. Patients with urodynamically demonstrated urge incontinence and reduced bladder-filling sensation constitute or those with urodynamically demonstrated urge incontinence and normal bladder-filling sensation were the largest abnormal groups.

tiple sclerosis, or overt infrapontine or peripheral neuropathy were excluded. The median age was 79 years. Approximately one-half had a score below 24/30, the conventional criterion for dementia, on the Mini-Mental State Examination (MMSE). Clinical diagnoses of type of dementia are unreliable, but a clinical diagnosis of possible primary degenerative dementia was reported in 20 patients and of possible multi-infarct dementia in 8 patients.

After discontinuation of any medication intended to influence bladder function, patients underwent comprehensive investigations, including 24-hour monitoring of incontinence and voiding, videourodynamic examination, cognitive testing, and single photon emission computed tomography (SPECT) of the brain [13]. Twenty-four-hour monitoring included measurement of total urine loss by weighing of pads, recording of fluid intake, recording of all voids with a uroflowmeter, and performance of three ultrasonographic measurements of postvoid residual urine volume at different times of day. Videourodynamic testing was used to establish type of incontinence and bladder-filling sensation; urge incontinence was considered objectively demonstrated only if actual urine leakage, associated with an involuntary detrusor contraction, was observed during the test. Bladder-filling sensation was classified as reduced if the sensation of bladder fullness was denied until an involuntary contraction, leading to leakage, started to develop.

The types of incontinence found on urodynamic testing in these patients are shown in Figure 17.1. Genuine stress incontinence and overflow incontinence were rare. Urge incontinence was objectively demonstrated during urodynamic testing in approximately one-half of the patients, and in approximately one-half of these, bladder-filling sensation was reduced. In patients with urge incontinence and reduced bladder sensation, the overactive detrusor function responsible for the incontinence was of the uninhibited overactive bladder type (see earlier)—that is, just one involuntary contraction occurred that led to urine leakage and terminated bladder filling.

The 24-hour monitoring showed that patients with urge incontinence objectively demonstrated on urodynamics experienced large amounts of urine leakage. Leakage was even more severe if bladder-filling sensation was reduced.

Established Urge Incontinence in the Frail Elderly: Evidence for a Cerebral Etiology

Incontinent geriatric patients often have some cognitive impairment, either because of cerebrovascular accidents or because of degenerative diseases. Sometimes, such people are assumed to be incontinent *because* they are cognitively impaired—that is, they forget to go to the bathroom until it is too late, or they void in inappropriate places because they do not know any better. However, not all cognitively impaired elderly people are incontinent, and not all incontinent elderly are cognitively impaired. Some studies have failed to show any association between cognitive impairment and incontinence [14].

In the study referred to in the section Urodynamic Findings in the Frail Elderly with Established Incontinence [6, 12], cognitive testing was carried out using the MMSE [15] and also the Cambridge Cognitive Examination (CAMCOG) [16], which provides a global score and subscores for different aspects of cognitive function. Functional SPECT scans, showing regional brain perfusion, were interpreted blindly by an experienced radiologist. His written reports were independently coded for underperfusion of each of 14 brain regions (7 on each side), and also for global underperfusion of the left and right cortical hemispheres (cortical thinning) [17].

Another 27 continent elderly patients who attended the same institution and who were similar in age, sex ratio, and cognitive status underwent cognitive testing with the MMSE and SPECT scanning of the brain as part of a workup for memory problems. They were used as a comparison group.

A significant but weak association was found between urge incontinence objectively demonstrated on urodynamics and overall cognitive impairment as demonstrated by the MMSE or the total CAMCOG score [18]. The association with one particular aspect of cognitive function—orientation, as measured by the CAMCOG—was much stronger (Figure 17.2), suggesting either that good orientation is important for bladder control or, more probably, that a specific region of the brain is important for both functions.

The SPECT brain scanning demonstrated that the perfusion of the cortex as a whole and of the frontal lobes in particular was reduced in patients with objectively demonstrated urge incontinence and reduced bladder sensation [17]. The reduced perfusion was particularly marked in the right superior frontal part of the cortex (Figure 17.3).

Possibility of Sex Differences

A striking difference was found between the sexes in the frequency of objectively demonstrated urge incontinence with reduced sensation (37% in men versus 16% in women; $P = .007$). Correspondingly, the association of this type of incontinence with reduced perfusion of the right frontal cortex was much clearer in men than in

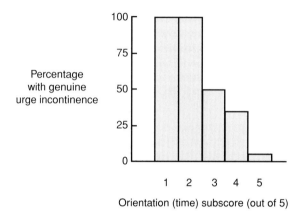

Figure 17.2 Bar graphs showing the relationship between urge incontinence and temporal orientation. Each bar shows, for those patients testing at a given value of the Cambridge Cognitive Examination subscore for temporal orientation, the percentage in whom urge incontinence was demonstrated urodynamically (as shown in Figure 17.1). (Reprinted with permission from DJ Griffiths, PN McCracken, GM Harrison, KN Moore. Urinary incontinence in the elderly: the brain factor. Scand J Urol Nephrol Suppl 1994;157:83–88.)

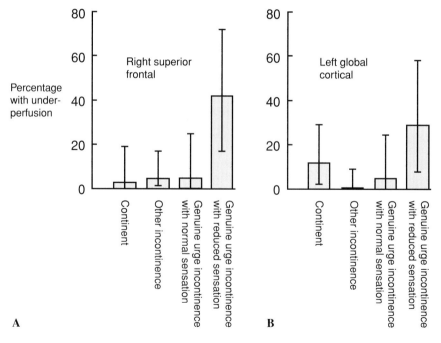

Figure 17.3 Percentage of patients in each of four patient groups (see Figure 17.1) with underperfusion of the right superior frontal region (**A**) and the left cortex as a whole (**B**). Vertical bars indicate 95% confidence intervals calculated from the binomial distribution. (Reprinted from DJ Griffiths, PN McCracken, GM Harrison, et al. Cerebral aetiology of urinary urge incontinence in elderly people. Age Ageing 1994;23:246–250. By permission of Oxford University Press.)

women. This difference may reflect a difference in the characteristic patterns of cortical dysfunction in the two sexes, or possibly a difference in cortical organization of bladder control, although the latter explanation seems unlikely in view of the positron emission tomography (PET) results reported in the following paragraph.

Results of Functional Brain Scanning in Young Men

PET scanning of the brains of young right-handed male volunteers has shed further light on these observations [19]. In these men, surprisingly, voiding control is localized on the right side from the cortex down to the brain stem, even though (in cats) the structures responsible for voiding control are present and functional on both sides of the brain [20]. A small area in the right inferior frontal region of the cortex is active when there is a voluntary intention to void; another area in the right superior frontal region is active during postponement of voiding when the bladder is full (see Figure 14.2). Further studies in younger women have confirmed these results [21], which are consistent with earlier, less detailed observations [11]. Presumably, in the elderly, lesions in these areas of the cortex may cause loss of voluntary control (urge incontinence) and reduced bladder sensation, as well as impaired orientation.

FACTORS THAT DETERMINE THE SEVERITY OF INCONTINENCE IN THE ELDERLY

In the group of incontinent elderly patients referred to in the previous section, many individual factors showed some statistical association with the severity of incontinence, as measured by the amount of urine leakage during 24-hour monitoring [22]. These include the urodynamic type of the incontinence, bladder sensation on urodynamics, previous urinary tract infection, activities of daily living score (related to mobility), fluid intake, number of voids during 24-hour monitoring, cognitive status, and regional brain underperfusion. Medications also appear to have some influence. A multiple regression analysis, intended to identify the most important of these interrelated factors, demonstrated the following.

On initial investigation, the behavioral factors of fluid intake and voiding frequency were among the most important. For each additional void per 24 hours, the amount of incontinence decreased by 31 ml. For each 100 ml less of fluid intake, the amount of incontinence decreased by 41 ml. Impaired orientation also affected the severity of incontinence. When patients were reinvestigated after several weeks of rehabilitation (and after any medical or behavioral intervention had been instituted), behavioral factors were less important; impaired orientation and reduced perfusion of the cortex as a whole both had significant effects on the amount of urine loss. Thus, both cortical and behavioral factors can be important determinants of severity of incontinence.

POSTVOID RESIDUAL URINE AND DETRUSOR HYPERACTIVITY WITH IMPAIRED CONTRACTILE FUNCTION

In the same group of patients, the volume of postvoid residual urine showed a diurnal variation and was largest in the early morning [23]. No clear association was found with cognitive impairment or regional brain perfusion [18]. Residual urine was associated with bladder capacity as measured during videourodynamics. Because the factors leading to poor bladder emptying (residual urine) are different from those associated with uninhibited overactive bladder and urge incontinence, the combination of detrusor overactivity and impaired detrusor contractility (detrusor hyperactivity with impaired contractile function) appears to be a fortuitous coincidence of two common conditions with different causes, rather than a single condition.

SUMMARY AND IMPLICATIONS OF THE FINDINGS

Urinary incontinence that develops in later life is characteristically of the urge type, and it is often accompanied by reduced sensation of bladder filling. This type of incontinence leads to particularly severe urine loss. The underlying urodynamic abnormality appears to be the uninhibited overactive bladder, as described by Geirsson et al. [10].

At least some proportion of this incontinence is associated with cortical changes, manifested as impaired orientation on cognitive testing and as cortical underperfusion, both globally and regionally in the frontal cortex, especially on the right side. These changes may be a consequence of cerebrovascular accidents or of degenerative disease. The right frontal part of the brain is involved in voluntary voiding. Lesions in this region probably impair voluntary control of voiding and lead to uninhibited overactive bladder and urge incontinence with reduced bladder sensation.

Because this type of incontinence depends on cortical changes, it is more common when cognitive impairment exists. However, cognitive impairment itself is unlikely to be the cause of the incontinence.

The combination of poor voluntary control and reduced sensation makes this type of incontinence particularly frustrating for caregivers, because the elderly patient has little warning of the impending need to void and may deny it only a short time before becoming wet. Realization that this behavior has an organic basis and is a characteristic part of the condition may make caregivers more tolerant of it.

Although established urge incontinence in the elderly clearly is unlikely to be curable, that behavioral factors are associated with its severity provides a scientific foundation for methods of management, such as fluid intake adjustment and regular or prompted voiding or toileting. Unfortunately, cognitive impairment and impaired mobility may make it difficult to use such behavioral measures successfully.

REFERENCES

1. International Continence Society. Standardisation of terminology of lower urinary tract function. Neurourol Urodyn 1988;7:403–426.
2. Urinary Incontinence in Adults: Clinical Practice Guideline. Rockville, MD: US Department of Health and Human Services, Public Health Service, Agency for Health Care Policy and Research, 1992;3. AHCPR publication 92-0038.
3. Van Mastrigt R. Quantification of lower urinary tract function and dysfunction. Neurourol Urodyn 1993;12:263–266.

4. El Badawi A, Yalla SV, Resnick NM. Structural basis of geriatric voiding dysfunction. IV. Bladder outlet obstruction. J Urol 1993;150:1681–1695.
5. Herzog H, Fultz N. Urinary incontinence in the community: prevalence, consequences, management, and beliefs. Top Geriatr Rehabil 1988;3:1–12.
6. Griffiths DJ, McCracken PN, Harrison GM, Gormley EA. Characteristics of urinary incontinence in elderly patients studied by 24-hour monitoring and urodynamic testing. Age Ageing 1992;21:196–201.
7. Resnick NM, Yalla SV. Detrusor hyperactivity with impaired contractile function: an unrecognized but common cause of incontinence in elderly patients. JAMA 1987;257:3076–3081.
8. International Continence Society. Fourth report on standardisation of terminology of lower urinary tract function. Terminology related to neuromuscular dysfunction of lower urinary tract. Br J Urol 1981;53:333–335.
9. Robertson AS, Griffiths CJ, Ramsden PD, Neal DE. Bladder function in healthy volunteers; ambulatory monitoring and conventional urodynamic studies. Br J Urol 1994;73:242–249.
10. Geirsson G, Fall M, Lindstrom S. Subtypes of overactive bladder in old age. Age Ageing 1993;22:125–131.
11. Morrison JFB. Bladder Control: Role of Higher Levels of the Central Nervous System. In M Torrens, JFB Morrison (eds), The Physiology of the Lower Urinary Tract. London: Springer-Verlag, 1987;237–274.
12. Griffiths DJ, McCracken PN, Harrison GM. Incontinence in the elderly: objective demonstration and quantitative assessment. Br J Urol 1991;67:467–471.
13. Hooper HR, McEwan AJ, Lentle BC, et al. Interactive three-dimensional region of interest analysis of HMPAO SPECT brain studies. J Nucl Med 1990;31:2046–2051.
14. Resnick NM, Yalla SV, Laurino E. The pathophysiology of urinary incontinence among institutionalized elderly persons. N Engl J Med 1989;320:1–7.
15. Folstein MF, Folstein SE, McHugh PR. "Mini-mental state": a practical method for grading the cognitive state of patients for the clinician. J Psychiatr Res 1975;12:189–198.
16. Roth M, Huppert FA, Tym E, Mountjoy CQ. CAMDEX: The Cambridge Examination for Mental Disorders of the Elderly. Cambridge, UK: Cambridge University Press, 1988.
17. Griffiths DJ, McCracken PN, Harrison GM, et al. Cerebral aetiology of urinary urge incontinence in elderly people. Age Ageing 1994;23:246–250.
18. Griffiths DJ, McCracken PN, Harrison GM, Moore KN. Urinary incontinence in the elderly: the brain factor. Scand J Urol Nephrol Suppl 1994;157:83–88.
19. Blok FMB, Willemsen ATM, Holstege G. A PET study on brain control of micturition in humans. Brain 1997;120:111–121.
20. Griffiths D, Holstege G, Dalm E, De Wall H. Control and coordination of bladder and urethral function in the brainstem of the cat. Neurourol Urodyn 1990;9:63–82.
21. Blok FMB, Sturms LM, Holstege G. Brain activation during micturition in women. Brain 1998;121:2033–2042.
22. Griffiths DJ, McCracken PN, Harrison GM, Moore KN. Urge incontinence in elderly people: factors predicting the severity of urine loss before and after pharmacologic treatment. Neurourol Urodynam 1996;15:53–57
23. Griffiths DJ, Harrison GM, Moore KN, McCracken PN. Variability of post-void residual urine volume in the elderly. Urol Res 1996;24:23–26.

18
Spinal Cord Injury

E. P. Arnold

A broad, interdisciplinary approach to the whole patient and to clinical decision making is central to good medical practice, but it is especially important in the management of those who have sustained the devastating experience of a spinal cord injury. Since the 1950s, a dramatic improvement has been seen not only in survival but also in the quality of life that such patients can expect. This improvement has been achieved by the establishment of designated spinal cord injury units; by improvements in general nursing care, particularly in lowering the risk of pressure areas; in improved quality and skill in all areas of rehabilitation, including mental, physical, social, and work areas; and by advances in the standards and scope of orthopedic and urologic care. Above all are the improved standards, enthusiasm, and cooperation of those dedicated to rehabilitation, including nurses, physiotherapists, occupational therapists, social workers, medical staff, and, of course, those who fund health care. Quality care must be patient-focused and crafted to meet patients' realistic goals and expectations.

In orthopedics, enormous progress has been made not only in spinal surgery techniques but also in improvement of hand function by techniques such as deltoid-to-triceps tendon transfers and improvement of wrist extension by rerouting of the brachioradialis tendon to the wrist extensors. These improvements mean that patients with C6 and C7 lesions can be provided with a key grip that permits some patients to undertake intermittent self-catheterization, which would not have otherwise been possible.

Although patients' problems with control of bladder, bowel, and sexual function after spinal cord injury are neurogenic, these patients are unlikely to be under the care of a neurologist. Their problems are quite different from those of patients with progressive neurologic disease for two reasons. First, as explained in this chapter, they are at significant risk of developing upper urinary tract damage and renal failure and must therefore remain under close urologic supervision. Second, whereas patients with progressive neurologic disease face the prospect of increasing disability, those who have suffered spinal cord injury are often otherwise fit and are younger. Thus, they require that their bladder dysfunction in particular

275

be dealt with once and for all, often by surgical means. However, a chapter about the problems of spinal cord injury is included here for interest and also because many of the techniques that have been developed to manage these patients can also be applied in patients with progressive neurologic disease.

CLASSIFICATION OF NEUROGENIC BLADDER DYSFUNCTION

Neurogenic bladder dysfunction can be categorized and described, but assigning it labels such as *upper motor neuron* or *autonomous* is counterproductive, because doing so assumes that we understand the site and nature of the pathologic lesion. Furthermore, the viscera are supplied by second-order neurons from sympathetic or parasympathetic ganglia, which confuses the definition of what is the upper or lower motor neuron. Approximately 10% of quadriplegic patients have an areflexic bladder. In some of these patients, specific neurophysiologic studies have identified a second lesion at the level of the conus or cauda equina that was not initially recognized [1]. Similarly, the term *autonomous bladder* is best avoided, as it does not specify the functional abnormality in the bladder, nor does it infer a level of the lesion. In the author's view, a better approach is to describe the particular bladder and urethral function and the ways in which bladder behavior is abnormal along the lines established by the International Continence Society, as shown in Table 18.1.

SPINAL SHOCK AND BLADDER MANAGEMENT

Spinal shock refers to the sudden cessation of spinal reflex activity in areas below the level of the injury and sometimes also in segments immediately above it. It lasts a variable time after trauma, from days to weeks. The striated muscles are hence flaccid, and the visceral smooth muscle activity is depressed, so that the bladder, rectum, and anus are all areflexic, and the pelvic floor is flaccid. Depending on the level of the lesion, hypotension may result because of lack of visceromotor reflexes.

After injury inflicted experimentally, sections of the spinal cord show hemorrhage followed by some hemorrhagic necrosis. Cellular and mitochondrial injury from impact can exaggerate the effects of the trauma. Cystic degeneration often follows and may extend to produce a post-traumatic syringomyelia ascending and descending from the level of the lesion, even years after the injury [2].

Acute urologic management therefore includes regular bladder drainage. In many spinal cord injury patients, such drainage is accomplished via a temporary suprapubic or urethral catheter to avoid overdistension of the bladder induced by the diuresis of the metabolic response to trauma and intravenous fluid administration and blood transfusions that may be required. Use of an indwelling suprapubic catheter rather than a urethral one can avoid the risk of urethritis or prostatitis, which, once established, can be difficult to eradicate. Our practice is to leave the bladder on continuous drainage until reflex activity reappears and then to convert most patients to intermittent self-catheterization. Some units can

Table 18.1   Categorization of bladder and urethral function

Detrusor activity
  Normal
  Overactive
    Hyperreflexic with or without failure to sustain contraction until the bladder is empty
    Low compliance
  Underactive
    Inappropriately low pressures, or pressures initially adequate but unsustained
    Areflexic
Bladder neck sphincter
  Normal
  Open
  Dyssynergic; instead of relaxing and funneling open when the detrusor contracts, the
    bladder neck becomes tighter and obstructs emptying
External urethral sphincter
  Normal
  Paralyzed
  Dyssynergic, indicating spastic contractions occurring while the detrusor is contracting
  Urethral instability, indicating urethral relaxations occurring spontaneously
Sensation
  Bladder
    Normal
    Abnormal—filling appreciated as an abdominal distension mediated by
      sympathetic fibers
  Urethra
    Normal
    Reduced or absent
    Hyperesthetic

institute sterile intermittent catheterization from the beginning if they have adequate numbers of staff available to do this as often as would be required to cope with the diuresis. Once through the initial phases of rehabilitation, the patient is instructed in the techniques of intermittent clean self-catheterization.

AUTONOMIC DYSREFLEXIA

Dangerous hypertensive episodes causing headache and risking cerebrovascular accidents are not uncommon. An episode can be triggered reflexively by any noxious stimulus from below the level of the spinal lesion. The stimulus may be somatic in origin, as in pressure areas or a fractured limb bone; or visceral, as in constipation, manual evacuation of bowel or enema, urethral catheterization, or even a bladder contraction. Such an episode is more likely in cases with upper thoracic lesions.

The pathogenesis of this syndrome is not well understood. The noxious stimulant is believed to lead to mass sympathetic overactivity within the cord. The result is intense vasospasm in skin and viscera supplied by segments of the cord that remain intact below the level of the lesion, and this causes the hypertension.

Skin pallor, sweating, and piloerection in these segments are seen. The hypertension is signaled by receptors in the aortic arch and carotid sinus that relay to the vasomotor center, which causes bradycardia and attempts to turn off the vasomotor spasm, resulting in vasodilation and redness in skin segments accessible to it above the level of the lesion.

Treatment is to withdraw the noxious stimulus if possible, raise the head of the bed, and give drugs to lower the blood pressure. Calcium-channel antagonists are often used.

For those who develop the syndrome or who experience increased frequency of it, a possible site of the noxious stimulus must be sought. This is not always easy in patients without sensation and may require intensive investigations, including abdominal computed tomography to detect cases in which an acute intra-abdominal process, such as appendicitis or cholecystitis, is the trigger.

To avoid precipitating autonomic dysreflexia, patients with spinal cord injuries who require bladder manipulations are given either a general anesthetic or a spinal anesthetic, despite their being unaware of any sensory input below their lesions. Patients who are catheterized or undergo urodynamic studies and who have a history of autonomic dysreflexia are monitored carefully during the procedures, which must be terminated if the blood pressure rises. Appropriate antihypertensive drugs should always be available and, if necessary, administered before the procedure.

RENAL DAMAGE IN PATIENTS WITH SPINAL CORD INJURY

Renal damage was common among patients with spinal cord injury in the early part of the twentieth century; together with sepsis and pressure sores, it was responsible for the high mortality, which approached 100%. Much of this risk can be avoided by meticulous management of lower urinary tract dysfunction. Renal damage can arise from stone formation, reflux, or obstruction.

Renal Stones

Patients are predisposed to renal stones by immobilization, which causes calcium reabsorption from the skeleton and muscle wasting from disuse, with purine degradation that increases uric acid excretion, as well as by the frequent incidence of urinary tract infections combined with urinary stasis.

Renal stones can be managed using the wide array of options now available, including electrohydraulic shock wave lithotripsy, percutaneous nephrolithotomy, and ureterorenoscopy.

Reflux Nephropathy

Reflux nephropathy is caused by post–spinal cord injury vesicoureteric reflux combined with intrarenal reflux of infected urine at high pressures. The risk of reflux seems greatest in the first 1–2 years after injury and occurs in approximately 10% of cases. Intrarenal reflux can lead to reflux nephropathy. The risk of reflux nephropathy seems to be related to high detrusor pressures [3]. The coarse pattern of scarring has been shown to be similar to that which occurs in cases of childhood reflux and reflux nephropathy [4].

Vesicoureteric reflux can be managed by ensuring a low-pressure system using anticholinergic medication and one or more of the methods listed in the section Bladder Management.

Obstructive Uropathy

The ureters may become dilatated because of resistance to drainage from the ureter via the ureteric orifice when the bladder wall is thickened, sacculated, and diverticulated, or when the resting pressures within the bladder are high due to low compliance or multiple phasic contractions.

Such dilation or obstruction responds in most cases to measures taken to lower bladder pressures and improve bladder emptying, as outlined in the following sections.

The key to reducing the risk of renal damage is to focus on lower urinary tract dysfunction, and this focus can be achieved by regular reassessment of patients, including performance on urodynamic studies.

BLADDER MANAGEMENT

The primary goals of bladder management are to achieve continence and to ensure satisfactory bladder emptying, which reduces the risk of urinary infection. The goal of any intervention should be to improve the patient's independence and at the same time to reduce the risk of upper urinary tract damage.

Bladder Emptying

Bladder emptying can be improved in many ways in spinal cord injury patients.

Shaped Wheelchair Cushion

Patients with spinal cord injury often have a lumbar lordosis, so that when they are seated in a wheelchair they effectively sit on the bulbar urethra; this can impede drainage. Such patients often notice that bladder drainage is better when they are lying down, although diuresis also increases when blood pressure, which is low in some patients while seated, returns to normal when they lie down. This pressure on the urethra can be avoided by using a U-shaped cushion.

Intermittent Self-Catheterization

If the patient has sufficient hand function, as do paraplegic patients and some patients with low-level quadriplegia, then intermittent self-catheterization can be useful. The aim is to achieve bladder emptying and reduce the risk of urinary tract infection. A clean intermittent self-catheterization technique is used. The catheter should be well lubricated and should be passed gently, particularly if any spasm occurs. After use, the catheter is washed without soap, dried, and kept in a clean plastic bag until next required. The same catheter can be used for a week. Some recommend use of a fresh catheter each time, but we have found this unnecessary.

Intermittent self-catheterization can also lead to continence in both areflexic and hyperreflexic bladders. If leakage occurs between catheterizations, use of an anticholinergic drug, such as oxybutynin chloride, may help. If leakage persists between catheterizations despite these measures, bladder emptying and continence must be addressed in other ways, as discussed in the section Continence.

Continuous Catheter Drainage

Continuous bladder drainage not only empties the bladder but also produces continence, unless hyperreflexic bladder spasms cause contraction around the balloon of the catheter and urethral leakage results.

In cases where continuous drainage is the method selected, use of a suprapubic catheter appears superior to use of a urethral catheter because of the decreased risk of urethritis and prostatitis, which can be difficult to eradicate. Suprapubic catheters for long-term drainage have been used regularly in our unit for the past 15–20 years. The advantages are that this method works well and offers less interference during sexual stimulation or intercourse, which is important when sexual functioning is possible [5].

The disadvantage of an indwelling catheter is that, as with any foreign body in the urinary tract, it can cause infection. In addition, when a balloon catheter is used, eggshell calculi can develop on the surface of the balloon; these can then drop off when the catheter is changed and form the nidus for bladder stone formation. An occasional complication of suprapubic catheters is that the tip can abut against the trigone, causing edema and vesicoureteric reflux. Many of these difficulties can be overcome by regular catheter care, including weekly bladder washouts and regular changing of the catheter every 2 weeks.

The risk of squamous cell carcinoma in spinal cord injury patients is small; however, the risk is considerably higher in this group than in the general population [6]. Whether the increased incidence is due to the presence of the catheter or to longstanding chronic infection is debated [7]. We now advise an annual cystoscopy after the first 5 years.

Medication

Striated muscle relaxants such as baclofen, which is a γ-aminobutyric acid antagonist acting at cord level, have been useful for reducing muscle spasms in limb muscles and to some extent in the pelvic floor as well. The aim is to reduce detrusor-sphincter dyssynergia and to improve bladder emptying.

Finding a drug to produce effective bladder smooth muscle excitation has been elusive, and as yet no drug exists that improves contractility. Cisapride, which improves gastric motility and emptying by facilitating acetylcholine delivery, was not effective when administered to a group of 21 patients with spinal cord injury [8].

External Urethral Sphincterotomy

In patients whose hand function is insufficient for intermittent self-catheterization via the urethra (or via a suprapubic continent diversion in quadriplegic patients), and in paraplegic patients who lack motivation, endoscopic ablation of the external urethral sphincter can be undertaken to allow more complete bladder emptying at lower pressures. The urine is then collected in a condom-type external urethral collecting device. The bladder drains more efficiently when the bladder contracts, but at other times the bladder neck is shut. If continuous drainage is sought and if ejaculation function can be sacrificed, then combining an external sphincterotomy with a bladder neck incision can improve the drainage even further.

External sphincterotomy is not always successful, partly because the dyssynergia affects the bulbospongiosus muscles, and late failures at this level or higher are not uncommon. The procedure can be repeated or a urethral stent considered.

The procedure traditionally was performed with an electrical cautery incision at the 12 o'clock position, commencing below the bladder neck and continuing to 5 cm distal to the verumontanum. Laser techniques are now used. The results appear similar [9]. The advantage of the laser techniques is that less bleeding occurs and morbidity is lower.

Before external sphincterotomy is undertaken, future management options must be considered. If a suprapubic catheter or continent diversion or sacral anterior root stimulator insertion are possible options, ablation of the external sphincter is best avoided, or urethral leakage might still occur after those procedures.

Urethral Stent

The technique of endoscopic placement of a wire mesh stent across the striated sphincter has been used with some success [10]. The procedure is not without complications. Stent removal is necessary at times because of migration, erosion, blocking of the lumen by granulations, or stones. This option is probably therefore best reserved for cases in which primary sphincterotomy has failed. Fewer complications were seen in the series of 25 men studied by Abdill et al. [11].

Suprapubic Diversion

Some quadriplegics who find intermittent self-catheterization of the urethra difficult because of poor hand function, and some women who cannot easily adduct their hips, can catheterize a suprapubic stoma. This method can be useful if bladder capacity is reasonable. In patients with overactive bladders, it can be combined with augmentation cystoplasty using a segment of bowel, or with detrusor myectomy. In detrusor myectomy, a large cap of the hypertrophied bladder muscle is removed, leaving the mucosa intact and effectively creating a large iatrogenic diverticulum of the bladder, which lowers pressures and improves functional bladder capacity. Either of these procedures can produce continence. Bladder emptying can then be achieved either by intermittent self-catheterization of the urethra or of a continent stoma, produced by a Mitrofanoff procedure, or a continent vesicostomy.

Ileal conduit urinary diversions were popular in the 1960s and 1970s, but in the long term this procedure led to upper urinary tract dilatation, and caution is now used in advising this procedure. It may still have a place in selected cases.

Continence

In men, an external condom-type urethral collecting device is often used to collect urinary drainage when the bladder contracts with high bladder pressures or when it leaks due to sphincter incompetence.

In women, no satisfactory external collecting device exists, and other measures, as discussed later, must be considered with the patient.

High Bladder Pressures

High bladder pressures develop because of a lack of coordinated urethral relaxation at the time that the detrusor contracts, so that a high isometric pressure rise occurs. This dilates the prostatic ducts; if infection is present, then the result can be chronic prostatitis, often with intraprostatic calculus formation.

The high pressure also results in bladder smooth muscle hypertrophy, trabeculation, sacculation, and diverticula formation. Vesicoureteric reflux can begin and does so in approximately 10% of cases after spinal cord injury. This carries the risk of renal damage due to reflux nephropathy. Bladder hypertrophy and high bladder pressures can also cause relative obstruction to ureteric drainage and ureteric dilatation without reflux. Hydronephrosis can ensue.

Incontinence is associated with overactive bladder dysfunction; therefore, the consensus is that every effort should be made to ensure that the neurogenic bladder does not function at high pressure.

Medication

Anticholinergic medication—for example, oxybutynin chloride—is often used on the basis that acetylcholine is the neuromuscular transmitter in the bladder. Its unwanted antimuscarinic side effects of dry mouth, blurred vision, and so forth can be avoided in some cases by administering the drug through intravesical instillation [12,13].

The α-adrenergic blockers, such as terazosin hydrochloride and phenoxybenzamine hydrochloride, have been used to reduce urethral smooth muscle tone and improve bladder emptying. In addition, some evidence exists that parasympathetic denervation leads to a change in the intramural ganglia in which dominance shifts to adrenergic stimulation of the intramural ganglion cell; alpha-blockers might then inhibit this ganglion cell and reduce contractility [14].

Overdistension

Deliberate, prolonged overdistension of the bladder with idiopathic detrusor instability has been used to reduce unstable activity. It has been noticed, but not well documented, that allowing the bladder to overfill in a patient recovering from spinal shock can delay the return of reflex activity. These observations were used in treating a group of quadriplegic patients by Iwatsubo et al. [15], who were able to convert 33 of 45 patients with quadriplegia to continence between intermittent self-catheterizations by that technique; however, the method is not often used.

Intravesical Instillation of Capsaicin

Capsaicin is a pungent ingredient of red chili peppers. It has a selective action on unmyelinated sensory neurons (C fibers) and has been used to reduce detrusor hyperreflexia [16]. In one study of 10 men with spinal cord injuries, capsaicin produced an increase in cystometric capacity in all but one; detrusor pressures were slightly lowered, and 3 patients were subjectively improved [17]. Because of its initial irritating effect on sensory neurons, capsaicin can produce autonomic hyperreflexia. More studies are required for adequate assessment of its place in therapy.

Sacral Deafferentation

Most centers that perform sacral anterior root stimulation for voiding in patients with spinal cord injury combine it with a sacral deafferentation performed at the same time that the electrodes are placed within the spinal canal. This procedure abolishes reflex activity in the detrusor and allows continence [18, 19]. The deafferentation of S2, S3, and S4 can be done at the level of the electrodes or higher up at the conus.

Deafferentation can be performed without electrode placement to achieve a flaccid bladder and reliable continence; bladder emptying is then achieved by intermittent self-catheterization or one of the other methods discussed here.

Detrusor Myectomy

Detrusor myectomy, or *bladder autoaugmentation*, refers to the removal of a patch of bladder muscle down to mucosa, across the dome and extending inferiorly so that approximately one-half the bladder wall muscle is removed. In effect, a diverticulum is created that bulges when the remaining detrusor muscle contracts, and this effectively lowers bladder pressures without the use of enteric segments. Although this procedure gives satisfactory results and increases bladder capacity at lower pressures, in some cases bladder compliance decreases with time.

Enterocystoplasty

Augmentation cystoplasty incorporates a detubularized segment of ileum or ileocecum, colon, or stomach into the bladder to produce a reservoir of larger capacity and low pressure. In patients with spinal cord injury, it is occasionally a useful adjunct to intermittent self-catheterization if bladder pressures are high and leakage is not controlled by intermittent self-catheterization and anticholinergics.

If the patient has difficulty performing intermittent self-catheterization via the urethra, an enterocystoplasty can be combined with creation of a suprapubic bladder diversion and surgical closure of the bladder neck. Intermittent self-catheterization can then be performed through the continent suprapubic stoma.

If the urethra and pelvic floor are weak, especially in women, then the procedure can be combined with implantation of an artificial urethral sphincter, or a cystourethropexy, such as a pubovaginal sling or colposuspension.

Bladder Emptying and Continence in Low-Pressure Areflexic Bladders

Intermittent self-catheterization is the preferable option for patients with low-pressure areflexic bladders. Some of these patients can void by Valsalva's maneuver and might even achieve reasonable emptying. However, this is not advised, as the chronic straining further stretches the paralyzed pelvic floor and eventually risks the occurrence of leakage in patients whose major problem initially was difficulty voiding.

If leakage due to sphincter weakness then supervenes, an appropriate step would be to perform a colposuspension or pubovaginal sling procedure; the patient would then achieve bladder emptying by intermittent self-catheterization.

Artificial urethral sphincter cuff placement is appropriate for some of these patients if other measures fail, but the risk of cuff erosion is high.

In some cases, formal closure of the bladder neck can be undertaken and a suprapubic catheterizable stoma into the bladder created—with a Mitrofanoff procedure, for example. Bladder neck closure is not always easy to achieve, and breakdown sometimes occurs.

SACRAL ANTERIOR ROOT STIMULATION AND DEAFFERENTATION

Electrically driven micturition accomplished via electrodes placed around the anterior roots of S2, S3, and the combined roots of S4 and S5 can be used to produce satisfactory bladder emptying. Reflex detrusor contractions can be abolished by dividing the posterior roots of S2, S3, and S4, or dividing the similar outflow at the conus level. From the electrodes placed intradurally, cables are led subcutaneously to a buried radio receiver positioned over the lower anterior chest wall. When micturition is required, a mirror-image radio transmitter is placed over the receiver, and a current is induced in the underlying diodes. The transmitter is connected to a hand-held battery control box.

The pelvic floor and urethral sphincter share the same sacral roots as the bladder and rectum. The detrusor is slower to develop a contraction than is the rapidly acting striated muscle; however, when the current is switched off, the sphincter relaxes rapidly while the detrusor does so more slowly, and voiding occurs post-stimulation. The sacral anterior root stimulation is carried out in bursts.

Bladder emptying is very satisfactory in the majority of patients, and the continence rate has been improved by the introduction of deafferentation via sacral posterior root rhizotomy [18, 20].

Methods are being refined to allow selective detrusor activation while blocking concomitant sphincter contraction. These refinements have focused on anodal block techniques. Reasonable results in 8 of 12 patients were described by Rijkhoff et al. [21, 22].

To be considered suitable for sacral anterior root stimulation, patients must have reflex bladder contractions proven on cystometry or provoked by transrectal electrical stimulation. They should also have sufficient hand function to manipulate the transmitter controls and sufficient mobility to get to the toilet unaided. The procedure is therefore suitable for most paraplegic patients but only some quadriplegic patients. The lesion should be complete, as the electrical stimulation might prove painful in those with incomplete lesions.

To summarize, patients undergoing sacral anterior root stimulation can expect the following outcomes:

1. Good bladder emptying is achieved in the majority with negligible postvoid residual urine. The incidence of urinary tract infection is much lower postoperatively than preoperatively.
2. Continence is achieved in most cases because of abolition of reflex bladder contractions by the deafferentation. Some leakage might occur remote from surgery in some patients, due to loss of reflex activity in the pelvic floor.

   If a fault should develop in the sacral anterior root stimulator, the patient should still remain dry but would need to empty the bladder by intermittent self-catheterization until the fault is repaired. Repair can be done successfully in most cases.
3. Bowel function is often improved. The settings used to stimulate the bladder also cause the upper colon to empty down into the rectum, from whence feces are more readily evacuated manually. In some patients, a program of electrical stimulation can be set that causes rectal evacuation as well.
4. Deafferentation does lead to loss of reflex erections. For most patients with spinal cord injury, reflex erections are insufficiently firm or sustained to enable useful function. If such function is adequate and is important to the patient, the patient should not have the deafferentation, particularly of the S2 root. After deafferentation, electrically driven erection can be achieved in approximately 30% of men, but often it cannot be relied on and pharmacologic means to drive an erection are required.

BOWEL FUNCTION

The pelvic parasympathetic nerves supply the rectum and the left colon as high up as the splenic flexure. The striated sphincter of the anus is supplied predominantly by S4 and partly by S3.

Constipation is almost universal in those with spinal cord injuries, and in many the bowel becomes distended and loaded with feces. Bowel emptying is achieved by the use of laxatives, usually in suppository form, to stimulate the passage of the bowel content from the upper left colon down to the rectum, from whence it is removed by manual evacuation.

For some patients, the antegrade colonic enema procedure is useful. The appendix is brought out to the skin surface as a catheterizable stoma for intermittent bowel irrigation (see Figure 12-2).

Those who have a sacral anterior root stimulator are able to achieve the emptying of the left colon into the rectum simply by using parameters set for bladder emptying. Setting a special program for defecation is helpful for some patients, who are then able to evacuate the bowel using electrical stimulation.

SEXUAL FUNCTION

The three main areas of sexuality are interpersonal relationships, sexual erotic satisfaction, and procreation. Although interpersonal relationships are clearly the most satisfying aspect, lack of sensation, difficulty in achieving and maintaining an erection, and difficulty in achieving a posture that allows intercourse can all add to anxiety and inhibition. Male fertility is often reduced after spinal cord injury because of poor semen quality or infection. All of these factors need to be openly addressed with patients by staff skilled in counseling.

Erection

The neurologic control of erections is mediated primarily via S2 and partly by S3, with neural impulses reaching the pelvic plexus and from there the erectile tissue via the nervi erigentes. Evidence is found that some control can also travel via sympathetics and allow some patients with cauda equina injuries to achieve psychogenic erection [23].

Pharmacologic erections can be achieved by intracavernosal injection of a variety of drugs. Often, the dosage needs to be lower in patients with neurologic problems than in those without such problems. The various treatments described in Chapter 13 are used. Sildenafil citrate has been found to be effective in patients with spinal cord injury.

Prostheses are not widely recommended because of the risk of erosion due to unrecognized pressure.

Ejaculation

Ejaculation can occur in some patients during penetrative intercourse. In patients who have had a bladder neck incision, transurethral resection of the prostate, or external sphincterotomy, semen might proceed retrogradely into the bladder and require that postejaculation urine be centrifuged and washed and the recovered sperm used for artificial insemination of the wife.

Vibratory stimulation of the glans can produce a satisfactory semen sample in some men. However, the procedure does carry the risk of inducing autonomic dysreflexia. Therefore, some patients must be given a general anesthetic so that a satisfactory semen sample can be obtained. Forty to 70% of men can achieve ejaculation by the vibration methods when the spinal cord lesion is above T11 [24].

Transrectal electrical nerve stimulation of the nervi erigentes can also produce electroejaculation in some patients in whom the vibration method is not satisfactory.

Semen quality appears better after vibratory stimulation than when electroejaculation is used [25]. Infection is common and needs to be cleared before the specimen is obtained, but antibiotics are also added to the specimen during preparation for either artificial insemination or assisted fertilization.

Sexuality in Women with Spinal Cord Injuries

As is well known, women with spinal cord injuries can menstruate, conceive, and give birth with few problems. Those with a paralyzed pelvic floor, however, do risk worsening of the condition due to overstretching during vaginal delivery; they also risk perineal tears. For patients with lesions at T10–T12, caesarean section may be needed. There is a risk of autonomic dysreflexia in those with lesions above T6.

Until the late 1990s, the physiologic aspects of intercourse and orgasm in the female have received little attention. The subject has been addressed by Whipple and Komisaruk [26]. The major neural pathways for orgasm seem to be via the pudendal nerve and pelvic afferents. Fibers also travel via the sympathetics to T10–T12, and some women with apparently complete lesions can still achieve orgasm. With higher lesions, some neurologic pathways travel via the vagus from the cervix in experimental animals, and this, too, may be a further neurophysiologic mechanism for maintenance of orgasm.

LOGISTICS AND UROLOGIC FOLLOW-UP

Because preservation of the kidneys depends on lower urinary tract function, patients with spinal cord injuries must be carefully followed up. Such follow-up includes standard radiography and renal ultrasonography to check for stones and dilatation. This is particularly important in the first 2 years. The key to preserving the integrity of the upper urinary tract is surveillance of the lower tract by urodynamics; this surveillance is particularly important in the child.

The urologist has many options for intervening to preserve upper urinary tract function while helping the patient to achieve continence and bladder emptying and to enjoy a life that is as normal as possible given the function remaining after the spinal cord injury.

REFERENCES

1. Light JK, Faganel J, Berri A. Detrusor areflexia in suprasacral spinal cord injuries. J Urol 1985;134:295–297.
2. Atkinson PP, Atkinson JLD. Spinal shock. Mayo Clinic Proc 1996;71:384–389.
3. Arnold EP, Cowan IA. Clinical significance of ureteric diameter on intravenous urography after spinal cord injury. Br J Urol 1988;62:131–135.
4. Bailey RR, Lynn KL, Swainson CP, et al. Vesico Ureteric Reflux and Reflux Nephropathy. In RW Schrier and CW Gottschalk (eds), Diseases of the Kidney. Boston: Little, Brown, 1987;747–783.
5. MacDiarmid SA, Arnold EP, Palmer NB, Anthony A. Management of spinal cord injured patients by indwelling suprapubic catheterisation. J Urol 1995;154:492–494.
6. El-Masri WS, Fellows G. Bladder care after spinal cord injury. Paraplegia 1981;19:265–270.
7. Dolin PJ, Darby SC, Beral V. Paraplegia and squamous cell carcinoma of the bladder in young women with findings from a case-control study. Br J Cancer 1994;70:167–168.

8. Wyndaele JJ, van Kerrebroeck PEV. The effects of 4 weeks treatment with Cisapride on cystometric parameters in spinal cord injury patients: a double-blind, placebo controlled study. Paraplegia 1995;33:625–627.
9. Perkash I. Contact laser sphincterotomy: further experience and longer follow-up. Spinal Cord 1996;34:227–233.
10. Shah NC, Foley SJ, Edham I, Shah PJ. Use of Memokath temporary urethral stent in treatment of detrusor-sphincter dyssynergia. J Endourol 1997;11:485–488.
11. Abdill CK, Rivas DR, Chancellor MB. Transurethral placement of external sphincter wire mesh stent for neurogenic bladder. Sci Nurs 1997;11:38–41.
12. Madersbacher H, Jilg G. Control of detrusor hyperreflexia by the intravesical instillation of oxybutynin hydrochloride. Paraplegia 1991;29:84–90.
13. Szollar SM, Lee SM. Intravesical oxybutynin for spinal cord injury patients. Spinal Cord 1996; 34:284–287.
14. Sundin T, Dahlstrom A, Norlen L, Sveduyn N. Sympathetic innervation and adrenoceptor function of the human lower urinary tract in the normal and after parasympathetic denervation. Invest Urol 1977;14:322–328.
15. Iwatsubo E, Komine S, Yamashita H, et al. Overdistension therapy of the bladder in paraplegic patients using self-catheterisation: a preliminary study. Paraplegia 1984;22:210–215.
16. Fowler CJ, Jewkes D, McDonald WI, et al. Intravesical capsaicin for neurogenic bladder dysfunction. Lancet 1992;339:1239.
17. Geirsson G, Fall M, Sullivan L. Clinical and urodynamic effects of intravesical capsaicin treatment in patients with chronic traumatic spinal detrusor hyper-reflexia. J Urol 1995;154:1825–1829.
18. Sauerwein D. Die operative Behandlung der spastischen Blasenlahmung bei Querschnittlahmung. Urologe 1990;29:196–203.
19. Van Kerrebroeck PEV, Koldwijn EL, Rosier PFWM, et al. Results of the treatment of neurogenic bladder dysfunction in spinal cord injury by sacral posterior root rhizotomy and anterior sacral root stimulation. J Urol 1996;155:1378–1381.
20. Brindley GS. The first 500 patients with sacral anterior root stimulation: general description. Paraplegia 1994;32:795–805.
21. Rijkhoff NJM, Wijkstra H, van Kerrebroeck PEV, Debruyne FMJ. Urinary bladder control by electrical stimulation: review of electrical stimulation techniques. Neurourol Urodyn 1997;16:39–53.
22. Rijkhoff NJM, Wijkstra H, van Kerrebroeck PEV, Debruyne FMJ. Selective detrusor activation by electrical sacral nerve root stimulation in spinal cord injury. J Urol 1997;157:1504–1508.
23. Bors E, Comarr AE. Neurological disturbance of sexual function with special reference to 529 patients with spinal cord injury. Urol Surv 1960;10:191–222.
24. Beretta G, Chelo E, Zanello A. Reproductive aspects in spinal cord injured men. Paraplegia 1989;27:113–118.
25. Brackitt NL, Padron OF, Lynes CM. Semen quality of spinal cord injured men is better when obtained by vibratory stimulation versus electro ejaculation. J Urol 1997;157:151–157.
26. Whipple B, Komisaruk BR. Sexuality and women with spinal cord injury. Spinal Cord 1997;35:136–138.

19
Bladder and Sexual Dysfunction in Multiple Sclerosis

Christopher D. Betts

Disturbances of the bladder and of sexual function are common in patients with multiple sclerosis (MS) and can result in some of the most distressing symptoms of the disorder. A good deal has been learned about how bladder and sexual dysfunction are related to the more general neurologic features of MS. Clinicians can now give their patients a rational explanation for the genitourinary problems in MS.

Men and women with MS frequently experience difficulties in their sexual life. Many factors are likely to contribute to the sexual dysfunction, but in addition to physical disabilities and psychological problems, a disorder of the neurologic mechanisms controlling the sexual response almost always exists. Now, both patients and doctors are more at ease discussing problems of sexual function; the reasons may include greater freedom in society to debate sexual matters, improved understanding of the basis for sexual dysfunction, and development of successful treatments for male erectile failure. Patients with MS should not be under the impression that the disease necessarily means an end to their sexual pleasure. Even when treatment is not possible, most patients are likely to benefit from explanation and counseling.

The bladder symptoms in MS can be extremely troublesome, but clinicians now recognize that urinary frequency, urgency, and urge incontinence do not indicate any serious underlying urologic problem. Only in occasional circumstances are complex urologic investigations required. For very many MS patients who have urinary symptoms, effective medical therapy is available, and patients must be given access to professionals with a good knowledge of the modern management of the neuropathic bladder in MS.

SEXUAL DYSFUNCTION IN MULTIPLE SCLEROSIS

Sexual Dysfunction in Men with Multiple Sclerosis

Since the 1920s, male erectile dysfunction (MED) has become increasingly recognized as a complication of MS. Studies of general symptomatology in MS

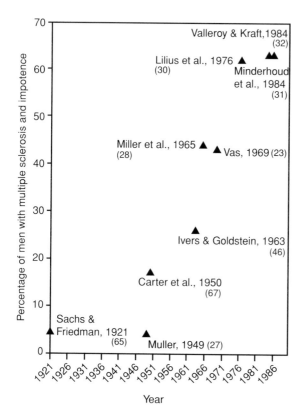

Figure 19.1 Reported incidence of erectile dysfunction in multiple sclerosis.

indicate that approximately 70% of men with MS develop erectile failure (Figure 19.1). MED and urinary symptoms occur with similar frequency in MS, but considerably more has been published about bladder dysfunction [1–22] than about erectile problems [23–26]. Intracorporeal injection therapy has proved highly successful for men with neurogenic MED, and this has stimulated a great deal of interest in neurogenic MED. Prostaglandin E_1 (PGE_1) is the most widely used drug for injection therapy. An interesting new development is the intraurethral PGE_1 pellet system or MUSE (medicated urethral system for erection), which may circumvent the natural reluctance to perform a penile injection (see Chapter 13).

Loss of ejaculatory function may complicate MS. Not only is this a problem for patients wishing to have children, but the loss can also undermine the benefits of intracorporeal injection therapy for MED. In some men with MS, treatment of the erectile failure is not appropriate, but most patients can benefit from an explanation of the basis for their sexual problems.

This section is particularly concerned with the neurologic basis for the erectile dysfunction in MS. The very important psychological aspects of MS that may contribute to the sexual difficulties are given little discussion. Chapter 7 covers the sexual problems of disabled patients from a psychological perspective.

The neural control of sexual function is discussed in detail in Chapter 5. The neural mechanisms important in penile erection are complex, and erection clearly can be mediated by psychogenic and reflex neurologic pathways. The pelvic parasympathetics arising from spinal cord segments S2 and S3 are thought to be the main effectors of erection, but in some circumstances hypogastric nerve pathways (sympathetic, T11–L2) can mediate erection in response to psychogenic stimuli. In normal erotic circumstances, both psychogenic and reflex mechanisms probably act synergistically in the mediation of erection, and important erector neural pathways must traverse the length of the spinal cord. In men with erectile failure due to central nervous system lesions, the dysfunction is generally thought to result from interruption of erector pathways to the penis. The importance of central lesions involving the sensory pathways from the penis in neurogenic MED is unknown.

Sexual Dysfunction and the Neurologic Features of Multiple Sclerosis

Müller [27] reported that MED was part of the presenting symptom complex of MS in 1% of males. Vas [23] studied 37 men with MS, 17 of whom had erectile failure. The mean duration of MS was 12 years in the men with total MED and 9 years in those with partial MED. We carried out a study of 48 men with MED due to MS, and only 1 man had erectile difficulties in association with the first symptoms of the neurologic disorder [25]. None of the patients had first presented with erectile symptoms alone and then developed other neurologic symptoms of MS. In our study series, the mean time between the onset of neurologic symptoms and the start of erectile problems was 9 years (median, 8 years; range, 1–30 years). The clinical data indicate clearly that MED without other neurologic features is extremely unlikely to be a heralding symptom of MS. The erectile dysfunction in MS tends to occur several years after the first symptoms of the neurologic condition.

Miller [28] reviewed the genitourinary symptoms of 297 MS patients from Newcastle, England. In this study, MED was always associated with urinary symptoms and usually occurred some time after the onset of the bladder dysfunction. In a later study, Vas [23] reported that the incidence of urinary symptoms was higher in men with MS and total MED than in men with normal erections or partial erectile failure. In our own series, only 1 man had MED and no urinary symptoms (Figure 19.2); in 18 men, the urinary symptoms and erectile problems began at approximately the same time; and in 21, the erectile failure developed after the onset of urinary symptoms (mean time between start of urinary symptoms and onset of MED was 3.3 years) [25]. In MS, MED is usually accompanied by bladder dysfunction, and the urinary symptoms often precede the erectile problems by several years [25, 28]. The neural mechanisms for erection seem to be more robust than the central pathways for bladder function. This might be due to the existence of both parasympathetic and sympathetic erector pathways. Also, erections may be mediated by reflex and psychogenic mechanisms, and this may account for normal erectile function in the presence of bladder symptoms.

Several authors have provided information about the findings of neurologic examination in patients with MS and disturbances of sexual function. Vas [23]

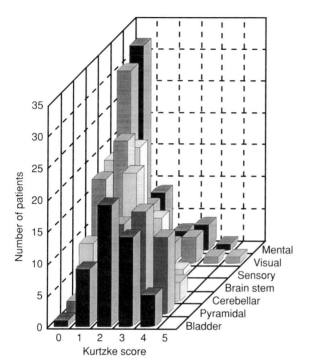

Figure 19.2   Kurtzke functional scores in 48 men with multiple sclerosis and erectile dysfunction.

found a higher overall Kurtzke disability score in patients with total MED compared to those with partial erectile failure. In the same study, Vas [23] described an association between anhidrosis and MED that was later confirmed by Cartlidge [29]. Sudomotor function was examined by spraying quinizarin powder on the whole body, front and then back. Patients with MS who had total MED did not sweat below the waist, whereas those with partial MED perspired normally on the face, upper limbs, trunk, groin, and perineum but not on the lower limbs. The absence of a dermatomal pattern for anhidrosis was attributed to the lesions' being in the central nervous system. Vas [23] proposed that the lesions responsible for erectile failure were situated in the lateral horns or connecting pathways in the dorsolumbar cord. Three questionnaire surveys of patients with MS have provided further information about the relationships between sexual dysfunction and the neurologic features of MS [30–32]. However, problems of male and female sexual function were considered together, and information about the neurologic deficits relating to MED and loss of ejaculation is not available. In one survey [30], 94% of the respondents with sexual problems had evidence of pyramidal tract dysfunction in their lower limbs. Lilius et al. [30] concluded that sexual dysfunction in MS was the result of spinal cord lesions and occurred in association with other symptoms of spinal origin. In a further study [32], an association was described between spasticity in the legs and sexual dysfunction, but Minderhoud et al. [31] found no relationship between sexual dysfunction and either pyramidal or cerebellar signs. Kirkeby et al. [24] also concluded that a poor relationship existed between sexual function and the Kurtzke disability scores. However, the data published by Kirkeby et al. [24] clearly show that most of the patients with MED and MS had moderately high Kurtzke disability scores (3 or higher). In our study [25], 48 patients with clinically definite MS and MED underwent a detailed neurologic examination and were assessed using the Kurtzke system [33]. The majority of the men were found to have unequivocal, bilateral pyramidal signs in their legs, and in only two were there no abnormal neurologic findings in the lower limbs (see Figure 19.2). The clinical studies clearly demonstrate that men with MS who have erectile dysfunction invariably have pyramidal impairment in their legs. No other neurologic finding in men with MS has been shown to be associated with sexual dysfunction.

Erectile Dysfunction and Neurophysiologic Tests

Neurophysiologic investigations have been used to test the neural pathways for erection in normal men and in those with erectile dysfunction [34, 35]. Haldeman et al. [36] first reported the recording of cortical somatosensory evoked potentials (CSEPs) in response to stimulation of the dorsal nerves of the penis. The cortical waveform and the latency of the response to dorsal nerve stimulation are similar to those of the evoked potentials recorded after posterior tibial nerve stimulation. The pudendal evoked potentials have been shown to be abnormal in a proportion of men with MS and erectile failure (Table 19.1). Kirkeby et al. [24] found abnormalities of the pudendal CSEPs in 26 of 29 patients with MS and MED; the bulbocavernosus reflex was also abnormal in 8. The abnormalities of the pudendal CSEPs are consistent with demyelination affecting the ascending pathways within the cord, whereas the abnormal bulbocavernosus reflex suggests a conus lesion. The fact that the bulbocavernosus reflexes were normal in most of the patients with abnormal pudendal responses suggests that the neurologic lesions were mainly suprasacral. We recorded the pudendal CSEPs and the right and the left tibial CSEPs in 44 men with erectile dysfunction [25]. The pudendal

Table 19.1   Abnormal pudendal cortical somatosensory evoked potentials in men with multiple sclerosis and erectile dysfunction

Study	*Number of patients*	*Number of patients with abnormal pudendal cortical evoked potentials*
Eretkin et al. [60]	11	6
Herman et al. [61]	1	1
Tackmann et al. [62]	7	5
Kirkeby et al. [24]	29	26
Ganzer et al. [63]	2	1
Betts et al. [25]	44	34
Pickard et al. [35]	16	13

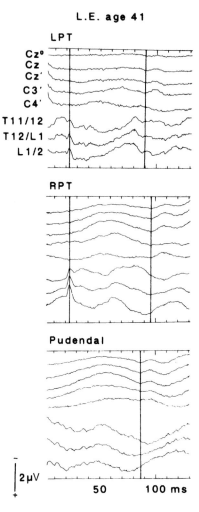

L.E. age 41

Figure 19.3   Left posterior tibial (LPT), right posterior tibial (RPT), and pudendal cortical evoked potentials in a man with multiple sclerosis and erectile failure. The waveforms are abnormal, and the latencies of the cortical responses are delayed.

and the tibial responses were abnormal in most of these patients. No patient had normal tibial responses with an abnormal pudendal evoked potential (Figure 19.3). A close correlation was also seen between the latencies of the pudendal CSEPs and the tibial CSEPs. If sacral cord lesions were a major factor in the etiology of MED in MS, then a dissociation would have been expected between the results of the pudendal and the tibial CSEPs. These results are further evidence that, in patients with MS and MED, the neural lesions are predominately above the sacral cord.

Whether the neural pathways tested by electrical stimulation of the dorsal nerves of the penis have any actual role in erection is unknown. The lesions causing the abnormalities of the pudendal CSEPs may have involved erector pathways in addition to afferent tracts from the penis.

Rodi et al. [37] reported greater sensitivity of the tibial than the pudendal evoked potentials in patients with MS and urinary symptoms. Ghezzi et al. [26] found neurophysiologic abnormalities as commonly in men with MS who did not have erectile dysfunction as in those who did. On the basis of our findings in patients with MS and MED, we concluded that testing the pudendal and tibial evoked potentials was of no greater value in recognizing spinal cord disease than clinical examination [25].

Ejaculatory Dysfunction

Little data have been published regarding disturbances of ejaculation in MS. In the series by Vas [23], all of the men with total erectile dysfunction had complete loss of ejaculation, and one-third of the patients with partial erectile failure also had ejaculatory dysfunction. In two questionnaire surveys, 37% [32] and 44% [31] of the men with MS complained of difficulty in achieving ejaculation. In our study, data about ejaculatory function was obtained from 40 patients [25]. Six men had complete loss of ejaculation, 19 reported that ejaculation had become difficult to achieve, and 15 had normal ejaculation. None of the men reported a dissociation between ejaculation and orgasmic sensation. The men with low Kurtzke pyramidal scores tended to have normal ejaculatory function, whereas the more disabled patients often had difficulty in achieving ejaculation. In the same study, a relationship between the cortical evoked potentials and ejaculatory dysfunction was suggested. Men with absent CSEPs often had the most severe neurologic lesions and usually showed accompanying loss of ejaculation (Figure 19.4). Again, whether the pathways tested by recording the cortical evoked potentials to dorsal nerve stimulation have any role in ejaculatory function is not known. Some have suggested that impairment in the transmission of afferent information from the penis might result in a failure to reach an orgasmic threshold within the postulated ejaculatory center. Also, spinal lesions could indirectly impair ejaculation by reducing perception of erotic penile sensation and so impair the facilitation of the ejaculatory center from higher centers [25].

Bladder Function in Men with Erectile Dysfunction

The majority of patients with MS and MED have bladder dysfunction. The most common urinary symptoms are irritative in nature (urgency, frequency, and urge incontinence) [18, 23, 28]. Tests of the detrusor function in patients with MS and MED should provide further knowledge of the underlying neurologic abnormalities. In our study, 41 of 45 men with MS and erectile failure were found on urodynamic testing to have detrusor hyperreflexia; the remaining 4 patients had stable bladder function [25]. The severity of the urinary symptoms was related to the degree of pyramidal impairment in the legs, a result consistent with previously reported findings [12, 18, 28]. In MS, the urodynamic finding of bladder hyperreflexia is thought to result from suprasacral spinal cord disease [9, 18], whereas conus lesions would be expected to cause detrusor areflexia [4, 38]. That individuals with MS and MED invariably have detrusor hyperreflexia indicates that the predominant disease is above the sacral cord.

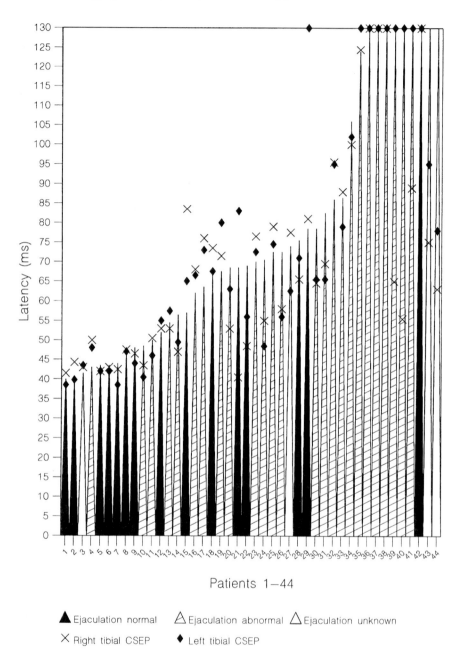

Patients 1–44

▲ Ejaculation normal   △ Ejaculation abnormal   △ Ejaculation unknown
✕ Right tibial CSEP   ◆ Left tibial CSEP

Figure 19.4   Latencies of the pudendal and tibial cortical evoked potentials in 44 men with multiple sclerosis and erectile dysfunction. (CSEP = cortical somatosensory evoked potential.)

Neuroendocrine Function, Psychiatric Morbidity, and Erectile Failure

Very little research has been conducted into the neuroendocrine aspects of erectile dysfunction in MS. Vas [23] measured the excretion of urinary gonadotrophins and reported indirect evidence of testosterone deficiency in approximately one-half of patients with MS and MED. However, Vas [23] acknowledged the deficiencies of the method used for gonadotrophin assay. Later, Kirkeby et al. [24] reported marginally elevated testosterone levels in 3 of 29 men with MS and erectile dysfunction; all the remaining patients had testosterone levels within the normal range. In our own series studying men with MS and erectile dysfunction, only one man was found to have an abnormally low serum testosterone value, but many of the men had testosterone values in the lower part of the normal range (CD Betts and CJ Fowler, unpublished data, 1991). The man with a low testosterone level had pyramidal signs in his legs, and testosterone therapy produced only partial improvement in his erectile function. Some patients with MED due to MS and low testosterone levels may not seek advice about their erectile difficulties because of low libido and a lack of concern for the problem. No studies have been published concerned primarily with neuroendocrine function in men with MS and sexual difficulties. This aspect of erectile failure in MS requires further research.

In MS, a small proportion of the patients with MED experience a spontaneous improvement in their erectile function [23, 25]. The neural lesions in MS may involve the pathways for psychogenic erection but spare the tracts for reflex erection. This situation may result in a history of a good erectile response to tactile stimulation but poor erections from psychogenic erotic stimuli. In view of these considerations, a history of varying erectile function should not be regarded as indicating that the problem is psychological. Psychiatric morbidity has been reported in almost 50% of patients with clinically definite MS and is more frequent than in disability-matched patients with neurologic disorders that do not affect the brain [39]. Depressive illness is one of the most frequently encountered problems in MS [40, 41]; MED may complicate the clinical situation. However, in patients with MS, MED, and pyramidal signs in the lower limbs, the erectile problem is most likely the result of spinal cord disease.

Management of Erectile Dysfunction

Intracorporeal injection therapy has proved to be a very significant advance in the treatment of neurogenic erectile dysfunction. Patients with MS and MED generally respond very well to these injections, and this treatment has probably been more successful in MS patients than in those with any other neurologic disorder. A good response to oral sildenafil citrate has been found in men with MS.

A detailed account of the management of neurogenic male sexual dysfunction is given in Chapter 13.

Summary

Erectile failure is a common problem in men with MS and is invariably associated with urinary symptoms and bladder hyperreflexia. The clinical findings and the neurophysiologic results indicate the presence of suprasacral spinal cord lesions in most patients with MS and MED. Difficulty in achieving ejaculation is a further problem in a significant proportion of this population and is also thought to result from spinal cord disease. The importance of neuroendocrine abnormalities in the etiology of male sexual dysfunction in MS remains uncertain and should be the subject of further research.

In MS, a considerable amount is known about the relationship between erectile failure, urinary symptoms, and impairment of pyramidal function in the lower limbs. Patients with MS and MED are likely to benefit from an explanation of the cause for their erectile difficulties, and this information can be given with reference to bladder symptoms and neurologic disability in the legs.

Sexual Dysfunction in Women with Multiple Sclerosis

Few reports exist of female sexual dysfunction in MS. Early questionnaire studies indicate that approximately 50% of women with MS have significant sexual problems [30–32]. The sexual troubles of women with MS include loss of libido, difficulty in achieving orgasm, lack of vaginal lubrication, pain during intercourse, dysesthesia, and lower limb spasticity.

Lundberg [42] studied 25 women with MS whose disability was not marked, and their responses were compared with those of a matched control group of women with migraine. Fifty-two percent of the women complained of sexual problems. None had experienced such difficulties before the onset of MS. A high proportion of the women recalled that the sexual difficulties had developed quite suddenly. Sixty-eight percent of the women with MS and sexual dysfunction had a history of urinary symptoms. Sexual problems were uncommon in the control group (12%). The investigators concluded that the sexual dysfunction in MS was a result of the neurologic disorder rather than due to psychological factors.

In a later study [43], 47 women with advanced MS were interviewed; 60% reported decreased libido; 40%, difficulty achieving orgasm; and 36%, reduced lubrication. The symptoms were more severe in the women with bladder and bowel dysfunction. In this study group, one-third of the females with MS had separated from their former sexual partners, and two-thirds of these women thought that their MS had been influential in the separation. In the same study, most of the women reported that they had never previously been asked about sexual function in relation to their MS.

Little specific treatment exists for the female sexual dysfunction in MS, but many women are likely to benefit from counseling by a knowledgeable individual.

BLADDER DYSFUNCTION IN MULTIPLE SCLEROSIS

The neural pathways that are important in bladder function traverse the length of the spinal cord between the pons and the sacral spinal cord, and they are particularly vulnerable in diseases involving the cord. In the dorsal tegmentum of the pons, an area is found that is thought to act on a spino-bulbo-spinal pathway and switch between the voiding and storage phases of micturition [44]. Also, the pontine micturition center is important during voiding in coordinating the detrusor muscle contraction with relaxation of the external urethral sphincter muscle. Higher centers, particularly the medial frontal lobes, act on the pontine micturition center in a mainly inhibitory manner. Lesions involving the neural pathways for bladder control may result in abnormal bladder storage or emptying, and often in a patient with spinal cord disease, both of the phases of micturition are disordered.

A detailed account of the neural control of micturition is given in Chapter 3.

Lower Urinary Tract Symptoms

Oppenheim [45] first recognized the high incidence of bladder symptoms in MS. Most study series since then have reported that approximately 75% of all patients with MS develop urinary symptoms. A few studies have reported a lower incidence of bladder problems in MS [46], but almost certainly the reason is that the patients had mild MS (Table 19.2). Miller et al. [28] found urinary symptoms in 75% of patients with MS, and in 50% they were persistent and troublesome.

Much of the data about urinary symptoms in the early stages of MS is probably unreliable, because formerly the diagnosis of MS was established only after several years, and information about bladder problems would depend largely on patient recall. Miller et al. [28] and Goldstein et al. [10] stated that urinary symptoms were the sole presenting feature of MS in 2% of patients and 2.3% of patients, respectively. In our study [18], which included 170 patients with MS and bladder dys-

Table 19.2 Urinary symptoms in multiple sclerosis

Study	Number of patients with multiple sclerosis	Multiple sclerosis patients first presenting with only urinary symptoms (%)	Multiple sclerosis patients first presenting with urinary and other neurologic symptoms (%)	All patients with multiple sclerosis and urinary symptoms (%)
Oppenheim [45]	30	—	—	80
Kahleyss [64]	35	—	—	88
Sachs [65]	141	—	—	40
Brickner [66]	62	—	10	85
Langworthy [1]	157	—	—	62
Muller [27]	582	—	5	62
Carter et al. [67]	47	—	11	78
Adams et al. [68]	389	—	2.8	44.5
Ivers and Goldstein [46]	144	—	1	10
Miller et al. [28]	297	2*	12	78
Goldstein et al. [10]	86	2.3*	14	97
Betts et al. [18]	170	0	2.3	100

Note: Dash indicates no value was reported.
*See text for explanation.

function, none of the patients had first presented with urinary symptoms alone. In the past, urinary retention in young women was attributed to MS, and this could account for the reports that patients with MS had first presented with only urinary symptoms [18]. Urinary retention secondary to neuropathic bladder dysfunction is quite unusual in MS [9, 18]. Also, an alternative cause for urinary retention in young women [47] is now well recognized, and retention without other neurologic symptoms should probably not be regarded as indicative of MS [18].

The urinary symptoms may be part of the presenting symptoms of MS in conjunction with other neurologic features; this has been reported in 1–14% of patients with MS (see Table 19.2).

The most common urinary symptom in patients with MS is urgency of micturition; this is followed by frequency and urge incontinence (Table 19.3). Urodynamic studies have shown that the urgency of micturition is due to detrusor hyperreflexia [18, 48]. Hesitancy of micturition is common and has been reported in between 25% and 49% of patients. This symptom may result from an abnormality in the relaxation of the external urethral sphincter (detrusor sphincter dyssynergia); this is discussed further in the next section. The term *urinary retention* has been used in the literature concerning MS to describe both total retention and hesitancy of micturition, so that the incidence of complete retention in patients with MS is unclear. However, complete failure to void secondary to a neuropathic bladder disorder is thought to be unusual in MS [9, 18].

Urodynamic Studies

In normal micturition, the detrusor muscle of the bladder contracts only when a person wishes to empty the bladder in suitable circumstances. To facilitate emptying, the external striated urethral sphincter relaxes at the time of detrusor contraction. The pontine micturition center is known to have a key role in this coordinated action.

Bladder hyperreflexia [49] has been the most common urodynamic finding in patients with MS and urinary symptoms (Table 19.4). In this disorder, the bladder contracts in an abnormal involuntary manner, often when the volume in the bladder is low (Figure 19.5). At the onset of one of these contractions, the person experiences a feeling of imminent micturition. The patient may be able to avoid incontinence by tightly contracting the pelvic muscles until the toilet has been reached. However, the pressure within the bladder during the period of involuntary detrusor hyperreflexia can be so great that, despite tight contraction of the external sphincter, urine escapes from the bladder, resulting in urge incontinence.

In our study [18], the urodynamic finding of hyperreflexia correlated well with the symptoms of urgency, frequency, and urge incontinence. All of the patients who had moderate or severe pyramidal dysfunction in their legs (Kurtzke pyramidal scores of 3 or higher) and complained of frequency and urgency or urge incontinence were found to have detrusor hyperreflexia [18]. The argument has been made that urodynamic studies (cystometry) are not necessary in a patient with urinary urgency and mild or moderate paraparesis, because in MS the bladder symptoms can be reasonably assumed to be due to detrusor hyperreflexia, and this condition is generally treated by anticholinergic medication [18].

Table 19.3   Urinary symptoms in patients with multiple sclerosis and bladder dysfunction

Study	Number of patients	Patients with urgency (%)	Patients with frequency (%)	Patients with urge incontinence (%)	Patients with hesitancy (%)	Patients with retention* (%)
Sachs and Freidman [65]	57	31	—	37	49	—
Langworthy [1]	97	54	33	34	40	—
Carter et al. [67]	36	24	17	50	—	17
Miller et al. [28]	231	60	50	36	33	2
Bradley [4]	90	86	60	—	28	20
Philp et al. [9]	52	61	59	47	25	8
Goldstein et al. [10]	86	32	32	49	—	—
Awad et al. [12]	47	85	65	72	36	—
Gonor et al. [16]	64	70	48	56	30	—
Betts et al. [18]	170	85	82	63	49	—

Note: Dash indicates no value was reported.
*See text for explanation.

Table 19.4   Urodynamic findings in multiple sclerosis patients with bladder dysfunction

Study	Number of patients	Detrusor function		
		Hyperreflexia (%)	Hyporeflexia/ areflexia (%)	Normal (%)
Bradley et al. [2]	99	59	40	0
Andersen et al. [3]	52	63	33	4
Bradley [4]	302	62	34	4
Summers [5]	50	52	12	18
Schoenburg et al. [6]	39	69	5	15
Piazza and Diokno [7]	31	74	6	9
Blaivas et al. [8]	41	56	40	4
Philp et al. [9]	52	99	0	1
Goldstein et al. [10]	86	76	19	—
Van Poppel et al. [11]	160	66	24	10
Awad et al. [12]	57	66	21	12
Hassouna et al. [13]	37	70	18	11
Petersen and Pedersen [14]	88	83	16	1
McGuire and Savastano [15]	46	72	28	0
Gonor et al. [16]	64	78	20	2
Weinstein et al. [17]	91	70	16	12
Betts et al. [18]	70	91	0	9
Sirls et al. [19]	113	70	15	6
Hinson and Boone [21]	70	63	28	9

Note: Detrusor hyperreflexia is the most common urodynamic abnormality; the occurrence of areflexia in multiple sclerosis has now been questioned [9, 18].

In addition to bladder hyperreflexia, interruption of the pathways between the sacral cord and pons may also cause a loss of the coordinated action of the detrusor and external sphincter, a disorder known as *detrusor sphincter dyssynergia* (DSD). Bladder hyperreflexia and DSD often coexist in the same patient. In DSDs the external sphincter contracts in an involuntary manner, simultaneously with the detrusor contraction. Hesitancy of micturition, an interrupted urinary stream, and incomplete bladder emptying in a patient with spinal cord disease suggest DSD (Figures 19.6 and 19.7). The reported incidence of DSD in MS varies from 18% to 66% [17, 50]. Technically, DSD is difficult to demonstrate because it requires a combination of pressure/flow recordings and urethral sphincter electromyography. In our study, 63% of patients had postmicturition residual volumes of more than 100 ml; most of these patients probably had DSD to varying degrees [18]. In the management of patients with MS and bladder problems, complex tests for DSD are not required, but measurement of the postmicturition residual volume is essential. Such measurement can be made either by insertion of a urethral catheter or by ultrasonography after voiding.

The occurrence of detrusor areflexia in MS has been questioned, and the suggestion has been made that some of the earlier studies may have included patients who did not have MS [9, 18].

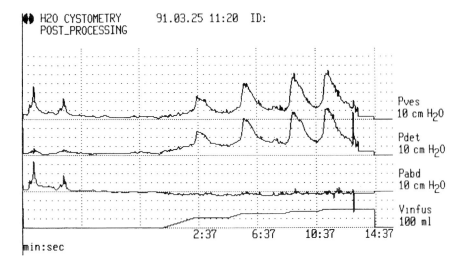

Figure 19.5   Filling cystometric study showing detrusor hyperreflexia. The rises and falls in detrusor pressure (Pdet) and intravesical pressure (Pves) are due to involuntary contractions of the bladder muscle. As the pressure rises, the patient experiences a sense of impending micturition and urgency to void (see text). The spikes at the beginning of the trace represent patient coughs and indicate that the catheters are recording correctly. (Pabd = intra-abdominal pressure measured via rectal catheter; Vinfus = volume of fluid instilled into the bladder.)

Bladder Dysfunction and the Neurologic Features of Multiple Sclerosis

Bladder symptoms were reported by Miller et al. [28] to be associated with the presence of pyramidal signs in the lower limbs. Awad et al. [12] compared patients' Kurtzke scores with their urinary symptoms and found that the presence of urge incontinence, urgency, nocturia, and frequency correlated with the scores for pyramidal and sensory dysfunction and with the total disability scores. The findings of our own study were in agreement with those of Miller et al. [28] and Awad et al. [12]; the occurrence and severity of the urinary symptoms were related to the degree of pyramidal dysfunction in the lower limbs (Figures 19.8 and 19.9) [18]. Figure 19.8 is a compilation of the Kurtzke scores for 186 patients with MS and urinary symptoms; only 2 patients with bladder dysfunction had no pyramidal signs in their legs. Few patients with moderately severe paraparesis did not experience urge incontinence (see Figure 19.9).

Upper Urinary Tract

In the past, emphasis was placed in the literature on the risk that the neurogenic bladder in MS would cause serious renal impairment [50–52]. In two large study series examining the causes of death in MS, no patient was reported to have died

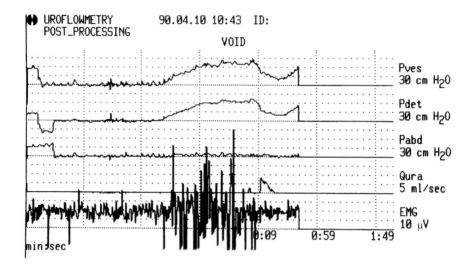

Figure 19.6   Voiding cystometric study showing detrusor sphincter dyssynergia (DSD). External urethral sphincter activity is recorded with an electromyographic (EMG) needle positioned in the striated sphincter muscle. Sphincter muscle activity increases (EMG) when the detrusor muscle contracts (Pdet), and voiding only occurs (Qura) when the activity in the sphincter declines. DSD can be anticipated in a patient with spinal cord disease who reports hesitancy and an interrupted flow (see Figure 19.7); often, a significant postmicturition residual volume is found. (Pabd = intra-abdominal pressure measured via rectal catheter; Pdet = detrusor pressure; Pves = intravesical pressure; Qura = flow of urine.)

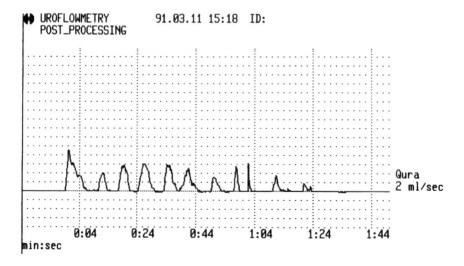

Figure 19.7   Urinary free flow test in a man with multiple sclerosis and lower limb pyramidal signs. The interrupted flow pattern is highly suggestive of detrusor sphincter dyssynergia. The postmicturition residual volume was 160 ml. (Qura = flow of urine.)

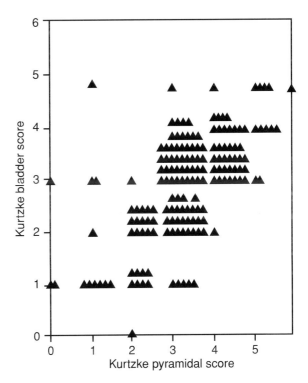

Figure 19.8   Kurtzke pyramidal and bladder scores of 186 patients with multiple sclerosis (see text).

of renal failure [53, 54]. The findings in more recent urologic studies confirm that renal failure in MS is extremely uncommon [11, 18, 48, 55].

Management of Urinary Symptoms

The two main bladder problems in patients with MS are detrusor hyperreflexia and incomplete emptying. Hyperreflexia can be anticipated in MS patients who have irritative urinary symptoms (urgency, frequency, and urge incontinence). The postmicturition residual cannot be predicted from the urinary symptoms and must be measured [56, 57].

If the postmicturition residual is raised (more than 100 ml is generally taken to be significant), then treatment to improve bladder emptying should be instituted. For many patients, clean intermittent self-catheterization is the most effective means of achieving bladder emptying.

At present, the first line of treatment for hyperreflexia is administration of the anticholinergic drug oxybutynin chloride. If bladder emptying is a problem, it must be corrected to obtain maximum benefit from anticholinergic medication.

If nocturia persists despite the outlined measures, then use of desmopressin acetate (DDAVP) can provide very useful symptomatic relief [58, 59].

Considerable ongoing research is investigating new agents to control bladder hyperreflexia, and the results of intravesical instillation of capsaicin are most promising. A full discussion of the treatment of bladder dysfunction in neurologic disease, including the newer modalities, is given in Chapter 11.

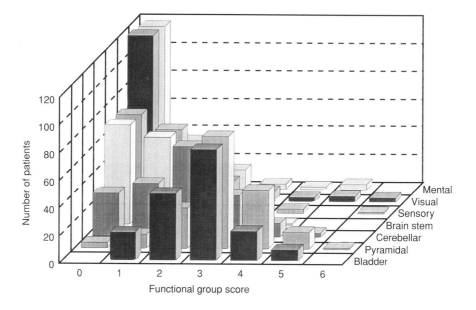

Figure 19.9   Kurtzke functional group scores of 186 patients with multiple sclerosis and urinary symptoms. Only two patients with urinary symptoms had no pyramidal signs.

Summary

In MS, bladder symptoms can be the cause of most distress to the patient, the caregiver, and the family, but with good advice the symptoms can be managed successfully.

In the past, particular emphasis was placed on urinary tract imaging and full urodynamic assessment in the management of urinary symptoms in MS. This teaching was probably at least partly responsible for the natural reluctance of neurologists to be responsible for the treatment of the neurogenic bladder in MS. There is now a general acceptance that the urinary symptoms are a further manifestation of the spinal cord disease and do not reflect a serious urologic problem. With this change, more neurologists are likely to become involved in the management of the bladder dysfunction in MS.

REFERENCES

1. Langworthy OR. Disturbances of micturition associated with disseminated sclerosis. J Nerv Ment Dis 1938;88:760–770.
2. Bradley WE, Logothetis JL, Timm GW. Cystometric and sphincter abnormalities in multiple sclerosis. Neurology 1973;23:1131–1139.
3. Andersen JT, Bradley WE. Abnormalities of detrusor and sphincter function in multiple sclerosis. Br J Urol 1976;48:193–198.
4. Bradley WE. Urinary bladder dysfunction in multiple sclerosis. Neurology 1978;28:52–58.

5. Summers JL. Neurogenic bladder in women with multiple sclerosis. J Urol 1978;120:555–556.
6. Schoenburg HW, Gutrich J, Banno J. Urodynamic patterns in multiple sclerosis. J Urol 1979;122: 648–650.
7. Piazza DH, Diokno AC. Review of neurogenic bladder in multiple sclerosis. Urology 1979;14:33–35.
8. Blaivas JG, Bhimani G, Labib KB. Vesicourethral dysfunction in multiple sclerosis. J Urol 1979;122:342–347.
9. Philp T. Read DJ, Higson RH. The urodynamic characteristics of multiple sclerosis. Br J Urol 1981;53:672–675.
10. Goldstein I, Siroky MB, Sax S, et al. Neurogenic abnormalities in multiple sclerosis. J Urol 1982;128:541–545.
11. Van Poppel H, Vereecken RL, Leruitte A. Neuro-muscular abnormalities multiple sclerosis. Paraplegia 1983;21:374–379.
12. Awad SA, Gajewski JB, Sogbein SK, et al. Relationship between neurological and urological status in multiple sclerosis. J Urol 1984;132:499–502.
13. Hassouna M, Lebel M, Elhilali M. Neurourologic correlation in multiple sclerosis. Neurourol Urodyn 1984;3:73–77.
14. Petersen T, Pedersen E. Neurourodynamic evaluation of voiding dysfunction in multiple sclerosis. Acta Neurol Scand 1984;69:402–411.
15. McGuire EJ, Savastano JA. Urodynamic findings and long-term outcome management of patients with multiple sclerosis–induced lower urinary tract dysfunction. J Urol 1984;132:713–715.
16. Gonor SE, Carroll DJ, Metcalf JB. Vesical dysfunction in multiple sclerosis. Urology 1985;25:429–431.
17. Weinstein MS, Cardenas DD, O'Shaughnessy EJ, Catanzaro ML. Carbon dioxide cystometry and postural changes in patients with multiple sclerosis. Arch Phys Med Rehabil 1988;69:923–927.
18. Betts CD, D'Mellow MT, Fowler CJ, et al. Urinary symptoms and the neurological features of bladder dysfunction in multiple sclerosis. J Neurol Neurosurg Psychiatry 1993;56:245–250.
19. Sirls LT, Zimmern PE, Leach GE. Role of limited evaluation and aggressive medical management in multiple sclerosis: a review of 113 patients. J Urol 1994;151:946–950.
20. Koldewijn E, Hommes O, Lemmens W, et al. Relationship between lower urinary tract abnormalities and disease-related parameters in multiple sclerosis. J Urol 1995;154:169–173.
21. Hinson JL, Boone TB. Urodynamics and multiple sclerosis. Urol Clin North Am 1996;23:475–481.
22. Porru D, Campus G, Garau A, et al. Urinary tract dysfunction in multiple sclerosis: is there a relation with disease-related parameters? Spinal Cord 1997;35:33–36.
23. Vas CJ. Sexual impotence and some autonomic disturbances in men with multiple sclerosis. Acta Neurol Scand 1969;45:166–184.
24. Kirkeby HJ, Poulsen EU, Petersen T, et al. Erectile dysfunction in multiple sclerosis. Neurology 1988;38:1366–1371.
25. Betts CD, D'Mellow MT, Fowler CJ. Erectile dysfunction in multiple sclerosis: associated neurological and neurophysiological deficits, and treatment of the condition. Brain 1994;117:1303–1310.
26. Ghezzi A, Malvestiti G, Baldini S, et al. Erectile impotence in multiple sclerosis: a neurophysiological study. J Neurol 1995;242:123–126.
27. Müller R. Studies on disseminated multiple sclerosis. Acta Med Scand 1949;222:67–71.
28. Miller H, Simpson CA, Yeates WF. Bladder dysfunction in multiple sclerosis. BMJ 1965;1: 1265–1269.
29. Cartlidge NEF. Autonomic function in multiple sclerosis. Brain 1972;95:661–664.
30. Lilius HG, Valtonen EJ, Wikstrom J. Sexual problems in patients suffering from multiple sclerosis. Scand J Soc Med 1976;4:41–44.
31. Minderhoud JM, Leehuis JG, Kremer J, et al. Sexual disturbances arising from multiple sclerosis. Acta Neurol Scand 1984;76:299–336.
32. Valleroy ML, Kraft GK. Sexual dysfunction in multiple sclerosis. Arch Phys Rehabil 1984;65:125–128.
33. Kurtzke JF. Rating neurological impairment in multiple sclerosis: an expanded disability status scale. Neurology 1983;33:1444–1452.
34. Fowler CJ, Betts CD. Clinical Value of Electrophysiological Investigations of Patients with Urinary Symptoms. In AR Mundy, TP Stephenson, AJ Wein (eds), Urodynamics: Principles, Practice and Application. Edinburgh, UK: Churchill Livingstone, 1994;165–181.
35. Pickard RS, Powell PH, Schofield IS. The clinical application of dorsal penile nerve cerebral evoked response recording in the investigation of impotence. Br J Urol 1994;74:231–235.
36. Haldeman S, Bradley WE, Bhatia N. Evoked responses from the pudendal nerve. J Urol 1982;128:974–980.
37. Rodi Z, Vodusek D, Denislec M. Clinical uro-neurophysiological investigation in multiple sclerosis. Eur J Neurol 1996;3:574–580.
38. Taylor MC, Bradley WE, Bhatia N, et al. The conus demyelination syndrome in multiple sclerosis. Acta Neurol Scand 1984;69:80–89.

39. Ron MA, Logsdail SJ. Psychiatric morbidity in multiple sclerosis: a clinical and MRI study. Psychol Med 1989;19:887–895.
40. Thompson AJ, McDonald WI. Multiple Sclerosis and Its Pathophysiology. In AK Asbury, GM McKhann, WI McDonald (eds), Diseases of the Nervous System: Clinical Neurobiology. Philadelphia: Saunders, 1992;1209–1228.
41. Feinsrein A. Multiple sclerosis, depression, and suicide. BMJ 1997;20:691–692.
42. Lundberg PO. Sexual dysfunction in female patients with multiple sclerosis. Int Rehabil Med 1981;3:32–34.
43. Hulter B, Lundberg PO. Sexual function in women with advanced multiple sclerosis. J Neurol Neurosurg Psychiatry 1995;59:83–86.
44. De Groat WC. Central Neural Control of the Lower Urinary Tract. In G Bock, J Whelan (eds), Neurobiology of Incontinence. Chichester, UK: Wiley, 1990;27–56.
45. Oppenheim H. Weitre notizen zur pathologie der disseminerten sklerose. Charite-ann 1889;14:412–418.
46. Ivers RR, Goldstein NP. Multiple sclerosis: a current appraisal of symptoms and signs. Proc Mayo Clin 1963;38:457–466.
47. Fowler CJ, Kirby RS. Abnormal electromyographic activity (decelerating bursts and complex repetitive discharges) in the striated muscle of the urethral sphincter in 5 women in urinary retention. Br J Urol 1985;57:67–70.
48. Chancellor MB, Kaplan SA, Blaivas JG. Detrusor-External Sphincter Dyssynergia. In G Bock, J Whelan (eds), Neurobiology of Incontinence. Chichester, UK: Wiley, 1990;195–213.
49. International Continence Society Committee. The standardisation of terminology of lower urinary tract function. Scand J Urol Nephrol 1988;114(suppl):5–19.
50. Blaivas JG, Holland NJ, Geisser B, et al. Multiple sclerosis bladder. Studies and care. Ann N Y Acad Sci 1984;436:328–346.
51. Samellas W, Rubin B. Management of upper tract complications in multiple sclerosis by means of urinary diversion to an ileal conduit. J Urol 1965;93:548–552.
52. Blaivas JG, Barbalias GA. Detrusor sphincter dyssynergia in men with multiple sclerosis: an ominous urologic condition. J Urol 1984;131:91–94.
53. Poskanzer DC, Schapira K, Miller H. Epidemiology of multiple sclerosis in the counties of Northumberland and Durham. J Neurol Neurosurg Psychiatry 1963;26:368–376.
54. Phadke JG. Survival pattern and cause of death in patients with multiple sclerosis: results from an epidemiological survey in north east Scotland. J Neurol Neurosurg Psychiatry 1987;5:523–531.
55. Sliwa JA, Bell HK, Mason KD, et al. Upper urinary tract abnormalities in multiple sclerosis patients with urinary symptoms. Arch Phys Med Rehabil 1996;77:247–251.
56. Fowler CJ. Investigation of the neurogenic bladder. J Neurol Neurosurg Psychiatry 1996;60:6–13.
57. Kornhuber H, Schutz A. Efficient treatment of neurogenic bladder disorders in multiple sclerosis with initial intermittent catheterisation and ultrasound-controlled training. Eur J Neurol 1990;30:260–267.
58. Hilton P, Hertogs G, de Wall H, Dalm E. The use of desmopressin (DDAVP) for nocturia in women with multiple sclerosis. J Neurol Neurosurg Psychiatry 1983;46:854–855.
59. Kinn A-C, Larsson P. Desmopressin: a new principle for symptomatic treatment of urgency and incontinence in patients with multiple sclerosis. Scand J Urol Nephrol 1990;24:109–112.
60. Ertekin C, Akyurekli O, Gurses AN, Turget H. The value of somatosensory evoked potentials and bulbocavernosus reflex in patients with impotence. Acta Neurol Scand 1985;71:48–53.
61. Herman CW, Weinberg HJ, Brown J. Testing for neurogenic impotence: a challenge. Urology 1986;27:318–321.
62. Tackmann W, Porst H, van Ahlen H. Bulbocavernosus reflex latencies and somatosensory evoked potentials after pudendal nerve stimulation in the diagnosis of impotence. J Neurol 1988;235:219–225.
63. Ganzer H, Madersbacher H, Rumpl E. Cortical evoked potentials by stimulation of the vesicourethral: clinical value and neurophysiological considerations. J Urol 1991;146:118–123.
64. Kahleyss. In discussion of Müller R. Studies on disseminated sclerosis. Acta Med Scand 1949;222:22–23.
65. Sachs B, Freidman ED. The general symptoms of multiple sclerosis and the mode of development of the symptoms of multiple sclerosis. Assoc Res Nerv Ment Dis 1921;2:49–55.
66. Brickner RM. Sensory and other aspects of multiple sclerosis. Bull Neurol Inst N Y 1936;5:16–20.
67. Carter S, Sciarra D, Merritt HH. The course of multiple sclerosis as determined by autopsy proven cases. Res Publ Assoc Nerv Ment Dis 1950;28:471–559.
68. Adams DK, Sutherland JM, Fletcher WB. Early clinical manifestations of disseminated sclerosis. BMJ 1950;2:431–436.

20
Bowel Dysfunction in Multiple Sclerosis

Clare J. Fowler and Michael Henry

PREVALENCE

Patients with multiple sclerosis (MS) frequently complain of problems with bowel function. Sullivan and Ebers [1] reported that 53% of their patients with MS complained of constipation. A study of a large number of patients with MS found that 43% had constipation and 51% had fecal incontinence; overall, 68% had some form of bowel symptoms [2]. A study of 77 patients receiving treatment for bladder symptoms due to MS found that 52% complained of some form of bowel dysfunction [3]. Among a group of 209 patients with MS who were surveyed, 78% reported some major bladder dysfunction and 41% reported bowel dysfunction [4]. Clearly, the prevalence of bowel dysfunction is very much higher in patients with MS than in the general population.

SYMPTOMS

In health, the lower bowel acts under voluntary control and performs two main functions: the storage and elimination of feces. In neurologic disease, both these functions may be affected either separately or together. Disorders of elimination produce complaints of constipation; disorders of storage, fecal incontinence. A combination of constipation and incontinence is not uncommon in patients with MS.

PATHOPHYSIOLOGY

Whereas bladder dysfunction in MS is known with some certainty to be due to spinal cord involvement [5], little is known about the cause of bowel disorders in the disease. The importance of spinal cord function is probably less critical. The

Table 20.1   Symptoms of colorectal dysfunction in multiple sclerosis and possible pathophysiologic causes

Constipation
Slow colonic transit
Abnormal rectal function
Intussusception
Fecal incontinence
Absent or decreased sensation of rectal filling
Poor voluntary contraction of anal sphincter and pelvic floor
Reduced rectal compliance
Obstetric injury causing weakness of the anal sphincter

innervation of the bladder arises from the sacral segments of the cord and thus has more caudal innervation than that of the lower limbs. The controlling centers for the bladder are situated in the dorsal tegmentum of the pons [6], so that any lesion of the spinal cord causing paraparesis is likely also to interrupt connections between the pons and the sacral part of the cord. If spinal cord disease were to be a major factor in causing the bowel disorders of MS, the incidence of these symptoms might be expected to be higher in patients who have a paraparesis and bladder dysfunction than in an unselected population. However, this has not been found to be the case; 32% of patients with clinical evidence of spinal cord disease and significant bladder symptoms had no complaints of bowel dysfunction [3].

It seems unlikely that a single identifiable neurologic deficit is associated with bowel symptoms. The research carried out suggests that a number of possible pathophysiologic mechanisms exist for the main symptoms; these are shown in Table 20.1.

CONSTIPATION

Constipation in MS can vary from being quite minor to being a severe and disabling problem. This complaint probably has several causes.

Abnormalities of colonic activity and a slow transit time have been shown in patients with MS [3, 7–9]. In some patients, reduced fluid intake, general poor mobility, and anticholinergic use may contribute to the problem. Chia et al. [10] speculated that slow transit is due to an autonomic nervous system deficit, such as occurs with a central nervous system lesion rostral to the thoracic cord; but severe constipation can occur in patients with little general neurologic disability due to MS. A highly speculative hypothesis is that it is due not to a specific neurologic lesion in the central nervous system but rather to some mechanism similar to that which causes fatigue in the disease.

A complaint that does appear to be associated with paraparesis in severely disabled patients is a difficulty in voluntarily switching on the mechanism of defecation. The normal process involves a complex series of neurologically controlled actions that are initiated in response to the conscious sensation of a full rectum. When this fullness is sensed, and if defecation is judged to be appropriate, it is initiated by raising the intra-abdominal pressure and straining down, which causes descent of the pelvic floor. The internal anal sphincter pressure falls due to the rectoanal inhibitory reflex, and the pubococcygeal muscle and the striated external sphincter relax. In patients with severe paraparesis and spasticity of the pelvic floor, difficulty with relaxation of the pubococcygeal muscle may be expected. In a small group of patients with severe constipation and paraparesis, a failure of effacement of the puborectal muscle during attempts to empty the rectum was demonstrated [11]. Several of these patients found that digitation assisted evacuation. When this maneuver was performed, it could be seen that they needed to hook the index finger over the puborectalis impression and pull the muscle downward until effacement was achieved, and then rectal emptying proceeded. Paradoxical contraction of the puborectal muscle has been proposed as a feature of constipation in patients with MS [10].

In a study by Gill et al., 3 of 11 patients with severe constipation were found to have developed an intussusception, and in one case this had produced an intrarectal obstruction [11]. Intussusception is thought to be the result of chronic straining, and such an abnormality should be suspected in patients with very severe difficulty with rectal emptying. In another study, a rectocele was thought to contribute to the failure to empty the bowel in two out of four patients with defecatory difficulties [9].

INCONTINENCE

In spinal health, defecation can be delayed if it is inappropriate by contraction of the external anal sphincter and pelvic floor. Many patients with MS who have fecal incontinence can be demonstrated either clinically or manometrically to have very poor voluntary squeeze pressure [9, 12, 13]. An association of this condition with spinal cord disease and a paraparesis might logically be expected.

A study by Nordenbo et al. [13] found a close association between absent or impaired rectal sensation and fecal incontinence. Rectal fullness was poorly sensed, and these authors suggested that loss of this normal sensation could well result in patients' being unaware of impending defecation.

The rectoanal inhibitory reflex has a local intramural pathway [14] and remains intact in spinal cord disease, enabling relaxation of the internal and external sphincters to occur in response to rectal filling without the need for voluntary input or conscious sensation. Nordenbo et al. also demonstrated a decreased rectal compliance in patients with MS, which might tend to result in early initiation of the rectoanal inhibitory reflex [13].

Some have also suggested that a lower motor neuron component due to anal sphincter weakness after obstetric injury may be a factor contributing to incontinence in some multiparous women with MS [15].

INVESTIGATIONS

Most studies have shown that fecal incontinence in MS is associated with constipation. As a general rule, a patient with MS who has incontinence without constipation should be investigated for other causes of lower bowel dysfunction.

Colonic transit times can be estimated by getting the patient to swallow radiopaque markers and taking a series of abdominal radiographs. Pressure studies of the rectum and sphincter contractions can be performed using manometry and are appropriate in patients whose predominant complaint is of incontinence.

Defecography is the most valuable investigation in patients complaining of difficulties with defecation. Defecography is a radiologic investigation that allows the process of defecation to be visualized. A barium-containing contrast agent is introduced into the rectum, and the function of the pelvic floor and sphincters can be studied as the patient attempts to defecate. When this method is used, a failure of effacement of the pubococcygeal muscle can be demonstrated and an intussusception can be identified.

MANAGEMENT

No published studies exist on the effect of medication on bowel symptoms in MS. Patients with MS who smoked cannabis rated improvement in their bladder and bowel control to be relatively small [16].

In general, most patients have tried enemas and laxatives themselves before complaining of their problem to their neurologist. If constipation is a complaint and lactulose has not been tried, the use of 10 ml of this medication daily should be recommended. An enema may assist in clearing the rectum, and if given in the morning, it may reduce the risk that fecal incontinence will occur at some other time during the day.

In a study that examined the value of using a vibrating device primarily to assist bladder emptying in patients with MS, a proportion of the patients reported the procedure to be helpful in assisting effective bowel emptying as well [17].

If rectal intussusception is demonstrated, surgical treatment may be necessary.

In general, however, little can be currently offered to the large number of patients with disturbed bowel function, which troubles both them and their caregivers greatly. New approaches to and new treatments for this problem are much needed.

REFERENCES

1. Sullivan S, Ebers G. Gastrointestinal dysfunction in multiple sclerosis. Gastroenterology 1983;84: 1640–1646.
2. Hinds J, Eidelman B, Wald A. Prevalence of bowel dysfunction in multiple sclerosis: a population survey. Gastroenterology 1990;98:1538–1542.
3. Chia Y-W, Fowler C, Kamm M, et al. Prevalence of bowel dysfunction in patients with multiple sclerosis and bladder dysfunction. J Neurol 1995;242:105–108.
4. Bakke A, Myhr K, Gronning M, Nyland H. Bladder, bowel and sexual dysfunction in patients with multiple sclerosis—a cohort study. Scand J Urol Nephrol 1996;179(suppl):61–66.
5. Betts CD, D'Mellow MT, Fowler CJ. Urinary symptoms and the neurological features of bladder dysfunction in multiple sclerosis. J Neurol Neurosurg Psychiatry 1993;56:245–250.
6. De Groat W. Central Neural Control of the Lower Urinary Tract. In G Bock, J Whelan (eds), Neurobiology of Incontinence. Chichester, UK: Wiley, 1990;27–56.
7. Glick E, Meshkinpour H, Haldeman S, et al. Colonic dysfunction in multiple sclerosis. Gastroenterology 1982;83:1002–1007.

8. Weber J, Grise P, Roquebert M, et al. Radiopaque markers transit and anorectal manometry in 16 patients with multiple sclerosis and urinary bladder dysfunction. Dis Colon Rectum 1987;30:95–100.
9. Waldron D, Horgan P, Patel F, et al. Multiple sclerosis assessment of colonic and anorectal function in the presence of faecal incontinence. Int J Colorectal Dis 1993;8:220–224.
10. Chia Y, Gill K, Jameson J, et al. Paradoxical puborectalis contraction is a feature of constipation in patients with multiple sclerosis. J Neurol Neurosurg Psychiatry 1996;60:31–35.
11. Gill K, Chia Y, Henry M, Shorvon P. Defecography in multiple sclerosis patients with severe constipation. Radiology 1994;191:553–556.
12. Sorensen M, Lorentzen M, Petersen J, Christiansen J. Anorectal dysfunction in patients with urologic disturbance due to multiple sclerosis. Dis Colon Rectum 1991;34:136–139.
13. Nordenbo A, Andersen J, Andersen J. Disturbances of ano-rectal function in multiple sclerosis. J Neurol 1996;243:445–451.
14. Lubowski D, Nicholls R, Swash M, Jordan M. Neural control of internal sphincter function. Br J Surg 1987;74:668–670.
15. Swash M, Snooks SJ, Chalmers DHK. Parity as a factor in incontinence in multiple sclerosis. Arch Neurol 1987;44:504–508.
16. Consroe P, Musty R, Rein J, et al. The perceived effects of smoked cannabis on patients with multiple sclerosis. Eur Neurol 1997;38:44–48.
17. Dasgupta P, Haslam C, Goodwin R, Fowler C. The Queen Square bladder stimulator: a device for assisting emptying of the neurogenic bladder. Br J Urol 1997;80:234–237.

21
Tropical Spastic Paraparesis

Prokar Dasgupta and Iqbal F. Hussain

ETIOLOGY AND SEROPREVALENCE

HTLV-I–associated myelopathy/tropical spastic paraparesis (HAM/TSP) is caused by human T-cell lymphotropic virus type I (HTLV-I), a retrovirus belonging to the Oncovirinae family [1]. Infection, which is lifelong, is transmitted by sexual intercourse, breast-feeding, transfusion of infected whole blood, or sharing of equipment during intravenous drug use. HTLV-I infection is endemic in Japan, the West Indies, many areas of sub-Saharan Africa, parts of South, Central, and North America, the Seychelles, and in some isolated populations. Many migrants from these areas are now residents in Europe [2]. This infection, in addition to being associated with HAM/TSP, is linked with subsequent development of adult T-cell leukemia and lymphoma and other inflammatory conditions. Although relatively rare in European countries, these disorders have been reported in the United Kingdom, France, Belgium, Italy, Portugal, Spain, Greece, Sweden, and Russia, not only among immigrants from areas in which HTLV-I infection is endemic, but also among indigenous Europeans [2].

The growing incidence of HTLV infections has led to the establishment of the HTLV European Research Network, a concerted effort by participating nations to understand the distribution and spread of HTLV in Europe. This network has established an algorithm for serologic screening for HTLV infections [2].

The seroprevalence of HTLV among blood donors in European countries is reportedly low, ranging from less than 1 in 100,000 to 30 in 100,000; these cases primarily represent infection with HTLV-I. However, screening in antenatal clinics in France and the United Kingdom have shown the seroprevalence of HTLV-I to be approximately 0.2%. HTLV-I clearly is now spreading into indigenous European populations, particularly women, through sexual transmission [2].

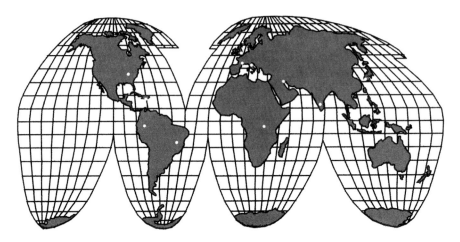

Figure 21.1 Geographic distribution of neurogenic bladder in tropical spastic paraparesis.

GEOGRAPHIC DISTRIBUTION OF NEUROGENIC BLADDER DUE TO TROPICAL SPASTIC PARAPARESIS

Neurogenic bladder dysfunction occurs in 75–100% of patients with HAM/TSP [3]. The bulk of the literature on this subject originates in Japan, where the infection is quite common [4, 5]. A few similar studies have been conducted among diverse populations in the West Indies [6], Brazil [7, 8], Colombia [9], Martinique (French West Indies) [10], Ethiopia [11], the United Kingdom [6, 12], the United States [13, 14], Italy [15], and other nations [16, 17] (Figure 21.1).

PATHOPHYSIOLOGY

The nerves to the bladder emerge from the S2–S4 segments of the spinal cord, whereas those to the lower limbs are immediately above them. These nerves are mainly under the inhibitory influence of the pontine micturition center through ascending and descending pathways. A suprasacral spinal cord lesion, as seen in TSP, causes a loss of this inhibitory control, leading to detrusor hyperreflexia with varying degrees of detrusor sphincter dyssynergia, along with spasticity of the lower limbs due to involvement of the pyramidal tracts.

Shibasaki et al. have described TSP as a "chronic diffuse leukomyelitis" [18]. The lesions comprise a chronic inflammatory disorder with perivascular lymphocyte cuffing. The spinal white matter is primarily involved, and the gray matter is relatively spared. The lateral and, to some extent, the posterior columns of the spinal cord are affected in a bilaterally symmetric fashion [18]. The pathology was described in detail by McMenemy before the discovery of HTLV-I; more recently, Iwasaki [19] has illustrated the main neuropathologic features in proven HTLV-I myelopathy.

Wu et al. detailed the neuroimmunologic features of TSP in a 73-year-old North American woman. They found tractal degeneration of the spinal cord, perivascular and meningeal fibrosis, demyelination, neuroaxonal spheroids, and neurofilamentous masses immunoreactive for phosphorylated neurofilament. This neuroaxonal dystrophy was characterized by a prevalence of CD8+ cells and class I major histocompatibility complex molecules and a paucity of CD4+ lymphocytes. Glial cells were also immunoreactive for cytokines, such as tumor necrosis factor-α, lymphotoxin, and interleukin 6 [20].

An ultrastructural study of TSP in a rat model showed separation of myelin lamellae in both the spinal cord and peripheral nerves. Axons were relatively spared, although some did have tuboreticular inclusions. Macrophages containing myelin were seen among demyelinated and remyelinated axons. Apoptosis of oligodendrocytes and Schwann cells with characteristic apoptotic bodies were also noticed. However, no virus particles themselves were identified within these lesions [21].

Peripheral neuropathy as against radiculopathy has also been described. Nerve biopsies may show perineural and perivascular infiltrates, loss of axons, wallerian degeneration, and demyelination of nerve fibers [22].

Some have suggested that infection of dendritic cells by the virus may be one of the first steps in altering the immune response [23], followed by "spontaneous" proliferation of CD8+ cells [24] and antibody formation and, later, by full-blown immunodeficiency [25]. The concentrations of neopterin within the cerebrospinal fluid are elevated, indicating intrathecal activation of cell-mediated immunity [26].

VESICAL PATHOLOGY IN TROPICAL SPASTIC PARAPARESIS

In TSP, the bladder is usually hyperreflexic and can become contracted as a result [27]. Rare cases of interstitial cystitis and persistent prostatitis have also been reported [28]. Nomata et al. found infiltration of the lamina propria with lymphocytes in some of these patients and suggested the possible involvement of immunologic mechanisms in the development of bladder dysfunction [27]. However, whether this is true is not yet established, because the presence of lymphocytes could merely reflect the propensity of these patients (as in other neurogenic bladder disorders) to urinary tract infections.

The curious appearance of Schwann cells and axons in the suburothelial layer of the bladder have been reported using immunohistochemical studies. These nerves are thought to have a sensory role and are clearly visible in biopsies taken with a flexible cystoscope when stained with S100 (a Schwann cell marker) and protein gene product (PGP) 9.5 (a nonspecific neuronal marker) [29]. Thickening of these neurons in TSP is quite marked, and in some of the bladder sections, the nerves appear as "sausage rolls" [30]. Such florid hyperplasia is not commonly seen in neurogenic bladders due to multiple sclerosis, transverse myelitis, or spinal cord injury, and certainly not in normal samples [31]. Perhaps they represent neurofilamentous masses in the bladder, such as have been described in the spinal cord. The cause for this finding is unexplained, and whether viral particles are responsible is yet to be ascertained (Figures 21.2 and 21.3).

Electron microscopy reveals relatively normal axons but large Schwann cell bands, the mean diameters of which are significantly greater than those in the bladders of patients with multiple sclerosis and in normal controls [31].

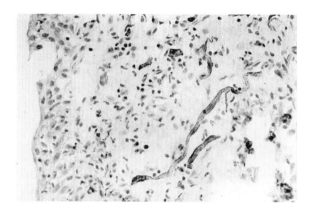

Figure 21.2   Thickened suburothelial nerves in a patient with tropical spastic paraparesis; S100 staining (×250).

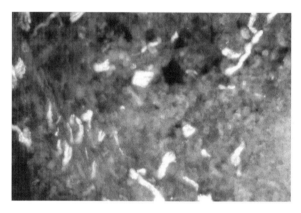

Figure 21.3   "Sausage roll" nerves in the lamina propria of the bladder in a patient with tropical spastic paraparesis; protein growth product (PGP) 9.5 staining (×250).

CLINICAL FEATURES

The usual urinary symptoms are urgency, frequency, urge incontinence, and sensation of incomplete emptying. The stream can be intermittent as a result of detrusor sphincter dyssynergia. These symptoms are associated with varying degrees of disability, which stabilizes after a period of time, unlike the progressive deterioration often seen in multiple sclerosis. Whereas some patients can walk with or without aids, others are wheelchair bound. Imamura et al., in a study series involving 25 patients, reported that the onset of urinary symptoms preceded other pyramidal symptoms in 24% of patients [32].

The majority of patients are women, but in the few male patients, voiding dysfunction can be accompanied by neurogenic erectile dysfunction.

INVESTIGATIONS

The following investigations are undertaken to establish the diagnosis:

1. Testing for serum antibodies to HTLV-I. These are usually present in high titer in patients with HAM/TSP. A variety of assays is available, including immuno-

fluorescence, gelatin particle agglutination, enzyme-linked immunoassay, radioimmunoprecipitation, and Western blot.
2. Testing for cerebrospinal fluid antibodies to HTLV-I.
3. Polymerase chain reaction (PCR). PCR testing is necessary if the diagnosis cannot be established by the above means [2]. A few cases of antibody-negative but PCR-positive HAM/TSP have been described.

The following studies can be performed to assess voiding dysfunction:

1. *Flow rate and assessment of postvoid residuals by ultrasonography.* The flow is typically interrupted as a result of detrusor sphincter dyssynergia. Postvoid residual volumes are easily assessed by ultrasonographic scanning; a volume of more than 100 ml is generally regarded as significant. Incomplete emptying in TSP is due either to detrusor hyperreflexia with associated external sphincter dyssynergia or to detrusor hyperreflexia with impaired contractility. In a few patients, the bladder may be hypocontractile.
2. *Cystometry.* Although the results of pressure-flow studies in TSP have been described on numerous occasions [5, 13, 33], such tests are not routinely necessary, as the irritative voiding symptoms can reasonably be assumed to be caused by detrusor hyperreflexia, which is present in the majority of patients [34]. Most investigators have also reported detrusor sphincter dyssynergia on electromyography [33, 35]. Urethral pressure profiles, when performed, are usually normal [36].

    Invasive urodynamic tests should be considered only if simple treatment measures, such as anticholinergic medication, fail to alleviate symptoms. The occasional patient in whom the voiding symptoms are obstructive rather than irritative also needs cystometry, as detrusor areflexia can sometimes be seen [33].

    The reason for detrusor underactivity in the presence of a suprasacral spinal cord infection is unclear, although some authors have suggested involvement of the posterior and anterior nerve roots by inflammatory exudate, as well as involvement of Onuf's nucleus by the disease process [19]. Komine et al. have suggested that patients with hyperreflexia have had the disease for a longer period than those with areflexia, possibly indicating that detrusor overactivity is not prominent in early stages of TSP [3].
3. *Neurophysiologic tests.* Motor and sensory nerve conduction studies of the median nerve are usually normal. Tibial somatosensory evoked potentials may show prolonged latencies in some patients [12, 18]. Sacral reflex latencies are mostly normal, and motor evoked potentials of the striated urethral sphincter after magnetic stimulation of the brain show delayed or absent responses in some patients [12]. Approximately one-third of patients may have evidence of denervation and reinnervation in the striated urethral sphincter on concentric needle electromyography, with prolonged duration of the motor unit responses [12]. These tests are not routinely necessary, except when the diagnosis is in doubt. They certainly do not alter decisions regarding bladder management if the diagnosis is already established.
4. *Upper urinary tract imaging.* This imaging is necessary to detect hydronephrosis due to high voiding pressures and should not be omitted in patients with a raised serum creatine level. Fortunately, renal impairment due to hydronephrosis is uncommon in TSP [5].

Table 21.1   Aims of treatment for tropical spastic paraparesis

To protect the upper urinary tract
To reduce detrusor hyperreflexia
To facilitate bladder emptying
To improve continence
To improve quality of life

MANAGEMENT

The aims of treatment for TSP are shown in Table 21.1. Specific therapeutic measures are detailed in the following sections.

Medication with Oral Anticholinergics

Oxybutynin chloride and probanthine are nonselective muscarinic receptor blockers; the tricyclic antidepressant imipramine is also known to have a similar effect. Oxybutynin chloride is the drug most commonly used to reduce detrusor hyperreflexia; it is started at a low dosage of 2.5 mg twice a day and increased to up to 5 mg three times a day orally. Patients must be warned about side effects, such as dry mouth, blurring of vision, and constipation.

The hope is that the introduction of selective muscarinic receptor blockers, such as tolterodine tartrate, will reduce the incidence of troublesome side effects and improve patient compliance.

Clean Intermittent Self-Catheterization

Since its introduction approximately 20 years ago, clean intermittent self-catheterization has revolutionized the management of the neurogenic bladder, particularly incomplete emptying. Not only does it improve continence, but it also protects the upper urinary tracts from dilation. The neurogenic bladder of TSP is no exception, and patients with postvoid residuals of more than 100 ml should be taught this technique before commencing anticholinergic therapy. The reason is that oxybutynin chloride worsens bladder emptying, and patients fail to notice symptomatic improvement if intermittent self-catheterization is not started concomitantly.

Approximately 60% of TSP patients need intermittent self-catheterization at some stage [5]. Those with smaller residuals can be managed on oxybutynin chloride alone; however, residuals must be checked periodically, particularly if the patient notices a deterioration in symptoms.

Intravesical Instillation of Capsaicin

Capsaicin, the pungent ingredient of red hot chilis, is available as a powder that can be dissolved in a solution containing alcohol and saline. The first report of its efficacy as an intravesical solution in TSP came from Fowler et al. in 1994

Table 21.2   Analysis of suburothelial nerve densities in human T-cell lymphotrophic virus type I–associated myelopathy/tropical spastic paraparesis patients before and after intravesical capsaicin treatment, using S100 and protein gene product (PGP) 9.5 staining

Stain	Nerve density	Control subjects: mean (range)	Patients with tropical spastic paraparesis: mean (range)	
			Precapsaicin	**Postcapsaicin**
S100	Nerves/square millimeter	78 (76-80)	142 (78–250)	86 (49–133)
PGP 9.5	Red %	2.5 (2.1–2.8)	7.9 (3.2–10.3)	5.8 (2.8–9.4)

Note: Mean value of five computerized readings of nerve density per patient and the ranges are shown.

[37]. Since then, its effects in TSP have been the subject of a further study that included patients with intractable urge incontinence unresponsive to anticholinergics. Patients had filling cystometries and flexible-cystoscope biopsies under local anesthesia (21SX forceps; Olympus, Tokyo, Japan) followed 2 weeks later by instillation of 100 ml of intravesical capsaicin, 1 mmol/liter in 30% alcohol in saline. Filling cystometries and flexible-cystoscope biopsies were repeated 6 weeks after instillation of capsaicin.

The same technique was used to obtain bladder biopsies from control patients with microscopical hematuria and normal bladders. The patients in the control group were not given intravesical capsaicin.

Ten-micrometer sections were stained with S100 and PGP 9.5, and nerve densities in the lamina propria were evaluated using sections stained with S100 (nerves per square millimeter) and computerized image analysis for those stained with PGP 9.5 (red %—the nerves appear red against a blue background).

All the TSP patients had improved continence after capsaicin instillations while performing clean intermittent self-catheterization. The symptomatic benefit lasted for a period of 4–6 months, following which patients had further doses of capsaicin with similar results. Objective evidence was found of an increase in bladder capacity on cystometry 6 weeks after capsaicin treatment. Capsaicin treatment caused a reduction in the nerve densities of the suburothelial nerves, which are thought to have a sensory function (Table 21.2) [30].

Although the rate of response to intravesical instillation of capsaicin is much higher in TSP patients [30] than in patients with multiple sclerosis (almost 100% versus 70%) [37], this form of treatment should be tried only in those who fail to respond to therapy with oral anticholinergics. The reason for this dramatic response in TSP is not known but may be related to the hyperplasia of suburothelial neurons described earlier.

Danazol Therapy

The anabolic steroid danazol, given orally in a dosage of 200 mg three times a day, has been found effective in resolving urinary incontinence in some patients [38, 39]. Gait disturbances seem to respond better than urinary symptoms [38], and women benefit more than men [39]. Side effects, such as hepatic dysfunction, amenorrhea, and fluid retention, can be controlled by reducing the dosage.

Miscellaneous Immunomodulatory Therapies

Nakagawa et al. have reported the beneficial effects of lymphocytapheresis, oral prednisolone, eperisone hydrochloride, intrathecal injection of hydrocortisone, intravenous administration of methylprednisolone, interferon-α, azathioprine, vitamin C, heparin sodium, salazosulfapyridine, erythromycin, fosfomycin trometh-amine, mizoribine, and thyrotropin-releasing hormone in a large number of patients [40, 41]. The sheer number of treatments reported suggests that they are not specific therapies directed toward bladder dysfunction, but improvement in urinary symptoms may be noticed during their use. A few patients show some response to high dosages of steroids or plasmapheresis.

SUMMARY

HAM/TSP is a myelitis caused by the retrovirus HTLV-I. What was initially described as *Jamaican neuropathy* [42] is now recognized worldwide, and the spread of the virus appears to be due to a movement of populations.

Detrusor hyperreflexia and incomplete bladder emptying occur in the majority of patients; however, detrusor acontractility should be suspected in those who present with reduction in urinary stream rather than urgency.

Interest has recently been shown in the vesical neuropathology of this disease. In TSP, the nerves in the lamina propria of the bladder have a striking, thickened appearance, the exact cause of which remains unclear.

The use of oral anticholinergics with or without clean intermittent self-catheterization is an effective first-line measure. In the few who fail to respond to this simple regime, intravesical instillation of capsaicin or danazol therapy can be offered as alternatives.

REFERENCES

1. Cruickshank JK, Rudge P, Dalgleish AG, et al. Tropical spastic paraparesis and human T-cell lymphotropic virus type 1 in the United Kingdom. Brain 1989;112:1057–1090.
2. The HTLV European Research Network. Seroepidemiology of human T-cell leukaemia/lymphoma viruses in Europe. J Acquir Immune Defic Syndr Hum Retrovirol 1996;13:68–77.
3. Komine S, Yoshida H, Fujiyama C, Masaki Z. Voiding dysfunction in patients with human T-lymphotropic-virus-type-1–associated myelopathy. Urol Int 1991;47(suppl 1):67–68.
4. Saito M, Kato K, Kondo A, Miyake K. Neurogenic bladder in HAM (HTLVI-associated myelopathy). Hinyokika Kiyo 1991;37:1005–1008.
5. Imamura A. Studies on neurogenic bladder due to human T-lymphotropic virus type-I associated myelopathy (HAM). Nippon Hinyokika Gakkai Zasshi 1994;85:1106–1115.
6. Cruickshank JK, Richardson JH, Morgan OS, et al. Screening for prolonged incubation of HTLV-1 infection in British and Jamaican relatives of British patients with tropical spastic paraparesis. BMJ 1990;300:300–304.

7. Araujo A de Q, Ali A, Newell A, et al. HTLV-I infection and neurological disease in Rio de Janeiro. J Neurol Neurosurg Psychiatry 1992;55:153–155.
8. Costa CM, Salgueiro MR, Carton H, et al. Tropical spastic paraparesis in Northeastern Brazil. Arq Neuropsiquiatr 1989;47:134–138.
9. Roman GC, Roman LN, Spencer PS, Schoenberg BS. Tropical spastic paraparesis: a neuroepidemiological study in Colombia. Ann Neurol 1985;17:361–365.
10. Vernant JC, Maurs L, Gessain A, et al. Endemic tropical spastic paraparesis associated with human T-lymphotropic virus type I: a clinical and seroepidemiological study of 25 cases. Ann Neurol 1987;21:123–130.
11. Abebe M, Haimanot RT, Gustafsson A, et al. Low HTLV-1 seroprevalence in endemic tropical spastic paraparesis in Ethiopia. Trans R Soc Trop Med Hyg 1991;85:109–112.
12. Eardley I, Fowler CJ, Nagendran K, et al. The neurourology of tropical spastic paraparesis. Br J Urol 1991;68:598–603.
13. Walton GW, Kaplan SA. Urinary disturbance in tropical spastic paraparesis: preliminary urodynamic survey. J Urol 1993;150:930–932.
14. Honig LS, Lipka JJ, Young KY, et al. HTLV-I associated myelopathy in a Californian: diagnosis by reactivity to a viral recombinant antigen. Neurology 1991;41:448–450.
15. Lugaresi A, Uncini A, Porrini AM, et al. HTLV-1 associated myeloneuropathy in an Italian. Acta Neurol Scand 1991;84:186–191.
16. Weber T, Hunsmann G, Stevens W, Fleming AF. Human retroviruses. Baillieres Clin Haematol 1992;5:273–314.
17. Montgomery RD. HTLV-1 and tropical spastic paraparesis. 1. Clinical features, pathology and epidemiology. Trans R Soc Trop Med Hyg 1989;83:724–728.
18. Shibasaki H, Endo C, Kuroda Y, et al. Clinical picture of HTLV-I associated myelopathy. J Neurol Sci 1988;87:15–24.
19. Iwasaki Y. Pathology of chronic myelopathy associated with HTLV 1 infection (HAM/TSP). J Neurol Sci 1990;96:103–123.
20. Wu E, Dickson DW, Jacobson S, Raine CS. Neuroaxonal dystrophy in HTLV-1-associated myelopathy/tropical spastic paraparesis: neuropathologic and neuroimmunologic correlations. Acta Neuropathol (Berl) 1993;86:224–235.
21. Abe M. Rat model of HTLV-I infection—ultrastructural study of HAM rat disease. Hokkaido Igaku Zasshi 1994;69:1399–1408.
22. Said G, Goulon-Goeau C, Lacroix C, et al. Inflammatory lesions of peripheral nerve in a patient with human T-lymphotropic virus type I—associated myelopathy. Ann Neurol 1988;24:275–277.
23. Ali A, Patterson S, Cruickshank K, et al. Dendritic cells infected in vitro with human T-cell leukaemia/lymphoma virus type-1 (HTLV-1); enhanced lymphocytic proliferation and tropical spastic paraparesis. Clin Exp Immunol 1993;94:32–37.
24. Macatonia SE, Cruickshank JK, Rudge P, Knight SC. Dendritic cells from patients with tropical spastic paraparesis are infected with HTLV-1 and stimulate autologous lymphocyte proliferation. AIDS Res Hum Retroviruses 1992;8:1699–1706.
25. Knight SC, Macatonia SE, Cruickshank JK, et al. Dendritic cells in HIV-1 and HTLV-1 infection. Adv Exp Med Biol 1993;329:545–549.
26. Ali A, Rudge P, Dalgleish AG. Neopterin concentrations in serum and cerebrospinal fluid in HTLV-I infected individuals. J Neurol 1992;239:270–272.
27. Nomata K, Suzu H, Yushita Y, et al. Bladder involvement in HTLV-I associated myelopathy. Nippon Hinyokika Gakkai Zasshi 1991;82:1161–1164.
28. Nomata K, Nakamura T, Suzu H, et al. Novel complications with HTLV-1-associated myelopathy/tropical spastic paraparesis: interstitial cystitis and persistent prostatitis. Jpn J Cancer Res 1992;83:601–608.
29. Dasgupta P, Chandiramani V, Beckett A, et al. Flexible cystoscopic biopsies for evaluation of nerve densities in the suburothelium of the human urinary bladder. Br J Urol 1997;80:490–492.
30. Dasgupta P, Fowler CJ, Scaravilli F, Shah J. Bladder biopsies in tropical spastic paraparesis and the effect of intravesical capsaicin on nerve densities. Eur Urol 1996;30(suppl 2):237A.
31. Dasgupta P. Bladder biopsies: a new diagnostic tool for tropical spastic paraparesis? Proc R Soc Med (Section of Neurology) December 1996;7.
32. Imamura A, Kitagawa T, Ohi Y, Osame M. Clinical manifestation of human T-cell lymphotropic virus type-I–associated myelopathy and vesicopathy. Urol Int 1991;46:149–153.
33. Saito M, Kondo K, Kato K, Gotoh M. Bladder dysfunction due to human T-lymphotropic virus type I associated myelopathy. Br J Urol 1991;68:365–368.

34. Yamashita H, Kumazawa J. Voiding dysfunction: patients with human T-lymphotropic-virus-type-1–associated myelopathy. Urol Int 1991;47(suppl 1):69–71.
35. Hattori T, Sakakibara R, Yamanishi T, et al. Micturitional disturbance in human T-lymphotropic virus type-1-associated myelopathy. J Spinal Disord 1994;7:255–258.
36. Sakiyama H, Nishi K, Kikukawa H, Ueda S. Urinary disturbance due to HTLV-1 associated myelopathy. Nippon Hinyokika Gakkai Zasshi 1992;83:2058–2061.
37. Fowler CJ, Beck RO, Gerrard S, et al. Intravesical capsaicin for the treatment of detrusor hyperreflexia. J Neurol Neurosurg Psychiatry 1994;57:169–173.
38. Harrington WJ Jr, Sheremata WA, Snodgrass SR, et al. Tropical spastic paraparesis/HTLV-1-associated myelopathy (TSP/HAM): treatment with an anabolic steroid danazol. AIDS Res Hum Retroviruses 1991;7:1031–1034.
39. Melo A, Moura L, Meireles A, Costa G. Danazol: a new perspective in the treatment of HTLV-1 associated myelopathy (preliminary report). Arq Neuropsiquiatr 1992;50:402–403.
40. Nakagawa M, Maruyama Y, Osame M. Therapy for HAM/TSP and AIDS. Nippon Rinsho 1994;52:3019–3025.
41. Nakagawa M, Nakahara K, Maruyama Y, et al. Therapeutic trials in 200 patients with HTLV-I–associated myelopathy/tropical spastic paraparesis. J Neurovirol 1996;2:345–355.
42. Montgomery RD, Cruickshank EK, Robertson WB, et al. Clinical and pathological observations on Jamaican neuropathy: a report of 206 cases. Brain 1964;87:425–460.

22
Cauda Equina Damage and Its Management

Iqbal F. Hussain

Because the spinal cord is shorter than the vertebral column, the most caudal roots arising from the lumbosacral segments of the cord travel a considerable distance in the cauda equina. Within this structure, they are at risk of damage. The mechanisms of injury are many; some are catastrophic and immediately recognizable, whereas others are insidious in onset with a variety of presentations. Diagnosis of a cauda equina lesion may be complicated and may require neuroradiologic imaging together with tests of bladder, bowel, sexual, and somatic function. Management may be difficult and require prolonged intensive and long-term rehabilitation.

ANATOMY OF THE CAUDA EQUINA

The spinal cord is often said to terminate at the level of the intervertebral disk between L1 and L2, but in fact this is true only in approximately one-half of all cases studied at postmortem. Depending on the length of the trunk and the degree of flexion, the spinal cord may terminate at a level anywhere from opposite the body of T12 to the disk between L2 and L3 or even between L3 and L4 [1, 2]. The cord is enclosed by the dura, arachnoid, and pia mater, which are separated by a potential subdural space and an actual subarachnoid space containing cerebrospinal fluid. The caudal spinal cord is termed the *conus medullaris* and is continuous with a filament of connective tissue known as the *filum terminale*. The dura and arachnoid meninges surround the filum terminale for 15 cm and extend to the level of the S2 vertebral body. A difference of approximately 5 vertebral bodies therefore exists between the conus and the distal extension of the meninges, and this is a good approximation to the length of the cauda equina (Figures 22.1 and 22.2).

In the cervical region, the spinal nerve roots exit from the vertebral column horizontally and above the respective vertebral segment. At the caudal end of the cord, the nerve roots descend for varying distances, beyond the conus medullaris in the case of S3 and S4, before reaching the corresponding neural foramen. In

325

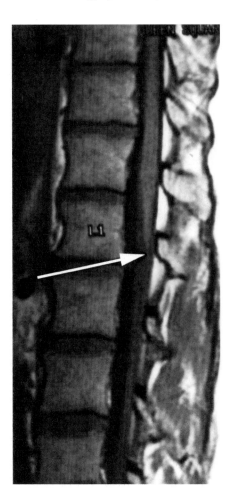

Figure 22.1 T₁SE magnetic resonance image of conus (sagittal view). The spinal cord terminates opposite the lower border of the L1 vertebral body (*arrow*).

this caudal region, the neural foramen is located below and medial to the respective neural arch, and the dorsal root ganglion lies at this point. The dorsal root ganglion is a sensory ganglion containing the cell bodies of the afferent nerves.

The bladder, bowel, and sexual organs receive important connections from the sacral part of the spinal cord by way of the pelvic plexus and pudendal nerve. The efferent parasympathetic outflow to the bladder, its main excitatory input, is provided via the pelvic nerves (S2–S4). They synapse on postganglionic neurons in the pelvic plexus or in ganglia located within the bladder wall itself. Parasympathetic innervation is also important for sexual function, such as reflex clitoral erection and vaginal lubrication in women, and is partly responsible for vasodilation of erectile tissue in men. The parasympathetic afferents have their cell bodies in the dorsal root ganglia of these same segments (S2–S4) before entering the dorsal horn. The urethral sphincter (rhabdosphincter) receives motor innervation from efferent somatic pathways via the pudendal nerve. The anterior horn cells that innervate it lie in the ventral horn of sacral segments S2-S4, in a region

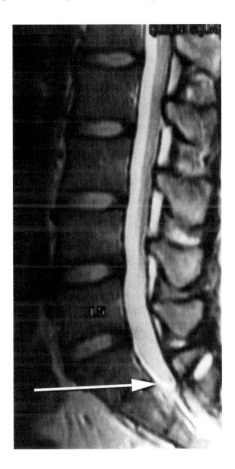

Figure 22.2 T$_2$FSE magnetic resonance image of thecal sac (sagittal view). The thecal sac terminates opposite the S2 vertebral body (*arrow*).

known as *Onuf's nucleus.* Sympathetic supply to the pelvic organs arises from T10–L1 and innervates the bladder neck and prostate (among the other male pelvic organs); it is important in both erection and ejaculation. The corresponding sympathetic afferents reside in the T11–L2 dorsal root ganglia.

The introduction of contrast-enhanced computed tomography (CT) and surface-coil magnetic resonance imaging (MRI) has allowed detailed visualization of the nerve roots within the thecal sac of the cauda equina. These roots are known to form a crescentic pattern that is arranged in pairs; the motor bundle is anterior and medial to its larger sensory bundle [3]. The cauda equina nerve roots were traced on CT and MRI scans and compared to the scans of cadaveric specimens by Cohen et al. [4]. They showed that, in the region of the proximal cauda equina (L2–L3), the roots occupy most of the space within the thecal sac, with the motor bundle lying anterior. More caudally, the nerve roots become separated in a crescentic distribution; there is more space within the thecal sac, and the L5 and S1 roots lie more anterior and lateral, whereas S2–S4 lie in the dorsal part of the thecal sac (Figure 22.3). Coronal sections can be obtained to show the location of the dorsal root ganglia within the neural canal (Figures 22.4 and 22.5). Note

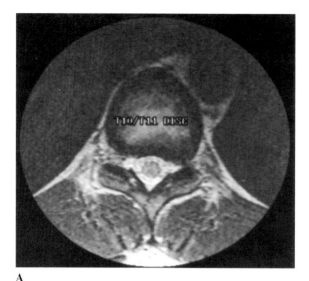

A

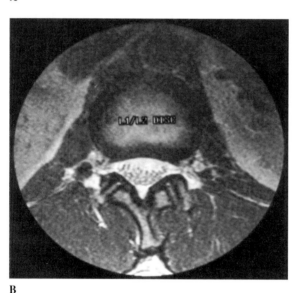

B

Figure 22.3 (**A–E**) T_2FSE magnetic resonance images (axial views) show serial sections taken through the intervertebral disk between T10–T11 (**A**), L1–L2 (**B**), L2–L3 (**C**), L5–S1 (**D**) and through the lower body of the S1 vertebra (**E**). Note that the spinal cord is circular in the most cranial section. With progressing caudal descent, individual roots become visible. This arrangement shows a crescentic shape (see text). (The author is grateful to the Queen Square Imaging Centre in London for carrying out the scans of the author's lower spine using a 1.5-Tesla magnetic resonance image scanner.)

that minimal space exists within the neural canal, and a lesion in this vicinity can cause considerable spinal nerve root compression.

CAUSES AND PRESENTATION OF CAUDA EQUINA DAMAGE

Severe damage to the cauda equina can occur after high-velocity impacts to the lumbosacral spine, as seen after road traffic accidents, falls from great height, or

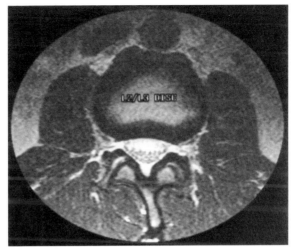

C

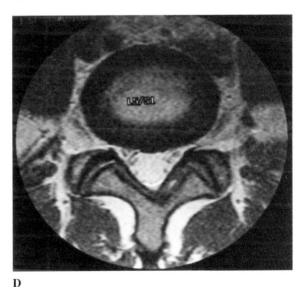

D

penetrating injuries from gunshot, shrapnel, or stabbing [5]. These injuries are likely to be associated with other local and more distant damage to soft tissue and bony structures. In one report, 85% of the spinal cord damage was found to occur preoperatively (all too often, at the time of the injury), approximately 10% in the early postoperative period, and the remainder as a late complication. Although these incidents are relatively rare, the increasing numbers and higher velocity of road traffic accidents, together with better emergency treatment, mean that patients with cauda equina injuries are more likely to survive and to require long-term care and rehabilitation.

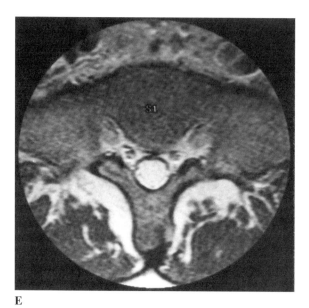

E   *Figure 22.3* (continued)

Abnormalities of the cauda equina may be developmental and may be evident at birth or even antenatally. The most common dysraphic anomaly of the lower cord is a tethered conus. The diagnosis is not always straightforward, although approximately 45% of patients show associated external signs, such as a skin dimple, angioma, or hairy patch [6]. Bladder dysfunction is common [7]. A meningocele is an extension of the dural sac outside the spinal canal (usually through a posterior defect), and such an abnormality may be seen on fetal ultrasonography. Although the diagnosis may be clear, very difficult management decisions may be involved, including the possibility of terminating the pregnancy. Fortunately, these and other congenital causes of cauda equina damage (Table 22.1) are rare, and their management tends to be referred to dedicated pediatric centers.

A much more common cause of cauda equina damage is prolapse of an intervertebral disk causing cord or root compression. The evolution of bipedality in humans is partly responsible for one of the most frequent reasons for seeking medical advice—back pain. In the lumbar vertebral segments, the most common site for disk herniation, the anterior spinous ligaments are immensely strong, so that anterior disk herniation is rare. The lumbar disks are particularly prone to herniation through the posterolateral projections with compression of neural structures, although, less frequently, midline posterior herniation may also occur [8]. Symptoms of cauda equina root compression include back pain, sciatica, saddle anesthesia, bladder and bowel dysfunction, and leg weakness. Considerable debate exists regarding the optimal timing of surgical decompression of an acute central disk prolapse, as is discussed in the section Management of Cauda Equina Damage.

Back pain is also frequently the presenting symptom of root compression from tumors of the cauda equina. These include neurofibromas; glial tumors, such as ependymomas and astrocytomas; and congenital midline tumors, such as dermoid, epidermoid, teratoma, and lipoma. Less common are meningiomas, arachnoid

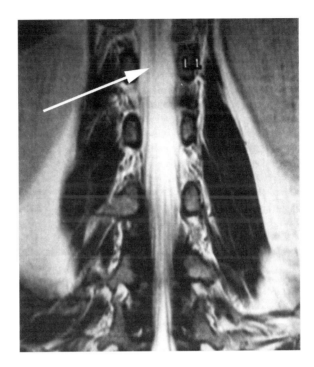

Figure 22.4   T$_2$FSE magnetic resonance image (coronal view) showing the collection of spinal nerve roots that make up the cauda equina after the cord terminates opposite the L1 vertebral body (*arrow*).

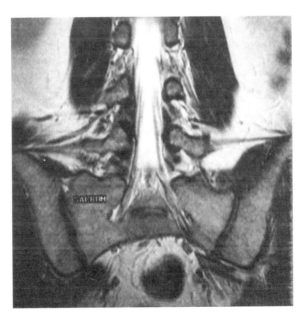

Figure 22.5   T$_2$FSE magnetic resonance image (coronal view) showing the dorsal root ganglia associated with the S1 nerve, which can be seen in the S1 foramina.

Table 22.1   Causes of cauda equina damage

Congenital	
Meningomyelocele	
Congenital dermoid sinus	
Congenital midline tumors: dermoid, epidermoid, teratoma, lipoma	
Acquired	
Infectious:	Neurosarcoidosis, schistosomiasis, abscess formation
Traumatic:	Road traffic accident, fall from height, penetrating injury (gunshot, stabbing)
Degenerative:	Central disk prolapse
Neoplastic:	Primary—ependymoma, neurofibroma, meningioma
	Secondary metastasis
Vascular:	Arteriovenous malformations
Iatrogenic:	Anesthetic, orthopedic, and neurosurgical procedures
	Lumbar arachnoiditis after radiculogram

cysts, meningeal cysts, and malignant melanoma [9]. The cauda equina may also be a site for metastatic disease; these metastases are commonly from an intracranial primary tumor, such as medulloblastoma and pinealoma [10]. Symptoms from cauda equina tumors are rarely specific, and such tumors are often insidious, resulting in late presentation and delayed diagnosis [11]. The common symptom of back pain may occasionally be ignored by the patient or medical practitioners until signs such as sensory loss, leg weakness, or, rarely, urinary retention develop. Pain that disturbs sleep is said to be characteristic of cauda equina tumor, whereas pain from disk disease is said to be eased by rest and recumbency, although this is not always the case. Sensory deficit in the perineal saddle region or sphincter disturbance should prompt investigation for cauda equina damage. Although rarely reported at presentation, sexual dysfunction in both men and women may occur [12, 13] and may feature prominently in legal settlements in cases in which negligence has been proven after cauda equina damage.

A rare cause of cauda equina damage is a spinal arteriovenous malformation (AVM). AVMs are a heterogeneous group of conditions that can produce neurologic deficit by direct cord compression or, more commonly, cause an alteration in the cord blood flow that leads to a secondary deficit. The cord receives its blood supply from the anterior and posterior spinal arteries, whereas the dural supply is segmental and comes from branches of the intercostal arteries. The presence of the malformation results in increased pressure in the draining coronal and medullary spinal veins, leading to a reduced arteriovenous pressure gradient, reduced blood flow, and cord ischemia. This may be one reason that the AVM presents as a cauda equina–type syndrome, despite the lesion's being considerably more rostral. In one report, Djindjian has shown that most AVMs are thoracolumbar (60%); only 12% are cervical, and the remaining 28% are thoracic [14].

In all causes of cauda equina damage, symptoms of bladder dysfunction can vary from complete urinary retention (either acute or chronic) to incontinence (both urge and stress incontinence). Because of the significant and predominant bladder symptoms, such patients may be referred to a urologic surgeon, and indeed some patients undergo urologic surgical intervention before the correct neurologic diagnosis is made. Predominant bowel symptoms are those of atonia with a variable degree of constipation, occasionally with overflow diarrhea. Men may present with erectile dysfunction, although decreased penile tactile sensation and ejaculatory dysfunction may be additional components. Women may report a loss of erotic sensation in the perineal region and an inability to appreciate sexual stimuli.

Somatic dysfunction is confined to the lower limbs and the perisacral region. Sensory deficit may be evident in the sacral, perineal, and scrotal area. Back pain is common, although, if solitary, the symptom is unlikely to be initially attributed to a cauda equina lesion. Lower limb weakness is often reported and confirmed on clinical examination. The ankle reflexes may be absent, and an extensor plantar response may be noted if cord or conus is also involved.

INVESTIGATION OF CAUDA EQUINA DAMAGE

Investigations are carried out to make a diagnosis, plan therapeutic intervention, or follow progression and allow a prognosis to be made. Cauda equina lesions give rise to bladder, bowel, sexual, and somatic dysfunction; the investigation of these is best carried out in a combined pelvic function laboratory.

Radiologic Investigations

Plain radiography of the spine is almost invariably carried out in the initial investigation of cauda equina lesions, although most useful information is obtained from CT or MRI. Excellent images of tissue contrast and discrete spatial resolution can be rapidly obtained noninvasively, and three-dimensional reconstructions can be carried out. Where AVMs are suspected, selective spinal angiography is helpful both in confirming the diagnosis and in planning interventional radiologic therapeutic strategies, such as embolization of fistulae. The features of relevance are the origin of the AVM, the number of feeding vessels, and the exact location of the AVM with respect to the spinal cord. Successful selective embolization has avoided open surgical intervention in some cases of spinal AVM presenting with cauda equina syndrome.

Urologic Investigations

The predominant urologic symptom in patients with cauda equina lesions is voiding difficulty. Patients report reduced flow, double and incomplete voiding, and, in severe cases, complete retention with overflow incontinence. These symptoms can be investigated by flow rate testing, measurement of residual volume, and cystometry. Patients with solitary cauda equina damage commonly demonstrate reduced urinary flow rate and incomplete voiding [15].

Assessment of the detrusor muscle by cystometry (Figure 22.6) may show a trace typical of the areflexic bladder, which has previously been reported in cauda equina lesions [16, 17]. However, reports of hyperreflexic cystometric findings after cauda equina damage also exist. Possible mechanisms for this include a direct and additional higher cord pathology, in which a large tumor of the cauda extends upward to cause unexpected cystometric findings or secondary ischemic damage to the cord at a higher level after the occurrence of a primary lesion affecting the cauda.

Additional information about the sphincter mechanism may be obtained if cystometry is combined with fluoroscopic examination of the bladder. Most

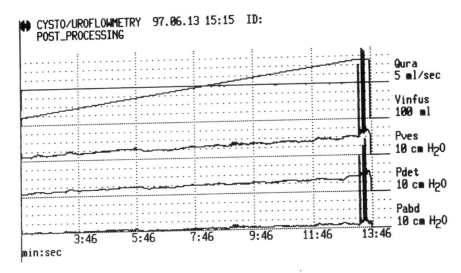

Figure 22.6　Cystometric recording from a female patient with a cauda equina lesion. The bladder was filled to nearly 700 ml; the patient had no sensation of bladder filling and was unable to void. She emptied her bladder by performing clean intermittent self-catheterization. (Pabd = intra-abdominal pressure measured via rectal catheter; Pdet = detrusor pressure; Pves = intravesical pressure; Qura = flow of urine; Vinfus = volume of fluid instilled into the bladder.)

studies confirm an incompetent bladder neck [18], although this is not a universal finding in cauda equina lesions, and the degree of incompetence may not correlate with the level of nerve injury [19]. Stress incontinence from bladder neck incompetence is a particularly troublesome symptom and, when it occurs in men, is almost always associated with a lower motor neuron injury.

Colorectal Investigations

Patients with cauda equina lesions may have troublesome bowel symptoms. Typically, they have an atonic bowel and are prone to developing severe and chronic constipation, although they may occasionally experience overflow fecal incontinence. This is thought to be possibly the result of parasympathetic denervation of the sigmoid and rectum. Incontinence of feces and flatus may also result from a denervated anal sphincter. Anatomic and functional investigations of colorectal disturbance may be helpful. Barium studies and colonoscopy can provide useful anatomic information. Functional studies include anorectal manometry and defecography, which may be performed in specialized combined pelvic function laboratories.

Investigations of Sexual Dysfunction

In cases of cauda equina damage, specific tests of sexual function rarely need to be performed. However, all symptoms reported by the patient should be clearly documented. Men may volunteer information regarding their loss of erectile function, whereas women may be more reluctant to report their symptoms. At a later date, this documentation may be required for medicolegal purposes.

In men, demonstrating that pharmacologically induced erection is possible (with intracavernosal injection or transurethral instillation of prostaglandin E_1) is important. This procedure rules out a vascular cause for the underlying pathology and can also be a useful therapeutic intervention. The introduction of sildenafil citrate (Viagra) has been a significant advance, not only in providing a new pharmacologic agent to aid male erectile dysfunction but also in publicizing sexual dysfunction in general. This is helping to initiate studies of the management of female sexual disorders, and clinical trials are being carried out to establish whether sildenafil citrate may be of benefit to women. The impact of sexual dysfunction on the quality of everyday life is unknown. Questionnaires are being validated that may become important tools in the assessment of sexual dysfunction in the future. As the therapeutic options increase with the development of safe and efficacious oral treatment, an urgent need exists for tools that may help the clinician establish the burden of sexual dysfunction in both men and women.

Neurophysiologic Investigations

Various neurophysiologic techniques may be used to demonstrate the root damage that occurs with a cauda equina lesion. These are reviewed in Chapter 9.

MANAGEMENT OF CAUDA EQUINA DAMAGE

A wide range of conditions can give rise to cauda equina damage, and the management reflects the underlying pathology. However, some general principles can be followed. An accurate assessment relying on history, examination, investigation, and special reports from personnel involved in the continuing care of the patient is very necessary. The immediate management of an acutely injured distal spinal cord often requires orthopedic or neurosurgical intervention. Instability of the spine must be accurately identified and promptly corrected. Root compression must be relieved; considerable debate (and medicolegal interest) exists regarding the expediency with which such surgical decompression is carried out. During the period of spinal shock, an indwelling catheter should be used to drain the bladder; clean intermittent self-catheterization can be introduced later.

Cauda equina damage from an acute compressive lesion raises an important issue: Is it the degree or the duration of compression that is clinically important? The classical teaching has always been that immediate decompression is vital for recovery. Two important animal studies have examined the problem. In a study involving female beagle hounds, Bodner et al. [20] demonstrated that neurologic function, as evaluated by cystometry, cortical evoked potentials, and histology, was dependent on the degree of compression of the cauda equina. Twenty-five percent compression resulted in minimal change to the cystometric findings and an increase in the cortical evoked potential mean latency of only 3.2%. However, with 75% compression, the cystometry trace was a flat line, the hallmark of an atonic bladder from lower motor neuron damage, and a 17.2% increase was seen in the mean latency of the cortical evoked potentials.

Delamarter [21], using a similar animal model for cauda equina syndrome, studied neurologic recovery after immediate, early, and late decompression after 75% compression to the cauda equina. Following compression, all the animals had significant lower extremity weakness, tail paralysis, and urinary incontinence. However, no statistically significant difference in recovery was found between the immediate, early, or late decompression groups. This information may be helpful in obtaining the consent of the patient before surgical intervention and may explain the residual neurologic deficit even after early decompression.

Ultimately, many patients with cauda equina lesions will be severely disabled and require a multidisciplinary management approach, which may involve occupational therapists, social workers, continence advisors, and sexual therapists in addition to medical personnel. Medicolegally, in cases of cauda equina damage in which negligence can be proven, large settlements can potentially be won. This is not surprising, because these patients are often young individuals who, as a result of their injuries, lose the capacity to maintain fecal and urinary continence, may have considerable loss of mobility, and also may suffer loss of sexual performance that can result in relationship disharmony. Symptomatic treatment of bladder, bowel, sexual, and somatic dysfunction may help to alleviate the distressing symptoms of a cauda equina lesion.

REFERENCES

1. Jit I, Charnalia VM. The vertebral level of the delimination of the spinal cord. J Anat Soc India 1959;8:93–101.
2. Bedorook GM. Injuries of the Thoracolumbar Spine with Neurological Symptoms. In PJ Vinken, GW Bruyn, R Braakman (eds), Handbook of Clinical Neurology (Vol 25). Injuries of the Spine and Spinal Cord. Part I. Oxford, UK: North-Holland, 1976;437–466.
3. Naidich TP, King DG, Moran CJ, Sagel SS. Computed tomography of the lumbar thecal sac. J Comput Assist Tomogr 1980;4(1):37–41.
4. Cohen SM, Wall EJ, Kerber CW, et al. The anatomy of the cauda equina on CT scans and MRI. J Bone Joint Surg Br 1991;73(3):381–384.
5. Robertson DP, Simpson RK. Penetrating injuries restricted to the cauda equina: a retrospective review. Neurosurgery 1992;31:265–270.
6. EB Hendrick, HJ Hoffman, RP Humphreys, RE McLaurin. Tethered Cord Syndrome. In R McLaurin (ed), Myelomeningocele. New York: Grune & Stratton, 1977.
7. Pang D, Wilberger J. Tethered cord syndrome in adults. J Neurosurg 1982;57:32–47.
8. Ransohoff J. Lesions of the Cauda Equina. In Clinical Neurosurgery. 1901;331–343.
9. Mathew P, Todd NV. Intradural conus and cauda equina tumours: a retrospective review of presentation, diagnosis and early outcome. J Neurol Neurosurg Psychiatry 1993;56:69–74.
10. J Greenwood, JE Rose. Spinal Cord Tumours. In RN Rosenberg (ed), The Clinical Neurosciences. New York: Churchill Livingstone, 1983;1381–1397.
11. Fearnside MR, Adams CBT. Tumours of the cauda equina. J Neurol Neurosurg Psychiatry 1978;41:24–31.
12. Comarr AE, Vigue M. Sexual counseling among male and female patients with spinal cord and/or cauda equina injury. Part I. Am J Phys Med 1978;57:107–122.
13. Comarr AE, Vigue M. Sexual counseling among male and female patients with spinal cord and/or cauda equina injury. Part II. Am J Phys Med 1978;57:215–227.
14. Djindjian R. Angiography of the spinal cord. Surg Neurol 1974;2:179–185.

15. Murayama N, Yasuda K, Yamanishi T, et al. Disturbances of micturition in patients with spinal arteriovenous malformations. Paraplegia 1990;27:212–216.
16. Nordling J, Meyhoff HH, Olesen KP. Cysto-urethrographic appearance of the bladder and posterior urethra in neuromuscular disorders of the lower urinary tract. Scand J Urol Nephrol 1982;16:115–124.
17. McGuire EJ, Wagner FCJ. The effect of sacral denervation on bladder and urethral function. Surg Gynec Obstet 1977;144:343.
18. Light JK, Beric A, Petronic I. Detrusor function with lesions of the cauda equina, with special emphasis on the bladder neck. J Urol 1993;149:539–542.
19. Barbalias GA, Blaivas JG. Neurologic implication of the pathologically open bladder neck. J Urol 1983;129:780.
20. Bodner DR, Delamarter RB, Bohlman HH, et al. Urologic changes after cauda equina compression in dogs. J Urol 1990;143:186–190.
21. Delamarter RB, Sherman JE, Carr JB. Cauda equina syndrome: neurologic recovery following immediate, early or late decompression. Spine 1991;16:1022–1029.

23
Peripheral Neuropathy

Prokar Dasgupta and P. K. Thomas

The peripheral nervous system comprises the somatosensory fibers in the cranial and spinal nerves and their accompanying autonomic components. The peripheral autonomic nervous system consists of the craniosacral parasympathetic outflow, the thoracolumbar sympathetic outflow, and the enteric nervous system. Visceral afferent fibers are of two types. Those that signal pain or other sensations, such as fullness, initially travel with the sympathetic nervous system, then traverse sympathetic ganglia without synapsing and enter the spinal nerves via the white rami communicantes. They have their cell bodies in the dorsal root ganglia. Physiologic afferents, involved in autonomic reflexes, travel either with the vagus or glossopharyngeal nerves and have their cell bodies in the inferior ganglia of these nerves.

For the somatosensory and autonomic components of the peripheral nervous system, disease processes can consist of generalized polyneuropathies with an approximately symmetric distribution on the two sides of the body, or focal and multifocal neuropathies, in which involvement is localized. Neuropathies can be functionally selective, so that motor, sensory, or autonomic function can be affected separately or in various combinations. They can also be selective in terms of the size of nerve fibers implicated, preferentially affecting large or small fibers or fibers of all sizes indiscriminately. In addition, they can give rise predominantly to axonal damage—that is, axonopathy—or to damage to the Schwann cells and myelin, leading to a demyelinating neuropathy with relative preservation of the axons. The clinical features of these different types of involvement have been considered by Thomas and Ochoa [1].

This chapter first considers the innervation of the genitourinary and lower alimentary tracts and then provides a selective review of the main neuropathies that affect bladder, bowel, and sexual function.

INNERVATION OF THE GENITOURINARY AND LOWER ALIMENTARY TRACTS

Lower Urinary Tract

The nerves supplying the bladder are derived from the inferior hypogastric (pelvic) plexus, which contains both sympathetic and parasympathetic components (see Chapter 2). The preganglionic sympathetic fibers arise from the sacral autonomic nucleus in the second to fourth sacral segments (mainly the latter two) of the spinal cord. The sympathetic fibers originate from cells in the intermediolateral column of the lower three thoracic and upper two lumbar segments of the spinal cord [2]. The inferior hypogastric plexus contains numerous small ganglia in which a proportion of both the sympathetic and parasympathetic fibers synapse and relay. Other preganglionic sympathetic fibers relay in the ganglia of the lumbar and sacral parts of the sympathetic chain.

The inferior hypogastric plexus lies in a fascial sheath that extends from the lateral wall of the pelvis to the base of the bladder and contains the ureters and the visceral branches of the internal iliac vessels. This fascia has been termed the *hypogastric sheath* [3], and its anterolateral aspect forms the posterior limit of the retropubic space of Retzius. In men, the posterior part of the hypogastric plexus lies in close relation to the anterolateral wall of the lower rectum, and the anterior part is related to the posterolateral aspect of the prostate and the seminal vesicles. In women, part of the plexus comes very close to the lower rectum near the anorectal junction, whereas the rest of it lies like a meshed band on the upper one-third of the vagina. Most of the plexus lies below the broad ligament, although the upper part extends into the cardinal ligament of Mackenrodt at the base of the broad ligament [4].

Nerve fibers from the anterior part of the inferior hypogastric plexus reach the bladder in the vesical plexus, which is composed of filaments that run along the vesical arteries. They enter numerous small ganglia distributed through the bladder wall, each consisting of 5–20 nerve cell bodies. In the detrusor, large numbers of nerve fibers are found both around and within the muscle bundles. Three categories of nerves have been defined: (1) The most widely recognized are presumed to be cholinergic, identified by their content of acetylcholinesterase [5]. (2) A few adrenergic nerve fibers represent a fairly meager sympathetic supply, mainly to blood vessels [6]. (3) A large noncholinergic nonadrenergic component has been described that represents part of the diffuse neurohumoral system of neuropeptide-containing nerves [2, 7].

The neurotransmitters that ultimately control detrusor behavior are released from vesicles contained in varicosities in the terminal branches of the efferent nerve fibers [2]. These vesicles are also mainly of three types: (1) clear small vesicles, which are thought to be cholinergic (approximately 5,000 vesicles are found per varicosity, with each vesicle containing approximately 5,000 molecules of the transmitter; each impulse causes approximately 50% of these vesicles to release acetylcholine; γ-aminobutyric acid [GABA] is also contained in small clear vesicles); (2) small dense core vesicles, which are presumptively nonadrenergic; and (3) large dense core vesicles, the nature of whose contents is unknown.

The intricate arrangement of the intramural ganglia in the human bladder, with a variety of fibers terminating in and emerging from them, represents an "intrinsic nervous system" [8] somewhat analogous to the plexuses within the intestines. Recent studies using colocalization techniques have demonstrated the presence of a wide variety of neuropeptides in this intrinsic system [8], but their exact interactions in this complex neuronal network are far from obvious.

Even less is known about the sensory innervation of the human bladder. The bulk of the sensory innervation is thought to lie in the suburothelial layer, as these nerves are unrelated to recognized neuroeffector target sites [5] and sometimes penetrate the urothelial basal lamina [9]. These can easily be stained with S100 (for Schwann cells) and protein gene product (PGP) 9.5 (for axons), and on electron microscopy they are found to be mainly unmyelinated nerve fibers with the axons containing both pale and dense core vesicles [10]. Sensory corpuscles resembling pacinian corpuscles (Timofeew's corpuscles) are present in the bladder wall of the fetus and neonate [11]. The sensory fibers, after leaving the bladder, run to the lower three thoracic and upper two lumbar segments, and the second to fourth sacral segments of the spinal cord, where some of them connect with preganglionic (efferent) neurons.

In males, the nonstriated muscle of the bladder neck is described as forming a circular collar around the preprostatic portion of the urethra [12], although no full agreement is found over this [13]. In females, the nonstriated muscle extends obliquely and longitudinally into the urethral wall and does not form a sphincter as in males. In males, the nonstriated muscle of the bladder neck has a rich nonadrenergic (sympathetic) innervation but a sparse cholinergic (parasympathetic) nerve supply [14]. In females, a sparse adrenergic but a rich cholinergic innervation is found.

Both sexes possess an external sphincter composed of striated muscle, situated around the membranous urethra in males and the distal urethra in females. The innervation of this sphincter is via the pelvic nerves and not from the pudendal nerves, as is often stated. Zvara et al. [15] demonstrated a dual nerve supply in men: from the inferior hypogastric plexus in an extrapudendal pelvic nerve (S2–S3) that runs close to the dorsolateral surface of the rectum, and from the pudendal nerve. Some small branches approach the sphincter after separating from the dorsal nerve of the penis. This is a purely sensory branch of the pudendal nerve, and these fibers may therefore represent part of the afferent pathway in the micturition reflex.

Genital Apparatus

Men

The prostatic plexus is the downward continuation of the inferior hypogastric plexus. It lies in the base and on the lateral aspect of the prostate and supplies the prostate, seminal vesicles, prostatic urethra, membranous and penile urethra, and bulbourethral glands. The lesser and greater cavernous nerves to the corpora cavernosa originate from the front of the plexus, are joined by branches from the pudendal nerve, and pass below the pubic arch [16]. The lesser cavernous nerves supply the penile urethra and the erectile tissue of the corpus spongiosum. The greater cavernous nerves connect with the dorsal nerve of the penis and supply the erectile tissue. The seminal vesicles are innervated from the vesical and prostatic plexuses and inferior hypogastric plexus. Extensions reach the ejaculatory ducts and vasa deferentia. The cutaneous supply of the external genitalia is outlined in Chapter 2.

Women

Uterine nerves originate from the inferior hypogastric plexus, particularly from the component in the broad ligament, the uterovaginal plexus. Branches traveling with arteries supply the vagina, cervix, and uterus and connect with a paracervical plexus containing small ganglia. Ascending branches connect with tubal nerves and with the ovarian plexus derived from the renal and aortic plexuses, as well as with branches from the superior and inferior hypogastric plexuses. The cutaneous innervation of the female external genitalia is described in Chapter 2.

Lower Alimentary Tract

The enteric nervous system possesses two principal plexuses that lie in the alimentary tract, extending from the esophagus to the rectum. The myenteric plexus (Auerbach's plexus) is situated between the outer longitudinal and inner circular muscle coats. The submucous plexus (Meissner's plexus) is situated between the inner muscle coat and the muscularis mucosae. Both plexuses consist of multiple small ganglia interlinked by fine bundles of unmyelinated axons. The total number of neurons in the enteric nervous system equals that in the spinal cord. Neurons of several types are present, embedded in a glial framework. Neurons of two types possess axons that end on smooth muscle and glands: One is excitatory and cholinergic, and the other is nonadrenergic and noncholinergic [7]. GABAergic inhibitory interneurons are also present, as are unipolar and bipolar neurons considered to have a sensory function.

The extrinsic innervation of the small intestine, cecum, colon, and rectum is derived from the vagal and sacral parasympathetic outflow and from the sympathetic nervous system. Intestinal branches of the vagus nerve reach the small intestine, cecum, colon, right colic flexure, and most of the transverse colon. The parasympathetic innervation of the remainder of the lower alimentary tract is derived from the pelvic splanchnic nerves. The sympathetic supply to the small intestine, cecum, and ascending and transverse colon arises from the superior mesenteric plexus, a downward continuation of the celiac plexus. A superior mesenteric ganglion lies near the origin of the superior mesenteric artery. Nerve bundles accompany branches of the artery. The inferior mesenteric plexus originates mainly from the aortic plexus with contributions from the second and third lumbar splanchnic nerves. An inferior mesenteric ganglion or isolated small ganglia lie adjacent to the origin of the inferior mesenteric artery. Branches travel with those of the artery to the left half of the transverse colon, the descending and sigmoid colon, and the rectum. The middle rectal plexus arises from the upper part of the inferior hypogastric plexus. Inferior rectal (hemorrhoidal) nerves arise from the pudendal nerve.

NEUROPATHIES AFFECTING BLADDER, BOWEL, AND SEXUAL FUNCTION

Metabolic Neuropathies

Diabetes Mellitus

Diabetes mellitus is the most common cause of polyneuropathy in developed countries. It gives rise to a variety of disturbances of peripheral nerve function, the most frequent being a distal symmetric polyneuropathy with relatively minor motor manifestations [17]. Indications are that small fiber sensory function is affected before that mediated by large myelinated fibers [18], which can lead to a pseudosyringomyelic picture with mutilating changes in the feet [19]. Autonomic neuropathy is a frequent accompaniment of diabetic sensory polyneuropathy and can be the dominant feature at times. Severe autonomic neuropathy is almost always associated with type 1 or insulin-dependent diabetes.

Cystopathy

That bladder function may be affected in diabetic neuropathy was recognized in early studies by Jordan and Crabtree [20], Rudy and Muellner [21], and Ellenberg [22]. It was evident in 14% of patients with diabetic neuropathy in the study series reported by Rundles in 1945 [23]. Frimodt-Møller [24] introduced the term *diabetic cystopathy*.

The onset of bladder dysfunction is usually insidious [25]. Initially, reduced bladder sensation occurs with increasing intervals between voiding. This is followed by slowing of the urinary stream and difficulty in voiding, so that the patient voids by abdominal straining. Postmicturition dribbling may occur. Differentiation from bladder neck obstruction can easily be made by pressure-flow studies [24]. Excess postmicturition residual urine, as determined by ultrasonography, correlates well with the presence of peripheral neuropathy and an increased incidence of urinary tract infections [26]. Cystometrograms show a significant increase in bladder capacity and retardation of the first desire to void accompanied by a decrease in detrusor contractility and increased residual volume in these patients compared with normal control subjects [27]. These findings may be present even in patients without urinary symptoms, indicating the presence of a subclinical diabetic cystopathy [27]. Paradoxically, detrusor hyperreflexia has also been noted, particularly in elderly diabetics [28]; it is probably related to concomitant lesions affecting the central nervous system.

Sympathetic skin responses in patients with diabetic cystopathy are either absent or of low amplitude and prolonged latency [27]. Cerebral potentials evoked by electrical stimulation of the vesicourethral junction through a bipolar electrode attached to a specially designed Foley catheter are prolonged or of low amplitude in more than 65% of these patients [29]. Sensory nerve conduction studies reveal abnormalities in the lower limbs in nearly all patients with diabetic cystopathy [30]. In a neuropathologic study of bladder wall biopsies obtained from 14 patients with severe cystopathy related to insulin-dependent diabetes, Van Poppel et al. [31] reported a decrease in acetylcholinesterase resulting from axonal loss and an increase in S100 positivity from Schwann cell proliferation.

The precise incidence of diabetic cystopathy is uncertain, because the results of community-based surveys are not available. The incidence in individual series has ranged from 5% to 71% [24, 32–34].

Bowel Dysfunction

Rundles [23] drew attention to constipation as a symptom of diabetic autonomic neuropathy. It is undoubtedly a common symptom [35], but its prevalence is difficult to assess. Maleki et al. [36], in a community-based study in the United States, found constipation to be more common in diabetic individuals than in the general population, and Janatuinen et al. [37], in a community-based study in Finland, found that diabetic individuals consumed more laxatives than control subjects. The mechanism of the constipation is uncertain, but autonomic neuropathy causing parasympathetic denervation is likely to be implicated. Battle et al. [38] found that the postprandial gastrocolic reflex was impaired in diabetic patients with neuropathy. Other non-neuropathic causes of course need exclusion in diabetic patients complaining of constipation.

Diabetic diarrhea is a more troublesome complication [39–41]. It typically occurs at night or after meals and is watery in nature. Nocturnal fecal incontinence may be a feature. The diarrhea is usually chronic but intermittent and alternates with bouts of constipation or normal bowel movements. It usually occurs in patients with long-standing diabetes [42]. Its pathophysiologic basis has not been established. Reduced vagal and sympathetic innervation may be involved, but detailed morphologic observations on the myenteric and submucous plexuses are not available. Inflammatory infiltrates have been demonstrated in relation to bundles of unmyelinated axons in the gut wall and in autonomic ganglia [43], raising the possibility of a superimposed autoimmune inflammatory component to the neuropathy. Reduced resting anal tone secondary to sympathetic denervation probably plays a part in the occurrence of nocturnal fecal incontinence. Impaired mucosal absorption of fluid could contribute to the watery diarrhea. The adrenergic innervation of the intestines stimulates water and electrolyte absorption. Experimentally, Chang et al. [44] have shown reduced α-adrenergic tone in enterocytes in diabetic rats.

Pancreatic enzyme and bicarbonate secretion in response to secretin and cholecystokinin is known to be impaired in patients with diabetes [45, 46], but frank pancreatic insufficiency or steatorrhea rarely develop.

Sexual Dysfunction

Sexual dysfunction has long been recognized to be common in diabetic men [47]; erectile dysfunction (ED) is more common than ejaculatory failure. Community-based prevalence studies are not available, but observations in several study series [47–50] have indicated a prevalence of 30–60%. Not all instances of ED in diabetic subjects are due to neuropathy, but this explanation is likely if other evidence of neuropathy is present. The possibility of psychogenic impotence can be investigated by recordings of nocturnal penile tumescence during rapid-eye-movement sleep, which may be preserved if the ED is psychogenic [51–53].

In patients with diabetic cystopathy, retrograde ejaculation may occur [54, 55]. During ejaculation, the internal sphincter of the bladder is normally closed by sympathetic activity. If this fails, semen passes retrogradely into the bladder instead of down the penile urethra.

Female sexual function in diabetes has been investigated only to a limited extent, but reduced vaginal secretion on sexual arousal has been reported [56].

Amyloidosis

Neuropathy due to deposition of amyloid in peripheral nerve can occur in patients with benign plasma cell dyscrasia (primary amyloidosis) or myeloma. The amyloid, referred to as *AL amyloid*, is derived from the variable portion of a monoclonal immunoglobulin light chain, more commonly lambda than kappa, or from the whole chain. The neuropathy is characteristically of small fiber type, initially giving rise to a predominant loss of pain and temperature sensation with later involvement of motor function and sensory modalities subserved by large myelinated fibers. Autonomic function is normally affected at an early stage. Reduced intestinal motility occurs, as may pseudo-obstruction [57]. Although amyloid deposition takes place in the gut wall, autonomic dysfunction is a more important cause for the troublesome diarrhea that may develop [58]. Amyloidosis can present with reduced urinary stream and infrequent voiding. Pressure-flow studies show reduced bladder contractility and significant postvoiding urine volume. Amyloid deposits may be observed in the bladder wall. ED is also a feature. The prognosis of primary amyloidosis is poor, largely because of the risk of development of renal or cardiac failure [59].

Neuropathy related to the inherited amyloidoses is considered in the section Inherited Neuropathies.

Toxic and Nutritional Neuropathies

Toxic neuropathies and neuropathies related to nutritional deficiency tend to affect predominantly large myelinated fibers; autonomic function, including bladder, bowel, and sexual function, is therefore relatively preserved. Neuropathy due to lead poisoning is occasionally associated with difficulty in voiding urine [60]; the abdominal pain (lead colic) and constipation that occur are presumably related to disturbances of intestinal motility, although this has not been investigated directly.

The chemotherapeutic drugs cisplatin and vincristine sulfate have been implicated in bladder dysfunction, giving rise to difficulty in voiding. Cisplatin causes a predominantly sensory neuropathy [61]. Treatment with vincristine sulfate predictably causes a neuropathy, often beginning with tingling paresthesia in the upper limbs, followed by distal weakness in the limbs. Bladder acontractility may be observed in cases of severe neuropathy [62, 63]. Paralytic ileus may develop after high initial doses. The neuropathy slowly recovers on discontinuation of the drug.

A distinctive neuropathy resulted from exposure to dimethylaminopropionitrile (DMAPN). It was used as a catalyst in a grouting mixture that also contained acrylamide, to which agent the neurotoxic effects were initially attributed. DMAPN was later introduced as a catalyst in the manufacture of polyurethane foam. Exposure led to the development of a neuropathy characterized by urinary hesitancy and abdominal discomfort, followed by difficulty in voiding and incontinence. Some individuals developed ED [64]. A mild distal sensorimotor neuropathy accompanied by sacral sensory impairment also occurred. Cystometrograms in affected individuals demonstrated an atonic bladder. Gradual improvement took place after removal from exposure, but mild residual bladder dysfunction and persistent ED were observed [64].

Infective Neuropathies

In tabes dorsalis, the lumbosacral roots are involved in an infection with *Treponema pallidum*. The predominant symptoms are a sensory ataxia and spontaneous neuropathic pains, but difficulty in voiding and urinary retention and ED may occur. Delay in the development of the sensation of bladder filling on cystometry has been reported [65], but some patients have been found to have detrusor hyperactivity and detrusor-sphincter dyssynergia, indicating that both sacral and suprasacral pathology may be present.

The most common neuropathy associated with infection with human immunodeficiency virus is a distal symmetric and often painful sensory neuropathy [66]. This sensory neuropathy may occasionally be accompanied by autonomic features, and, rarely, a predominantly autonomic neuropathy can occur. Guillain-Barré syndrome (see the following section, Immune-Mediated Neuropathies) may develop at the time of seroconversion. The cauda equina may be affected either by cytomegalovirus infection or by lymphoma, leading to urinary and fecal incontinence. The urodynamic findings are variable, but bladder acontractility may be demonstrable [60, 67].

Chancellor et al. [68] have reported the results of urodynamic investigations in seven patients with borreliosis (Lyme disease) caused by tick-borne infection with *Borrelia burgdorferi*. Two patients had detrusor areflexia, whereas the others were hyperreflexic. Both peripheral neuropathy and central nervous system lesions can occur in this condition. Archibald and Sexton [69] have recorded the long-term sequelae in nine patients with Rocky Mountain spotted fever, an infection caused by *Rickettsia rickettsii*. These included peripheral neuropathy and central nervous system deficits together with urinary and fecal incontinence. A flaccid bladder attributed to peripheral neuropathy has been reported in legionnaire's disease [70].

Immune-Mediated Neuropathies

The Guillain-Barré syndrome is an acute paralytic disorder that frequently follows infection with *Campylobacter jejuni* or an upper respiratory tract infection [71]. It is usually demyelinating, although some cases involve a primary axonal process (acute motor axonal neuropathy, acute motor and sensory axonal neuropathy) [72]. In the more severe cases, autonomic function may be affected and the bladder may be involved. Cystometry demonstrates delay in the initial sensation of bladder filling and detrusor areflexia [73]. Not all patients recover bladder function in the long term, and in those who do, this recovery may take months [67]. The frequency of bladder involvement is difficult to estimate, because a catheter is often inserted in severely ill patients as part of their intensive care. Constipation is common and is related both to weakness of the abdominal wall, which prevents straining, and to reduced intestinal motility [71]. Rarely, paralytic ileus is seen in the acute stage.

Involvement of bladder, bowel, and sexual function is not usually a feature in chronic inflammatory demyelinating polyneuropathy (CIDP), but in a personally observed case of sensory CIDP, ED related to loss of penile sensation recovered fully after treatment with corticosteroids.

Bladder involvement attributed to peripheral neuropathy has been described in systemic lupus erythematosus [74].

Inherited Neuropathies

Porphyria

A predominantly motor neuropathy may complicate the acute attacks in the autosomal dominant disorders of acute intermittent and variegate porphyria and hereditary coproporphyria as well as the recessively inherited condition δ-aminolevulinic acid dehydratase deficiency. All are disorders affecting hepatic heme metabolism. The proximal muscles tend to be affected to a greater extent than the distal ones. Attacks may be precipitated by drugs or alcohol. They are often ushered in by psychiatric features and abdominal pain before the muscle weakness appears. Constipation and hesitancy of micturition may occur.

Hereditary Amyloid Neuropathy

The familial amyloid polyneuropathies are a heterogeneous group of autosomal dominant disorders in which amyloid is precipitated in the peripheral nerves and other organs [75]. The amyloid is most frequently derived from transthyretin (TTR) but can also arise from apolipoprotein A-I or gelsolin. A large number of mutations in the gene for TTR have been described, the commonest being the methionine 30 (met 30) or Portuguese form, tyrosine 77 (tyr 77) or German form, and alanine 60 (ala 60) or Irish/Appalachian form. The age of onset is extremely variable, ranging from 17 to 78 years. The onset is commonly with painful dysesthesia in the lower limbs accompanied by pain and temperature sensory loss. The upper limbs are involved later. This often leads to a mutilating acropathy. Motor involvement and loss of large fiber sensory modalities follow. Autonomic manifestations are an early feature, causing orthostatic hypotension, gastric atony, alternating constipation and diarrhea, ED, urinary hesitancy, and infrequent voiding. Pressure-flow studies confirm reduced bladder contractility with significant postvoiding residual volumes. In addition to the small fiber neuropathy, amyloid may be deposited in the gut and bladder wall, which may contribute to the alimentary and urinary symptoms.

TTR familial amyloid polyneuropathy is steadily progressive, leading to death at an average of 10 years after the onset of symptoms, although some hope exists that liver transplantation may retard or arrest progress [76, 77]. Diarrhea can be improved, as was seen in personally observed cases.

Hereditary Sensory and Autonomic Neuropathies

The most common hereditary sensory and autonomic neuropathies are the dominantly inherited type I hereditary sensory neuropathy (HSN I), the recessively inherited type II hereditary sensory neuropathy (HSN II), and familial dysautonomia (Riley-Day syndrome), also recessively inherited. A pure sensory neurogenic bladder of large functional capacity with voluntary micturition remaining unaffected has been reported in HSN II [78]. Megacolon has been described in the Riley-Day syndrome, but urinary voiding problems and ED are not features of this disorder.

Mitochondrial Disorders

A recently defined syndrome combines mitochondrial myopathy, peripheral neuropathy, gastrointestinal disease, and encephalopathy and is designated *MNGIE* (*myo-neuro-gastrointestinal encephalopathy*) [79, 80]. The gastrointestinal disease presents with intermittent diarrhea and pseudo-obstruction.

Hirschsprung's Disease

In Hirschsprung's disease (congenital megacolon) ganglion cells are absent from the wall of the distal bowel. The rectum is always affected, and the rectosigmoid region is affected in 70% of cases. In 20% of cases, the aganglionosis involves the colon for a variable distance proximal to the sigmoid, and in 10%, the aganglionosis also affects the small intestine. Peristalsis is interrupted in the aganglionic segment, leading to obstruction and dilatation of the gut proximal to the affected region. Presentation is usually in the neonatal period with failure to pass meconium, but the disorder can present later with a history of constipation dating back to infancy.

Hirschsprung's disease is a neurocristopathy related to the abnormal migration, proliferation, or survival of particular neural crest cell lineages. It has been shown to be caused by heterozygous mutations in the RET proto-oncogene [81]. The RET gene encodes for a transmembrane tyrosine kinase receptor expressed in neural crest lineages. Its ligand is glial cell–derived neurotrophic factor. Hirschsprung's disease mutations lead to a loss of function of the mutant RET tyrosine kinase.

Multiple Endocrine Neoplasia Type 2B

Multiple endocrine neoplasia type 2B (MEN 2B) is a rare autosomal dominant disorder that combines medullary thyroid carcinoma, pheochromocytoma, and ganglioneuromatosis with various skeletal and connective tissue abnormalities. Affected individuals possess a marfanoid habitus and a distinctive facial appearance that includes everted eyelids because of thickening of the tarsal plates and multiple neuromatous nodules in the lips and tongue. A variety of gastrointestinal symptoms occur [82]. These include vomiting, diarrhea, constipation, megacolon, and dilatation of the small intestine and stomach. Pathologically, these symptoms are associated with ganglioneuromatosis involving a non-neoplastic proliferation of the nerve and ganglion cells of the gut and other organs. The alimentary symptoms may be the presenting feature. Recognition of their cause is important in view of the occurrence of medullary thyroid carcinoma and pheochromocytoma in this disorder.

As in Hirschsprung's disease, the MEN 2 syndromes are neurocristopathies related to mutations in the RET proto-oncogene [81]. The mutations in MEN 2 differ in that they lead to a gain of function with constitutive activation of the receptor.

Injury to Pelvic Nerves

Most injuries to the pelvic nerves are iatrogenic, although stretch injury to the spinal nerves and sacral plexus can occur as a result of pelvic fractures. Occasionally, the damage is intentional, as in the subtrigonal injection of phenol to reduce detrusor instability [83] or hyperreflexia refractory to conservative methods of treatment.

Voiding dysfunction is often reported after abdominoperineal resection for carcinoma [84] or radical hysterectomy [85], but a direct relation to the operation is more likely for abdominoperineal resection than for hysterectomy [4]. The pelvic parasympathetic nerves may be directly damaged during dissection of the lower aspect of the rectum, particularly in men. In addition, when the rectum, with its investing fascial coat, is pulled anteriorly to one side, the pelvic nerves are distracted away from the posterolateral pelvic wall, injuring the nerves supplying the bladder. During hysterectomy, the chances of injury to the pelvic nerves are lower because of the differing anatomic relationships, unless an unusually long cuff of the vagina is removed, or the operation is more radical and involves removal of the cardinal ligaments at the base of the broad ligament [4, 86].

Injury to the pelvic nerve supply to the internal sphincter of the bladder neck, above the pelvic floor, could be the cause of some cases of postprostatectomy incontinence or incontinence after abdominal perineal resection. The suggestion has also been made that incontinence after radical prostatectomy could occur from damage to the nerve supply to the sphincter arising from the dorsal nerve of the penis, which is purely sensory. Such patients would have normal functional urethral sphincteric length and closure pressure and yet suffer from stress incontinence in response to rise in urethral pressure during physical activity because of loss of normal sensation of the sphincter area [15].

Our understanding of the pathophysiology of these injuries is limited, but complete transection of both inferior hypogastric (pelvic) plexuses would be expected to decentralize rather than denervate the bladder, because most of the vesical ganglia are intraneural, and the postganglionic fibers would thus still be intact [86]. Neal et al. [87] found nerve terminal densities to be much lower in bladder biopsies of patients who had had excision of the rectum. Painless urinary retention is common in the early weeks after a pelvic plexus injury. Detrusor function may recover gradually and paradoxically be accompanied by urgency and stress incontinence. Injury to the pudendal nerve may result in loss of the bulbocavernosus and anocutaneous reflexes. Ultrasonographic examination confirms significant postvoiding residual urine. Urodynamic studies are best delayed for approximately 6 weeks after injury. Decreased bladder sensation, reduced compliance, and detrusor hypocontractility, along with an open bladder neck in a videocystometrogram, are the usual findings [86]. External sphincter electromyography may show evidence of denervation.

REFERENCES

1. Thomas PK, Ochoa J. Clinical Features and Differential Diagnosis. In PJ Dyck, PK Thomas, JW Griffin, et al. (eds), Peripheral Neuropathy (3rd ed). Philadelphia: Saunders, 1993;749–774.
2. Mundy AR. Clinical Physiology of the Bladder, Urethra and Pelvic Floor. In AR Mundy, TP Stephenson, AJ Wein (eds), Urodynamics, Principles, Practice and Application (2nd ed). Edinburgh, UK: Churchill Livingstone, 1994;15–27.
3. Uhlenhuth E, Day EC, Smith RA, Middleton EB. The visceral endopelvic fascia and the hypogastric sheath. Surg Gynaecol Obstet 1948;86:9–28.
4. Mundy AR. An anatomical explanation for bladder dysfunction following rectal and uterine surgery. Br J Urol 1982;54:501–504.
5. Dixon JS, Gosling JA. The Anatomy of the Bladder, Urethra and Pelvic Floor. In AR Mundy, TP Stephenson, AJ Wein (eds), Urodynamics, Principles, Practice and Application (2nd ed). Edinburgh, UK: Churchill Livingstone, 1994;3–14.
6. Sundin T, Dalhstrøm A, Norlen L, Svedmyr N. The sympathetic innervation and adrenoreceptor function of the human lower urinary tract in the normal state and after parasympathetic denervation. Invest Urol 1977;14:322–328.
7. Burnstock G. Innervation of bladder and bowel. Ciba Foundation Symp 1990;151:2–18.
8. Smet PJ, Edyvane K, Jonavicius J, Marshall VR. Neurochemically distinct classes of nerve terminals encircle intrinsic neurons in human urinary bladder. Neurourol Urodyn 1995;14:511.
9. Dixon JS, Gilpin S-A, Gilpin CJ. Presumptive sensory axons of the human urinary bladder: a fine ultrastructural study. J Anat 1987;151:199–207.
10. Dasgupta P, Chandiramani V, Beckett A, et al. Flexible cystoscopic biopsies for evaluation of nerve densities in the suburothelium of the human urinary bladder. Br J Urol 1997;80:490–492.
11. Dixon JS, Jen PYP, Gosling JA. Immunohistochemical characteristics of human paraganglion cell and sensory corpuscles associated with the urinary bladder. A developmental study in the fetus and neonate. J Anat 1998;192:407–415.
12. Williams PL (ed). Gray's Anatomy. Edinburgh, UK: Churchill Livingstone, 1995.
13. Woodburne RF. The sphincter mechanism of the urinary bladder and the urethra. Anat Rec 1961;141:11–20.
14. Gosling JA, Dixon JS, Lendon RG. The autonomic innervation of the human male and female bladder neck and proximal urethra. J Urol 1977;118:302–305.
15. Zvara P, Carrier S, Kour N-W, Tanagho EA. The detailed neuroanatomy of the human striated urethral sphincter. Br J Urol 1994;74:182–187.
16. Lepor H, Gregerman M, Crosby R, et al. Precise localization of the autonomic nerves from the pelvic plexus to corpora cavernosa: a detailed anatomical study of the male pelvis. J Urol 1985;133:207–212.
17. Said G. Diabetic neuropathy: an update. J Neurol 1996;243:431–440.
18. Guy RJC, Clark CA, Malcolm PN, Watkins PJ. Evaluation of thermal and vibration sensation in diabetic neuropathy. Diabetologia 1985;28:131–137.
19. Said G, Slama G, Selva J. Progressive centripetal degeneration of axons in small fibre type diabetic polyneuropathy: a clinical and pathological study. Brain 1983;106:791–807.
20. Jordan WR, Crabtree HH. Paralysis of the bladder in diabetic patients. Arch Intern Med 1935;55: 17–25.
21. Rudy A, Muellner SR. The neurogenic bladder in diabetes mellitus: early recognition and treatment with a report of cases. J Urol 1941;45:844–857.
22. Ellenberg M. Diabetic neurogenic vesical dysfunction. Arch Intern Med 1966;117:348–354.
23. Rundles RW. Diabetic neuropathy: general review with a report of 125 cases. Medicine (Balt) 1945;24:111–160.
24. Frimodt-Møller C. Diabetic cystopathy: I. A clinical study on the frequency of bladder dysfunction in diabetics. Danish Med Bull 1976;23:267.
25. Ellenberg M, Weber H. The incipient asymptomatic diabetic bladder. Diabetes 1967;16:331–335.
26. Beylot M, Marion D, Noel G. Ultrasonographic determination of residual urine in diabetic subjects: relationship to neuropathy and urinary tract infection. Diabetes Care 1982;5:501–505.

27. Ueda T, Yoshimura N, Yoshida O. Diabetic cystopathy: relationship to autonomic neuropathy detected by sympathetic skin response. J Urol 1997;157:580–584.
28. Kaplan SA, Alexis ET, Blaivas JG. Urodynamic findings in patients with diabetic cystopathy. J Urol 1995;153:342–344.
29. Sarica Y, Karatas M, Bozdemir H, Karacan I. Cerebral responses elicited by stimulation of the vesico-urethral junction (VUJ) in diabetics. EEG Clin Neurophysiol 1996;110:55–61.
30. Buck AC, Reed PI, Siddiq YK, et al. Bladder dysfunction and neuropathy in diabetes. Diabetologia 1976;12:251–258.
31. Van Poppel H, Stessens R, Van Damme B, et al. Diabetic cystopathy: neuropathological examination of urinary bladder biopsies. Eur Urol 1988;15:128–131.
32. Fagerberg S-E, Kock NG, Peterén I, et al. Urinary bladder disturbances in diabetics. I. A comparative study of male diabetics and controls aged between 20 and 50 years. Scand J Urol Nephrol 1967;1:19–27.
33. Ioanid CP, Noica N, Pop T. Incidence and diagnostic aspects of the bladder disorders in diabetics. Eur Urol 1981;7:211–214.
34. Nijhawan S, Mathur A, Singh V, Bhandari VM. Autonomic and peripheral neuropathy in insulin dependent diabetics. J Assoc Phys India 1993;41:565–556.
35. Feldman M, Schiller LR. Disorders of gastrointestinal motility associated with diabetes mellitus. Ann Intern Med 1983;98:378–384.
36. Maleki D, Camilleri M, Van Dyke CT, et al. Gastrointestinal symptoms in noninsulin-dependent diabetes mellitus (NIDDM) in a U.S. community: a pilot prevalence study. Gastroenterology 1996;110:A27.
37. Janatuinen E, Pikkarainen P, Laakso M, Pyörälä K. Gastrointestinal symptoms in middle-aged diabetic patients. Scand J Gastroenterol 1993;28:427–452.
38. Battle WM, Snape WJ Jr, Alava A, et al. Colonic dysfunction in diabetes mellitus. Gastroenterology 1980;79:1217–1221.
39. Muri JW. Nocturnal diarrhoea in diabetes mellitus. Acta Med Scand 1953;146:143–145.
40. Sheridan EP, Bailey CC. Diabetic nocturnal diarrhea. JAMA 1946;130:632–634.
41. Malins JM, French JM. Diabetic diarrhoea. QJM 1957;26:467–480.
42. Clouse RE, Lustman PJ. Gastrointestinal symptoms in diabetic patients: lack of association with neuropathy. Am J Gastroenterol 1989;84:868–872.
43. Duchen LW, Anjorin A, Watkins PJ, Mackay J. Pathology of autonomic neuropathy in diabetes mellitus. Ann Intern Med 1980;92:301–303.
44. Chang EB, Fedorak RN, Field M. Experimental diabetic diarrhea in rats: intestinal mucosal denervation, hypersensitivity and treatment with clonidine. Gastroenterology 1986;91:564–569.
45. Frier M, Saunders JHB, Wormsley KG, Bouchier IAD. Exocrine pancreatic dysfunction in juvenile-onset diabetes mellitus. Gut 1976;17:685–691.
46. El-Newihi J, Dooley P, Saad C, et al. Impaired exocrine pancreatic dysfunction in diabetics with diarrhea and peripheral neuropathy. Dig Dis Sci 1988;33:705–712.
47. Rubin A, Babbott D. Impotence in diabetes mellitus. JAMA 1958;168:498–500.
48. Kolodny RC, Kahn CB, Goldstein HH, Barnett DM. Sexual function in diabetic men. Diabetes 1974;23:306–309.
49. McCulloch DK, Campbell IW, Wu FC, et al. The prevalence of diabetic impotence. Diabetologia 1980;18:279–283.
50. Fairburn CG, Wu FC, McCulloch DK, et al. The clinical features of diabetic impotence: a preliminary study. Br J Psychiatry 1988;140:447–452.
51. Hosking DJ, Bennett T, Hampton JF. Diabetic impotence: studies of nocturnal erection during REM sleep. BMJ 1979;2:1394–1396.
52. Karacan I. Diagnosis of erectile impotence in diabetes mellitus: an objective and specific method. Ann Intern Med 1980;92:334–336.
53. Kaneko S, Bradley WE. Evaluation of erectile dysfunction with continuous monitoring of penile rigidity. J Urol 1986;137:1026–1029.
54. Greene LF, Kelalis PP, Weeks RE. Retrograde ejaculation of semen due to diabetic neuropathy: report of 4 cases. Fertil Steril 1963;14:617–625.
55. Ellenberg M, Weber H. Retrograde ejaculation in diabetic neuropathy. Ann Intern Med 1966;65:1237–1246.
56. Tyrer G, Steele JM, Ewing DJ, et al. Sexual responsiveness in diabetic women. Diabetologia 1983;24:166–171.
57. Legge DA, Carlson HC, Wollaeger EE. Roentgenologic appearance of systemic amyloidosis involving gastrointestinal tract. Am J Radiol 1970;110:406–413.

58. Battle WM, Rubin MR, Cohen S, Snape WJ Jr. Gastrointestinal-motility dysfunction in amyloidosis. N Engl J Med 1979;301:24–25.
59. Gertz MA, Kyle RA. Amyloidosis: prognosis and treatment. Semin Arthritis Rheum 1994;24: 124–138.
60. Nickell K, Boone TB. Peripheral neuropathy and peripheral nerve injury. Urol Clin North Am 1996;23:491–500.
61. Roelofs RI, Hrusjesky W, Rogin J, Rosenberg L. Peripheral sensory neuropathy and cisplatin chemotherapy. Neurology 1984;34:934–938.
62. Wheeler JS Jr, Siroky MB, Bell R, Babayan BK. Vincristine-induced bladder neuropathy. J Urol 1983;130:342–343.
63. Legha SS. Vincristine neurotoxicity: pathophysiology and management. Med Toxicol 1986;1: 421–427.
64. Keogh JP. Classical syndromes in occupational medicine: dimethylaminopropionitrile. Am J Ind Med 1983;4:479–489.
65. Hattori T, Yasuda K, Kita K, et al. Disorders of micturition in tabes dorsalis. Br J Urol 1990;65: 497–499.
66. Cornblath DR, McArthur JC. Predominantly sensory neuropathy in patients with AIDS and AIDS-related complex. Neurology 1988;38:794–796.
67. Khan Z, Singh VK, Yang WC. Neurogenic bladder in acquired immune deficiency syndrome (AIDS). Urology 1992;40:289–291.
68. Chancellor MB, McGinnis DE, Shenot P, et al. Urinary dysfunction in Lyme disease. J Urol 1993;149:26–30.
69. Archibald LK, Sexton DJ. Long-term sequelae of Rocky Mountain spotted fever. Clin Infect Dis 1995;20:1122–1125.
70. Bernardini DL, Lerrick KS, Hoffman K, Lange M. Neurogenic bladder: new clinical findings in legionnaires' disease. Am J Med 1985;78:1045–1046.
71. Hughes RAC. Guillain-Barré syndrome. London: Springer Verlag, 1990.
72. Griffin JW, Li CY, Ho TW, et al. Guillain-Barré syndrome in northern China: the spectrum of neuropathological changes in clinically defined cases. Brain 1995;118:577–596.
73. Kogan BA, Solomon MH, Diokno AC. Urinary retention secondary to Landry-Guillain-Barré syndrome. J Urol 1981;126:643–644.
74. Wada T, Yokoyama H, Ikeda K, et al. Neurogenic bladder due to peripheral neuropathy and a visual disturbance in an elderly man with systemic lupus erythematosus. Ann Rheum Dis 1992;51:547–549.
75. Harding AE, Reilly MM. Molecular Genetics of Inherited Neuropathies. In AK Asbury, PK Thomas (eds), Peripheral Nerve Disorders 2. Oxford, UK: Butterworth–Heinemann, 1995;119–139.
76. Holmgren C, Ericzon BG, Groth CG, et al. Clinical improvement and amyloid regression after liver transplantation in hereditary transthyretin amyloidosis. Lancet 1993;341:1113–1116.
77. Skinner M, Lewis WD, Jones LA, et al. Liver transplantation as a treatment for familial amyloidotic polyneuropathy. Ann Intern Med 1994;120:133–134.
78. Harris JD, Benson GS. Positive bethanecol chloride supersensitivity test in hereditary sensory neuropathy. J Urol 1980;124:923–924.
79. Bardosi A, Creutzfeldt W, Di Mauro S, et al. Myo-, neuro-, gastrointestinal encephalopathy (MNGIE syndrome) due to partial deficiency of cytochrome c-oxidase: a new mitochondrial multisystem disorder. Acta Neuropathol (Ber 1) 1987;748:248–258.
80. Blake D, Lombes A, Minetti C, et al. MNGIE syndrome: a report of 2 new patients. Neurology 1987;40(suppl 1):294.
81. Edery P, Eng C, Munnich A, Lyonnet S. RET in human development and oncogenesis. Bioessays 1997;19:398–395.
82. Carney JA, Hayles AB. Alimentary tract manifestations of multiple endocrine neoplasia type 2b. Mayo Clin Proc 1977;52:543–548.
83. Cox R, Worth PHL. Chronic retention after extratrigonal phenol injection for bladder instability. Br J Urol 1986;58:229–230.
84. Neal DE, Williams NS, Johnston D. A prospective study of bladder function before and after sphincter-saving resections for low carcinoma. Br J Urol 1981;53:558–564.
85. Smith PH, Turnbull GA, Currie DW, Peel KR. The urological complications of Wertheim's hysterectomy. Br J Urol 1969;41:685–688.
86. Thomas PJ. Pelvic Plexus Injury. In AR Mundy, TP Stephenson, AJ Wein (eds), Urodynamics, Principles, Practice and Application (2nd ed). Edinburgh, UK: Churchill Livingstone, 1994;345–358.
87. Neal DE, Bogue PR, Williams RE. Histological appearances of the nerves of the bladder in patients with denervation of the bladder after excision of the rectum. Br J Urol 1982;54:658–666.

24
Spina Bifida

Matgorzata Borzyskowski

Open and closed spina bifida are the most common causes of vesicourethral dysfunction in childhood and are significant causes of this problem in adults. There are many survivors with this condition from the late 1950s and onward, when shunting for hydrocephalus was first introduced, better antibiotics became available, and primary closure could be performed for all patients. After these advances, renal failure secondary to urologic problems became a significant cause of morbidity and death. Since the 1970s, however, a major change has occurred in the management of the neuropathic bladder, brought about by the combination of a greater understanding of the pathophysiology of the dysfunction, the introduction of clean intermittent catheterization (CIC) by Lapides et al. in 1972 [1], and the availability of various pharmacologic agents and newer surgical techniques. The result has been a reduction in renal damage, improved continence, and a better quality of life. In addition, spina bifida in itself is not a bar to renal transplantation, and each patient needs to be considered for treatment as would anyone else in renal failure.

The incidence of spina bifida has fallen as a result of prenatal diagnosis and termination of affected pregnancies. This is not the only reason for the decline, however, because the number of cases decreased before prenatal diagnosis became available, and the decline has been greatest in areas of highest prevalence, suggesting an environmental influence. An increasing number of adult survivors now exist who have varying problems, and among these patients, the most common reason for hospital admission is urologic problems. In 1991, a Medical Research Council trial showed clear evidence of the role of folic acid in preventing neural tube defects, and the recommendation is now that all women with a previously affected pregnancy take folic acid supplements before conception [2].

Spina bifida is a developmental defect due to failure of fusion of the neural tube on approximately the twenty-eighth day of gestation. The defect can occur anywhere along the length of the neural tube and results in an anencephaly if the forebrain does not develop. Failure of fusion of the neural tube causes defective closure of the vertebral canal. The most common lesion is thoracolumbar, and cervical lesions are the least common.

Open and closed spina bifida cover a wide spectrum of disorders, which range from myelomeningocele to a minor abnormality of the sacrum. Open spina bifida is the most common and includes those lesions in which the skin over the sac is incomplete. It includes myeloschisis and myelomeningocele, in which the spinal cord and nerve roots are outside the vertebral canal and are covered by a membrane centrally and by skin peripherally. Associated lipomata, tethered nerve roots, a split cord, and hydrosyringomyelia may be found. The cord is usually tethered at a low level, and associated hydrocephalus is common.

The term *closed spina bifida* is used to describe all significant lesions that are covered with skin and includes the split notochord syndrome, dorsal dermal sinuses, fibrolipomas of the filum terminale, and diastematomyelia, in which a sagittal cleft divides the cord into two. This condition should not be confused with simple failure of fusion of the vertebral arches of L5 or S1 (often referred to as *spina bifida occulta*), which is not regarded as significant [3] unless other abnormalities, such as bladder, bowel, or neurologic abnormalities, are present. Closed spina bifida may present with a cutaneous lesion, such as a hairy patch, dimple, nevus, or lumbosacral lipoma. The neural structures do not herniate through the mesenchymal defect. Asymmetric limb growth, contractures, pes cavus, sensory or reflex loss, bladder dysfunction, and constipation may be presenting features. Hydrocephalus is not usually a feature of closed spina bifida. Sacral agenesis occurs more commonly in children born to diabetic mothers. All patients with closed spina bifida require magnetic resonance imaging (MRI) of the spine to determine the pathology (Figures 24.1 and 24.2) and the need for neurosurgical intervention to free the spinal cord from its low and posterior attachment.

Spina bifida, like spinal cord injury but unlike progressive neurologic disease, is a potential cause of serious upper urinary tract damage despite improved management. One should never assume that all is well because the neurologic deficit is minor or no problems are apparent, for the kidneys can be slowly and progressively damaged with very few manifestations. This is demonstrated by the following case history:

Case 1: A 23-year-old man was referred to the adult urologic team in 1996. He was born with spina bifida, which was repaired at birth. He had had no subsequent orthopedic or urologic intervention and worked as a stock controller and lived alone. He had presented at his local hospital with tiredness. Investigations had shown a creatine level of 270 g/liter and gross bilateral hydronephrosis. The bladder was small and thick-walled. He was continually wet, wore diapers, and had recently noted that if he drank large volumes he passed a lot of clear fluid by rectum.

He looked well and was ambulant without aids. Examination revealed wasted calves, reduced anocutaneous reflex, absent perianal sensation, and a patulous anus. Rectal examination revealed a firm, irregular, scarred area in the region overlying the prostate and bladder.

Investigations confirmed gross hydronephrosis, a creatine level of 243 g/liter, and a glomerular filtration rate of 23 ml/1.73 m². A fistula between the prostate and rectum was found. Cystoscopy revealed a trabeculated bladder, fibril urethra, and tight distal urethral sphincter. He was found to have prostatitis. The proctorectal fistula was closed. He had a clam ileocystoplasty and loop sigmoid colostomy, which has subsequently been closed. He awaits

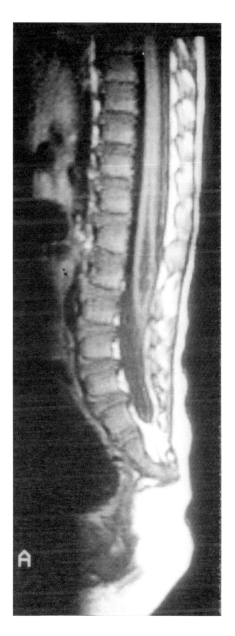

Figure 24.1   Low tethered cord. A cavity is
seen within the cord.

implantation of an artificial urinary sphincter to deal with his incontinence. His
renal function remains severely compromised.

In some of these patients, the neurologic deficit is minor, and the neuropathic
bladder is the major handicap. Incontinence may be the reason for referral, and
its investigation may reveal the underlying spinal cord abnormality. These chil-

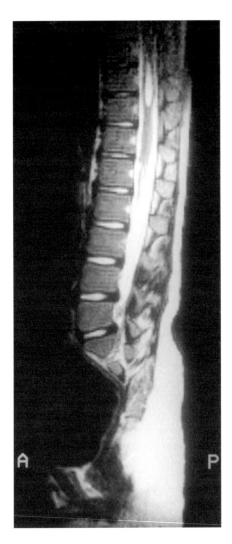

Figure 24.2   Abnormal spine with a very short sacrum.

dren often present with a combination of bladder and bowel problems, and examination may reveal a spinal abnormality or minor neurologic deficits in the lower limbs, which are often asymmetric, as demonstrated by the next two cases.

Case 2: A 7-year-old girl was referred to the neurourology service by her general practitioner because of incontinence and constipation. She had been under the care of a number of physicians and had undergone several procedures. She was born with bilateral talipes and had had three operations on her feet, the last a year before referral. She had suffered from severe constipation requiring hospitalization on two occasions and had a rectal biopsy to exclude Hirschsprung's disease. Her mother is an insulin-dependent diabetic. On examination, the girl was constipated and had a full bladder. She had a short spine with a fatty swelling at the base of it. Wasting of the left calf, brisk knee reflexes, absent left ankle jerk, and absent anal reflex were noted. MRI of the spine confirmed sacral agenesis with an expanded cavity in the distal thoracic cord that terminated at L1, and there was a fatty streak down to L4. Videourodynamics showed detrusor sphincter dyssynergia and incomplete bladder emptying. Her renal function was normal, and she is learning to self-catheterize to empty her bladder.

Case 3: A 4-year-old boy presented with lifelong urinary incontinence, urinary tract infection, and constipation. He had been found to have a thick-walled bladder and was referred because of the possibility of posterior urethral valves. His mother has diabetes. On admission, suspicions of a neurologic abnormality arose when he was found to have abnormal ankle reflexes. Radiography of the lumbosacral spine showed spina bifida occulta at L5 and sacral dysgenesis. MRI revealed a truncated distal cord that ended at T12, with a cavity from T3 to the distal cord. Videourodynamics showed a small, poorly emptying, hyperreflexic bladder. His renal function was normal. He is taking oxybutynin chloride and performing clean intermittent self-catheterization (CISC) and is now dry. His bowel problems were much more difficult to treat. However, an antegrade continence enema procedure (see Chapter 12) has been successful.

A high index of suspicion must therefore be maintained, particularly regarding patients who present with a combination of constipation and incontinence, and the appropriate investigations must be performed.

Patients with low lesions and minor neurologic problems often have the most dangerous bladders in terms of renal function; all should be fully investigated (with both neuroradiography and tests of bladder and renal function) and managed as indicated by these findings. Benign symptomatology may mask factors that put the kidneys at significant risk, for there appears to be little correlation between the neurologic findings and the bladder dysfunction [4–6]. Thus, all of these patients should have videourodynamic studies at the time of diagnosis so that abnormalities and risk factors can be detected early and the kidneys protected from damage.

Johnston and Borzyskowski [7] reviewed their findings regarding 51 patients with closed spina bifida at the time of referral to a specialist neurourologic clinic. Twenty-five patients were referred because of urinary tract problems and 12 because of neurologic deficits; the diagnosis of closed spina bifida had already been made in some, and 7 had had neurosurgical intervention. Thirty children had abnormal voiding behavior at the time of referral; however, videourodynamic studies were normal in only two, and 25% had evidence of renal scarring at initial referral. Thus, neither the clinical neurologic assessment nor the history of voiding behavior was a reliable indicator of bladder dysfunction and subsequent risk of renal damage.

Patients with spina bifida may have many associated problems, including hydrocephalus, orthopedic problems, constipation, and learning difficulties. Therefore, assessing the patient as a whole is important, because management may be affected by the intelligence, motivation, skeletal deformities, and manipulative skills of the patient.

CLASSIFICATION

The majority of spinal cord lesions are incomplete; therefore, classification of bladder dysfunction based on the type and level of neurologic deficit is very difficult and would be very complex. Predicting bladder and urethral abnormalities from the neurologic deficit is difficult, and, as already stated, individuals with low lesions and minor or absent neurologic deficits often have very aggressive bladders with a significant risk of renal damage [4, 7].

Videourodynamic studies have demonstrated three types of bladder dysfunction in spina bifida, based on the ability of the bladder to contract and the degree of emptying that occurs [8].

1. *Contractile.* All patients with this type of bladder dysfunction exhibit hyperreflexia; detrusor sphincter dyssynergia is found in most; detrusor compliance is normal. The majority have incontinence with reduced capacity and incomplete bladder emptying. The bladder neck is competent in 50% [9]. If vesicoureteric reflux is present, the risk of renal damage is significant [10].
2. *Intermediate.* This type of bladder dysfunction is the most common and the most dangerous for the upper urinary tract. Bladder wall compliance is reduced, and thus intravesical pressure is persistently raised. Detrusor contractions are ineffective, and this, combined with an incompetent bladder neck and a static or fixed distal sphincter (which is both incompetent and obstructive), leads to incomplete bladder emptying and incontinence, which may be almost continuous [9]. Surgery is often required, not only to achieve continence but also, more important, to protect the kidneys.
3. *Acontractile.* In this type of bladder dysfunction, no demonstrable detrusor contractions are found; an incompetent bladder neck and a static or fixed distal sphincter are present, leading to overflow and stress incontinence [9]. This type is a relatively safe bladder, although research has shown that, in some, implantation of an artificial sphincter may lead to poor bladder compliance or even hyperreflexia.

This classification is very useful in predicting which patients are at risk of renal damage and also in predicting the outcome of different treatment modalities in terms of establishing continence.

As is apparent, the urethra plays a significant role in the pathogenesis of this condition in spina bifida. This was confirmed by Mundy et al. [9] when they reviewed 402 studies involving 207 children (ranging in age from 1 month to 16 years). Detrusor behavior was classified as described above. The conclusions were that urethral dysfunction was almost universal. However, bladder neck obstruction did not occur in any of these patients, and it is now recognized that in patients with spina bifida, the obstruction occurs at the distal sphincter, which is either dyssynergic in the contractile group or fixed/static in the intermediate and acontractile groups. Incontinence occurs because of bladder neck weakness (stress incontinence) and the incompetent fixed/static distal sphincter. In the 73 children with contractile dysfunction, the bladder neck was incompetent in 50%, and detrusor sphincter dyssynergia was present in 95%. In the 82 children with intermediate bladders and the 52 children with acontractile bladders, the bladder neck was incompetent at their usual bladder volumes. The distal sphincter mechanism was both obstructive and incompetent due to the more or less fixed level of the sphincter.

INVESTIGATIONS

Investigations are aimed at assessing the problem and identifying the risk factors so that management can be tailored to the needs of each individual patient.

Assessment of Renal Function

All patients with spina bifida and neuropathic vesicourethral dysfunction should have regular assessment of renal function, particularly if they are known to have vesicoureteric reflux, symptomatic recurrent urinary tract infections, raised intravesical pressure (from detrusor sphincter dyssynergia, reduced bladder compliance, or hyperreflexia), or poor bladder emptying. The frequency of reassessment is governed by the severity of the bladder and renal problems.

Initial baseline investigations include plasma renal biochemistry assays, renal and bladder ultrasonography before and after bladder emptying (by whatever means is being used), and a dimercaptosuccinic acid scan to assess differential renal function and to look for renal scars. Although plasma creatine level is a good indicator of renal function in the able-bodied, caution is required in interpreting it in patients with abnormal muscle bulk, which commonly occurs in spina bifida. In this group, plasma creatine levels may be much lower than expected for the degree of renal impairment the patient may have; therefore, glomerular filtration rate uncorrected for surface area (because of difficulties of measuring this) is a much better indicator of renal function, and serial measurements over the years provide reliable information. Further investigations may be required based on the findings—for example, if vesicoureteric obstruction is suspected.

Intravenous urography is now carried out much less frequently than before the advent of ultrasonography. The latter has transformed the management of these patients, yielding useful information on the kidneys (size, shape, growth, scarring), collecting systems, and degree of bladder emptying and its effect on pelvicaliceal and ureteric dilatation. In those patients, particularly children, whose kidneys are known to be at risk because of raised intravesical pressure, detrusor sphincter dyssynergia, poor emptying, or reflux, ultrasonography can be performed very frequently (sometimes monthly) to allow early detection of problems.

Regular urine culture is important, particularly in those patients who have vesicoureteric reflux or symptomatic urinary tract infections. All patients with vesicoureteric reflux should be given prophylactic antibiotics, as should those who have recurrent symptomatic infections. Asymptomatic infections identified from routine culture in patients who do not have reflux usually do not require treatment. The bladder must be checked to ensure that it is being emptied regularly and completely in those in whom recurrent infections are a problem. This is easily done by ultrasonography.

Assessment of Bladder and Urethral Function

The best way of assessing bladder and urethral function is by videourodynamic study, which enables accurate evaluation of bladder and urethral function and identification of risk factors so that management can be tailored to the needs of each patient. Some clinicians prefer to combine cystometry with electromyographic measurements. However, such testing does not provide information on reflux and bladder emptying; a micturating cystourethrogram is required to obtain this additional information. Indirect radionucleotide studies to assess reflux are not accurate in these patients, who cannot void voluntarily.

In children, videourodynamic studies are carried out using standard techniques. Filling is adjusted to allow for the child's age; filling starts at 2–3 ml per minute and should not exceed 10 ml per minute. Catheter sizes also vary with the size of the child. Age is no bar to videourodynamic study; however, the child (when appropriate) and the caregivers must be well prepared for the test. We have found it useful to give the family written information before the investigation. The test should be carried out in a pediatric setting with personnel accustomed to dealing with children.

Information Obtained on Videourodynamic Study

Videourodynamic studies provide information on the following:

1. Bladder capacity
2. Bladder shape and outline
3. Detrusor pressure at rest, during filling, and during voiding
4. State of the bladder neck and distal urethral sphincter during filling, voiding, and detrusor contractions
5. Voiding or leak pressure
6. Bladder emptying
7. Vesicoureteric reflux

Videourodynamic studies should be performed as soon as the diagnosis of spina bifida, either open or closed, is made, so that factors known to be dangerous to the kidneys can be identified and the appropriate management instituted early. Raised intravesical pressure due to any cause (hyperreflexia, reduced bladder compliance, detrusor sphincter dyssynergia) in the presence of reflux, particularly if the urine is infected, is a very dangerous situation that must be identified [10–12].

Debate has occurred, however, about the timing of videourodynamic studies, particularly in babies with spina bifida, and about the predictive value of urodynamic evaluation. Bauer et al. [13] found that, among 36 newborn infants with myelodysplasia, 18 had detrusor sphincter dyssynergia and 13 of these later developed hydroureteronephrosis. This development occurred in only two of nine without reflux and in one of nine with no sphincter activity. The 16 infants with hydronephrosis improved after decompression with either vesicostomy or CIC. The authors concluded that those with detrusor sphincter dyssynergia were at great risk and needed close monitoring, and that CIC should be started early. Other workers have confirmed these findings [14]. All stressed the importance of regular monitoring, even in those with less dangerous bladders, as detrusor behavior may deteriorate [15]. The most vulnerable times for the kidneys are the first 5 years of life and adolescence, at which time the bladder and urethral behavior may deteriorate, putting the kidneys at greater risk. In addition, continence often worsens.

Workers in the United States have devised a hostility score based on the urodynamic findings [16]. The parameters used are reflux, bladder wall compliance, hyperreflexia, leak pressure, and activity of the distal sphincter during detrusor contraction. Each parameter is scored 0–2, with the maximum of 10 points (total of the five parameters) indicating the most hostile bladder; this score is used as an aid in timing intervention to protect the upper urinary tract. However, the investigators stress the importance of regular monitoring, because bladder behavior may change with time and become more hostile.

Our practice is to carry out videourodynamic study as soon as feasible in babies after spinal surgery has been performed and problems with hydrocephalus have been dealt with. Children who present later with closed spina bifida should have a videourodynamic study as soon as the diagnosis is suspected, as already indicated. These children or adults may have minimal symptomatology but significant abnormality on videourodynamic study. Continent children may have poorly emptying high-pressure bladders with vesicoureteric reflux (VUR). Satar et al. [17], in their report of 21 older children and adults with occult spinal dysraphism, stressed that such patients are more likely to present with irreversible urologic problems and that early identification, evaluation, and treatment prevents progression of the urinary dysfunction.

With the results of these investigations, management can be planned, taking into account the adverse factors for renal functions (detrusor sphincter dyssynergia, reflux, poor bladder compliance, or high bladder pressure) and those required to achieve continence (a reasonable bladder capacity and some degree of outflow resistance). The safest bladder is an empty, low-pressure bladder free of infection, without vesicoureteric reflux.

MANAGEMENT

The aims of management are, first and most importantly, to preserve renal function; second, to achieve continence; and third, to enable the individual to lead as normal a life as possible.

For these aims to be achieved, the pathophysiology of this condition must be understood. Renal, bladder, and urethral function must be accurately assessed so that risk factors can be identified. In addition, management must adopt a realistic approach that takes into account all the other problems the patient may have. Not all patients can be made completely dry; however, continence can be improved in the majority—surgically if this has not been achieved by other means.

NONSURGICAL MANAGEMENT

In general, nonsurgical management is based on increasing bladder capacity and improving bladder emptying so that the next void occurs before the functional bladder capacity is reached. The main limiting factor for continence is usually severe sphincter weakness. Bladder emptying can be achieved by using the following methods:

1. Bladder expression or Credé's maneuver, although it is often disliked by children, can be a useful way of emptying the bladder, particularly if urethral resistance is low. However, this method should never be advocated unless VUR and detrusor sphincter dyssynergia have been excluded.

2. Straining can prove useful in emptying, assuming that the innervation of bladder wall musculature is preserved.
3. CIC and CISC have greatly improved the quality of life in these patients, but these methods are not the answer for all. They are purely means of emptying the bladder; however, by doing so, the kidneys are protected and the risk of infection reduced [18–24]. Children aged 6 and older can be expected to catheterize themselves, and physical handicap is no bar to this [25]. The patient may still be wet between catheterizations because of hyperreflexia, reduced bladder capacity, or sphincter incompetence; thus, use of pharmacologic agents may be required in addition to CIC or CISC to improve continence between catheterizations.
4. Continuous catheterization is disliked by many as a means of management and is not without problems [26]. However, it may be the only way to manage a severely handicapped female patient. It is also the method of choice to decompress the upper urinary tracts in patients with hydronephrosis and can be used as a long-term measure in those presenting with severe renal damage to protect the kidneys from further damage. In the author's experience, it has been a useful way of getting children through their critical growth periods, although ultimately, renal transplantation has been required in some.

The pharmacologic agents used fall into two main groups:

1. Anticholinergics, such as oxybutynin chloride and propantheline bromide, which reduce intravesical pressure and thus indirectly improve bladder capacity. They are used to reduce hyperreflexia and thus can have a beneficial effect on reflux.
2. α-Adrenergic agents, such as ephedrine hydrochloride, that increase the tone in the bladder neck region if bladder neck weakness is present. However, these are not effective enough to prevent stress incontinence if the incompetence is severe.

These two drugs may be used alone or in combination with CIC, Credé's maneuver, or straining in patients with hyperreflexia, stress incontinence, and poor emptying. If they are used without CIC, bladder emptying must be monitored closely by ultrasonography.

Various aids are available to help the patient deal with incontinence. These include various types of pads, diapers, and pants, as well as penile appliances. The latter are fairly useless for young boys, because achieving a good fit is difficult and many boys do not like wearing them.

A nurse specialist is an essential member of the management team for patients with these problems. The nurse advises patients on the types of incontinence appliances and aids available, teaches CIC, counsels and advises patients and their families, and visits schools to advise personnel when necessary.

SURGICAL INTERVENTION

If, despite these measures, renal function deteriorates, the degree of incontinence is unacceptable, or both, then surgical intervention is required. The timing depends on the nature of the problem. If renal function is deteriorating despite optimum nonsurgical management, then there is no choice about surgical intervention; but if surgery is to be carried out for incontinence alone, then no immediate urgency exists. Deterioration of renal function is usually due to outflow obstruction at the distal sphincter and high intravesical pressure, and may be compounded by reflux. The problem may be made worse by persistent or recurrent infections in the presence of reflux.

The timing of surgery for incontinence can be tailored to the patient's needs, and in children and young adults should be at their request and not that of their caregivers. All patients undergoing reconstructive surgery must be able to intermittently catheterize before surgery, because the risk is high that this will be required to achieve emptying postoperatively. Thus, surgery solely for incontinence should not be offered to those not prepared to intermittently catheterize.

The surgical options used are the following:

1. Vesicostomy may be required in babies and infants to decompress and protect the kidneys when indwelling catheters or CIC is not a feasible option. This procedure allows for urinary drainage into a diaper. When the child is older, other forms of management, such as CIC, can be considered.
2. Sphincterotomy to overcome distal sphincter obstruction is now rarely performed, because the incomplete bladder emptying can be overcome by the use of CIC; occasionally in males, however, bladder emptying can be achieved without this if a limited sphincterotomy is performed.
3. The major advance has been reconstructive bladder surgery using the bowel, either in an augmentation procedure (clam cystoplasty) or in a substitution cystoplasty, in which most of the bladder is removed and replaced by bowel. The latter procedure is required if the bladder is small and very thick-walled. Often, the decision as to which procedure is required is made at the time of surgery itself. Nearly all parts of the gastrointestinal tract have been used, although a clam ileocystoplasty is the most common procedure [27]. This procedure reduces the intravesical pressure and increases bladder capacity, and it is used both to protect the kidneys and to improve continence. The procedure is not without problems, which include mucus production, infection, stone formation, metabolic problems (if renal function is compromised), perforation, and the possibility of malignancy [28]. Thus, careful selection is mandatory.

   In patients with sphincter weakness, continence can be further improved by the implantation of an artificial urinary sphincter, and often reconstructive bladder surgery is combined with the insertion of an artificial urinary sphincter cuff. The sphincter can be activated if required by a minor procedure at a later date. Approximately 60% of patients undergoing this procedure need to catheterize postoperatively, and complications may occur [29].

   In patients not able to catheterize by urethra, a continent urinary diversion can be created using the Mitrofanoff procedure. The appendix is reimplanted into the bladder wall to produce a continent catheterizable abdominal channel [30]. Other tubular structures are now used, and continence rates of 94% are reported [31]. Standard ileal loop urinary diversion is now rarely performed; however, it may be the only option and occasionally can be very successful.

NEUROPATHIC BOWEL

Neuropathic bowel patients frequently have associated bowel problems with constipation and soiling. The problem is secondary to deficient sensation of the lower bowel, rectum, and anus; a patulous or atonic anus is often present. This problem must be addressed early, with attention paid to diet and establishment of a regular toileting regime (preferably after meals). Bowel continence is often more difficult to achieve than urinary continence, and complex bladder surgery to treat urinary incontinence should not be considered until the bowel problem has been addressed.

For some, regular manual evacuation is the answer. However, a high-fiber diet and a regular toileting regime, with laxatives if required, is preferable. Some patients require regular use of suppositories or enemas of various types to achieve a regular bowel action without soiling in between. The well-motivated patient is able to work out a routine that suits him or her. However, in some patients, when all else has failed and the patient does not want to be reliant on others, surgical intervention may be required to provide a catheterizable colonic stoma to enable antegrade continence enemas. This is known as the *ACE procedure* (see Chapter 12) [32]. When there is no appendix, a tubulized fecal/colonic flap, small bowel tube, or percutaneously inserted catheter may be used. Although several weeks may be required to adjust to the enema regime, results are encouraging [33, 34].

Bladder reconstruction with or without a Mitrofanoff stoma can be combined with the formation of an ACE stoma [35].

As with all the methods of management described, careful selection of patients is vital. Sufficient motivation and manipulative skills are paramount to achieving success. These patients and their families require a great deal of encouragement and counseling, and the nurse specialist plays a vital role here. Long-term results are still being assessed for the newer procedures described.

CONCLUSION

Obviously, these patients must be cared for by a team expert in managing the complete range of problems these patients have. Close cooperation must be ensured between the urologist, pediatrician, neurologist, neurosurgeon, orthopedic surgeon, nephrologist, and nurse specialist. Ideally, the patients should be seen in some form of combined clinic, such as a spina bifida clinic. The problems are lifelong. Renal damage can occur at any age (including during adult life), and thus regular long-term reassessment is necessary in an appropriate setting to ensure continuing success in management.

REFERENCES

1. Lapides J, Diokno AC, Silber SJ, Lowe BS. Clean intermittent self-catheterization in the treatment of urinary tract disease. J Urol 1972;107:458–461.
2. Medical Research Council Vitamin Study Research Group. Prevention of neural tube defects: results of the Medical Research Council Vitamin Study. Lancet 1991;338:131–137.
3. Sutherland RS, Mevorach RA, Baskin LS, Kogan BA. Spinal dysraphism in children: an overview to prevent complications. Urology 1995;46:294–304.
4. Borzyskowski M, Neville BGR. Neuropathic bladder and spinal dysraphism. Arch Dis Child 1981;56:176–180.

5. Bauer SB, Atala A, Dyro FM, et al. Urologic manifestations in patients with diastematomyelia [abstract]. J Urol 1992;147:251A. Abstract 152.
6. Perez LM, Barnes N, MacDiarmid SA, et al. Urologic dysfunction in patients with diastematomyelia. J Urol 1993;149:1503–1505.
7. Johnston L, Borzyskowski M. Bladder dysfunction and neurological disability at presentation in closed spina bifida. Arch Dis Child 1998;79:33–38.
8. Rickwood AMK, Thomas DG, Philp NM, Spicer RD. Assessment of congenital neuropathic bladder by combined urodynamic and radiological studies. Br J Urol 1982;54:512–518.
9. Mundy AR, Shah PJR, Borzyskowski M, Saxton HM. Sphincter behaviour in myelomeningocoele. Br J Urol 1985;57:647–651.
10. McGuire EJ, Woodside JR, Borden TA, Weiss RM. Prognostic value of urodynamic testing in myelodysplastic patients. J Urol 1981;126:205–209.
11. Mundy AR, Borzyskowski M, Saxton HM. Videourodynamic evaluation of neuropathic vesicourethral dysfunction in children. Br J Urol 1982;54:645–549.
12. Gamal M, Ghoniem MB, Roach MB, et al. The value of leak pressure and bladder compliance in the urodynamic evaluation of meningomyelocoele patients. J Urol 1990;144:1440–1442.
13. Bauer SB, Hallett M, Khoshbin S, et al. Predictive value of urodynamic evaluation in newborns with myelodysplasia. JAMA 1984;252:650–652.
14. Sidi AA, Dysktra DD, Gonzalez R. The value of urodynamic testing in the management of neonates with myelodysplasia: a prospective study. J Urol 1986;135:90–93.
15. Spinder MR, Bauer SB, Dyro FM, et al. The changing neurourologic lesion in myelodysplasia. JAMA 1987;258:1630–1633.
16. Galloway NTM, Mekras JA, Helms M, Webster GD. An objective score to predict upper tract deterioration in myelodysplasia. J Urol 1991;145:535–537.
17. Satar N, Bauer SB, Shefner J, et al. The effect of delayed diagnosis and treatment in patients with occult spinal dysraphism. J Urol 1995;154;754–758.
18. Lapides J, Diokno AC, Lowe BS, Kalish MD. Follow-up on unsterile intermittent catheterization. J Urol 1974;111:184–186.
19. Lapides J, Diokno AC, Gould FR, Lowe BS. Further observations on self catheterization. J Urol 1976;116:169–171.
20. Borzyskowski M, Mundy AR, Neville BGR, et al. Neuropathic vesicourethral dysfunction in children. Br J Urol 1982;54:641–644.
21. Plunkett JM, Braren V. Clean intermittent catheterization in children. J Urol 1979;121:469–471.
22. Brock WA, So EP, Harbach L, Kaplan GW. Intermittent catheterization in the management of neurogenic vesicourethral dysfunction in children. J Urol 1981;125:391–393.
23. Kass EJ, McHugh T, Diokno AC. Intermittent catheterization in children less than 6 years old. J Urol 1979;121:792–793.
24. Diokno AC, Sonda LP, Hollander JB, Lapides J. Fate of patients started on clean intermittent catheterization therapy 10 years ago. J Urol 1983;129:1120–1122.
25. Robinson RO, Cockram M, Strode M. Severe handicap in spina bifida: no bar to intermittent self-catheterization. Arch Dis Child 1985;60:760–762.
26. Minns RA, Dag JC, Duffy SW, et al. Indwelling urinary catheters in childhood spinal paralysis. Zeitschrift für Kinderchirurgie 1980;31:387–397.
27. Woodhouse CR. Reconstruction of the lower urinary tract for neurogenic bladder: lessons from the adolescent age group. Br J Urol 1992;69:589–593.
28. Mundy AR, Nurse DE. Calcium balance, growth and skeletal mineralization in patients with cystoplasties. Br J Urol 1992;69:257–259.
29. Bosco PJ, Bauser SB, Colodny AH, et al. The long term results of artificial sphincters in children. J Urol 1991;141:396–399.
30. Mitrofanoff P. Cystostomie continente trans-appendiculaire dans le traitement des vessies neurologiques. Chir Paediatr 1980;21:297–305.
31. Woodhouse CRJ, Gordon EM. The Mitrofanoff principle for urethral failure. Br J Urol 1994;73:55–60.
32. Malone PS, Ransley PG, Kiely EM. Preliminary report: the antegrade continence enema. Lancet 1990;336:1217–1218.
33. Squire R, Kiely EM, Carr B, et al. The clinical application of the Malone antegrade colonic enema. J Pediatr Surg 1993;28:1012–1015.
34. Shandling B, Chait PG, Richards HF. Percutaneous cecostomy: a new technique in the management of fecal incontinence. J Pediatr Surg 1996;31:534–537.
35. Roberts JP, Malone PS. Treatment of neuropathic urinary and faecal incontinence with synchronous combined bladder reconstruction and ACE procedure. Br J Urol 1994;76:386–389.

25
Nonpsychogenic Urinary Retention in Young Women

Michael J. Swinn and Clare J. Fowler

Although isolated urinary retention affecting young women is not just a phenomenon of modern times, little was written about it in the early urologic literature and even less about its possible causes. Nevertheless, the urologist or urogynecologist is not infrequently faced with a young woman in urinary retention, and the differential diagnosis is likely to include a neurologic disorder. Subsequently, if no evidence of such a disorder is found, the assumption is often made that the problem is psychogenic. Indeed, the largest body of medical literature on the subject of urinary retention in young women refers to psychogenic or "hysterical" urinary retention [1–8]. Even some contemporary textbooks prompt the opinion that the problem has a psychogenic origin [9].

Viewed logically, in the absence of physical obstruction, urinary retention can occur either because of failure of detrusor contraction or because of failure of sphincter relaxation (or both). Clearly, this complaint may have a number of possible causes. Because of the prevalence of multiple sclerosis in young women and the frequent involvement of bladder function in that disease, this is often considered as a likely diagnosis. With the advent of magnetic resonance imaging, however, multiple sclerosis is relatively easy to exclude. Also, the clinical features of urinary retention in isolation are not typical of the bladder dysfunction encountered in multiple sclerosis. In multiple sclerosis, the evidence points to the fact that patients have bladder involvement because of their spinal cord disease, and that, in turn, is likely to produce concomitant neurologic signs in the lower limbs [10]. An alternative suggested diagnosis for retention is a cauda equina syndrome. Such a lesion may indeed cause a large atonic bladder, but the other associated clinical features, such as sacral anesthesia, are absent in these women. Thus, the history and clinical examination show that urinary retention is often unexplained and occurs as an isolated disorder.

In fact, for many years, a disorder of sphincter relaxation in young women has been recognized as an observable phenomenon. Moore described a series of women with difficulty in voiding and various degrees of urinary retention and in whom cystoscopic examination suggested hypertrophy of the urethral sphincter [11]. Raz and

367

Smith described exceptionally high urethral closure pressures in young women with complete urinary retention. They found that the maximal urethral pressure was consistently recorded from the mid-urethra and postulated that retention was due to spasticity of the striated urethral sphincter or pelvic floor [12].

Fowler et al. proposed the existence of a syndrome of urinary retention in young women due to impaired relaxation of the striated muscle of the urethral sphincter, which can be demonstrated using electromyography (EMG); the syndrome was associated with polycystic ovaries in a proportion of subjects [13]. The hypothesis is that, in these young women, a primary abnormality of the striated muscle of the urethral sphincter exists that impairs its ability to relax. This abnormality produces a characteristic EMG signal. When a concentric needle electrode is used to record from the striated muscle of the urethral sphincter, EMG activity that has two distinct components can be recorded. First, complex repetitive discharge activity occurs, which produces a sound like that of a motor bike or helicopter over the audio amplifier of an EMG machine. Second, a sound occurs that has a pronounced decelerating component. This latter activity bears a superficial resemblance to myotonia; however, on close examination, the activity is observed to be due to deceleration of one of the components of a complex repetitive discharge, and because of this, it has been described as a decelerating burst (Figure 25.1) [13]. The increase in sphincter tone and afferent activity from it are postulated to result in efferent inhibition of the detrusor. This explanation fits with the clinical observations that the retention, for the most part, is painless and that these young women present with bladder capacities in excess of one liter.

Single fiber EMG analysis has shown that, when a complex repetitive discharge activity is firing steadily, the jitter between component potentials is so low that the activity must be due to ephaptic—that is, direct muscle-to-muscle—transmission (Figure 25.2). Although each potential is presumably initiated by neuromuscular transmission, the direct spread of impulses throughout the muscle results in a self-perpetuating impairment of contraction or, in this instance, impaired sphincter relaxation. The hormonal imbalance inherent in polycystic ovary syndrome was postulated to cause an impairment of insulation of the striated urethral sphincter muscle membrane, thus allowing the ephaptic transmission to spread.

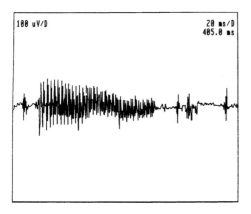

100 uV/D   20 ms/D
                            405.0 ms

Figure 25.1   Electromyographic (EMG) recording from the striated urethral sphincter of a woman in complete urinary retention. The activity shown is a "decelerating burst"; when many of these are heard together over the audio output of the EMG machine, the sound is reminiscent of the underwater singing of whales.

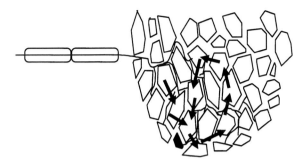

Figure 25.2 Diagrammatic representation of ephaptic transmission occurring in the striated urethral sphincter of a young woman in urinary retention. The impulse follows a disordered, circuitous route, and this is hypothesized to prevent the sphincter from relaxing. (Reprinted with permission from CJ Fowler. Pelvic Floor Neurophysiology. In JW Osselton, CD Binnie, R Cooper, et al. [eds], Clinical Neurophysiology: EMG, Nerve Conduction and Evoked Potentials. Oxford, UK: Butterworth–Heinemann, 1995;233–252.)

Abnormalities of sphincter behavior, however, are less commonly the cause of the symptoms; the symptoms are usually secondary to reactive changes in the detrusor. Some patients with abnormal sphincter EMG activity present with urgency and frequency and can be demonstrated to have detrusor instability with low flow and sometimes impaired emptying; however, the majority of young women have urinary retention, either complete or partial, as far as is known.

Since the original observation [13], various centers have reported corroborative evidence for the hypothesis. In one study of 477 patients referred for neurourologic evaluation, complex repetitive discharges were found in the urethral sphincter of 10%. The authors concluded that the activity is not uncommon, but that it appears to be associated with an increased postmicturition residual volume or a history of recurrent infections [14]. Webb et al. found the EMG abnormality in 8 out of 18 women in urinary retention, although these authors also found the abnormality in the anal sphincter [15]. The hypothesis that the activity causes impaired sphincter relaxation was confirmed by a study of Deindl et al., who used hooked-wire electrodes to record prolonged EMG activity from the urethral sphincter during voiding cystometry and demonstrated the presence of an intermittent stream together with bursts of complex repetitive discharge activity [16].

EMG of the urethral sphincter is a difficult diagnostic technique. The abnormality is not often found in the anal sphincter, and a needle electrode must be used to record directly from the striated muscle of the urethral sphincter. Various different techniques have been developed to carry out this procedure with minimal discomfort, but even a highly practiced operator may have difficulty locating the EMG abnormality in the muscle. Considerable determination on the part of the patient and the electromyographer is often required, and, because the needle placement and interpretation of the EMG signal require an uncommon combination of skills and interests, the test is not widely performed.

An attempt to define the natural history of this condition was undertaken by retrospective analysis of the cases of nearly 60 women with complete retention and an abnormal sphincter EMG [17]. This is a disorder that affects exclusively young, premenopausal women; the average age of onset is 26.3 years. In approximately one-half of the patients, urinary retention appears to have been precipitated by an operation or at least the use of a general anesthetic, but on direct questioning, abnormal voiding was revealed to predate the onset of retention in the majority (78%). The most common abnormality cited, present in more than two-thirds, was the lack of desire to void for long periods. It is not uncommon for women who subsequently develop retention to void just twice in a 24-hour period, and one-half experience intermittent urinary flow before their urinary retention. An underlying hormonal cause is suggested by the finding that, of the two-thirds of patients who had undergone pelvic ultrasonography, one-half were found to have polycystic ovaries.

Although this bladder disorder follows a benign course, there is rarely a spontaneous return to normal voiding. The only treatment that was shown to be consistently effective is neuromodulation of the sacral nerves via a permanently implanted sacral nerve stimulator. In this procedure, electrical stimulation is delivered unilaterally via the third sacral foramen. For a patient with long-standing complete urinary retention to be returned to normal voiding overnight through this procedure is not uncommon. The precise mechanism of action has yet to be defined, but recordings of the latency of the observed response to stimulation suggest that the effect is via an afferent mechanism, possibly a spino-bulbar-spinal pathway [18].

The delineation of an organic cause of urinary retention in women clearly has considerable importance in terms of correct patient management. Almost one-half of the young women in retention seen in our department were told that their retention was due to their psychological state or were at least left with this impression. The majority in whom the EMG abnormality has been demonstrated expressed tremendous relief at discovering that their problem had been shown to have a physical cause.

REFERENCES

1. Knox SJ. Psychogenic urinary retention after parturition resulting in hydronephrosis. BMJ 1960;5210:1422–1424.
2. Larson JW, Swenson WM, Utz DC, Steinhilber RM. Psychogenic urinary retention in women. JAMA 1963;184:697–700.
3. Margolis G. A review of the literature on psychogenic urinary retention. J Urol 1965;94:257–258.
4. Allen T. Psychogenic urinary retention. South Med J 1972;65:302–304.
5. Barrett D. Psychogenic urinary retention in women. Mayo Clin Proc 1976;51:351–356.
6. Montague DK, Jones LR. Psychogenic urinary retention. Urology 1979;13:30–35.
7. Bird J. Psychogenic urinary retention. Psychother Psychosom 1980;34:45–51.
8. Bassi P, Zattoni F, Aragona F, et al. Psychogenic urinary retention in women. Diagnostic and therapeutic aspects. J Urol 1988;94:159–162.
9. Siroky M, Krane R (eds). Clinical Neuro-Urology. Functional Voiding Disorders in Women. Boston: Little, Brown, 1991;445–457.
10. Betts CD, D'Mellow MT, Fowler CJ. Urinary symptoms and the neurological features of bladder dysfunction in multiple sclerosis. J Neurol Neurosurg Psychiatry 1993;56:245–250.
11. Moore T. Bladder-neck obstruction in women. Proc R Soc Med 1953;467:558–563.
12. Raz S, Smith RB. External sphincter spasticity syndrome in female patients. J Urol 1976;115:443–446.

13. Fowler CJ, Christmas TJ, Chapple CR, et al. Abnormal electromyographic activity of the urethral sphincter, voiding dysfunction and polycystic ovaries: a new syndrome? BMJ 1988;297:1436–1438.
14. Jensen D, Stein R. The importance of complex repetitive discharges in the striated female urethral sphincter and male bulbocavernosus muscle. Scand J Urol Nephrol Suppl 1996;179:69–73.
15. Webb RJ, Fawcett PRW, Neal DE. Electromyographic abnormalities in the urethral and anal sphincters of women with idiopathic retention of urine. Br J Urol 1992;70:22–25.
16. Deindl FM, Vodusek DB, Bischof LC, Hartung R. Zwei verschieddene formen von miktionsstorungen bei jungen frauen: dyssynerges verhalten im beckenboden oder pseudomyotonie im externen urethralen sphinkter? Aktuelle Urologie 1998;28:88–94.
17. Swinn MJ, Fowler CJ. The clinical features of non-psychogenic urinary retention in women (Fowler's syndrome). Neurourol Urodyn 1998;174:383–384.
18. Fowler CJ, Swinn MJ. The long latency of anal sphincter contraction on S3 stimulation shows the reflex is afferent-mediated. Neurourol Urodyn 1998;174:355–356.

Index

Note: Page numbers followed by *f* indicate figures; page numbers followed by *t* indicate tables.

Absorbent pads, for incontinence, 180, 180f
Acetylcholine, in cavernous relaxation, 52
Acute motor and sensory axonal neuropathy, 346
Acute motor axonal neuropathy, 346
Adolescent(s), influence of neurologic disability on sex and relationships in, 79–80
β-Adrenergic agents, for bladder dysfunction in spina bifida patients, 362
Alimentary tract, lower, innervation of, 342
Alprostadil, for erectile dysfunction, 210
Ambulatory urodynamics, 102
Amyloidosis, neuropathies associated with, 345
Anal canal, 6f, 8
  electrical stimulation of, 132
Anal manometry, in bowel problem evaluation, 187
Anal plug, for urinary incontinence, 202–203
Anal sphincter, damage to
  electromyography of, 150
  repair of, in bowel problem management, 197
Anal triangle, 8
Anal ultrasonography, in bowel problem evaluation, 188
Anejaculation, 220
Anismus, 111
Anococcygeal ligament, 8
Anorectal physiology tests, in bowel problem evaluation, 187–188

Anorectum
  control of during continence and defecation, 29f
  functions of, 21
Antegrade continence enema, in bowel problem management, 197, 198f
Anterior sacral root, stimulation of, 128–129, 129f
Anticholinergic(s)
  for bladder dysfunction in spina bifida patients, 362
  for detrusor hyperreflexia, 164–166, 165f
  oral, for tropical spastic paraparesis, 320
Anus, musculature of, 6f, 8
Anxiety, sexual response effects of, 74–75
Arterial inflow, evaluation of, in vasculogenic erectile failure, 154–156
Arteriography, selective pudendal, in vasculogenic erectile failure evaluation, 156
Arteriovenous malformations, spinal, cauda equina damage due to, 332
Artificial bowel sphincter, in bowel problem management, 199, 200f
Attitude(s), disorders of, effects of on sexual response, 78–79
Autonomic dysreflexia, in spinal cord–injured patients, 277–278
Autonomic function testing, in neurogenic erectile failure, 151–152
Autonomic nervous system responses, measurement of, 135–138, 137f

Autonomic neuropathies, hereditary, 348
Autonomous bladder, 276
Azathioprine, for tropical spastic paraparesis, 322

Back pain, cauda equina damage and, 330–331
Baclofen, use in spinal cord–injured patients, 280
Balloon distention, in bowel problem evaluation, 187
Balloon expulsion tests, in bowel problem evaluation, 188
Behavior
    bladder and bowel problems effects on, 66
    disorders of, effects of on sexual response, 74
Behavioral retraining, in incomplete bladder emptying, 177
Benign orgasmic cephalalgia, 44–45
Biofeedback, for constipation, 193–194
Bladder
    autonomous, 276
    disabilities associated with, 60
    electrical stimulation of, 132
    functions of, 20
    handicaps associated with, 61–62
    housework affected by, 62–63
    impairments of, 59–60
    low-pressure areflexic, bladder emptying and continence in, 284
    neural control of, 25f
    neuroanatomic sites in modulation of, 22, 23f
    neuroanatomic specialization of, 20–24, 23f
    neurogenic. *See* Neurogenic bladder
    neuropathic
        behavioral reactions to, 66
        consequences of, 57–67
        dependence on health services due to, 65
        employment affected by, 64–65
        nutrition affected by, 62
        parenting affected by, 63
        psychological issues affected by, 65–66
        residential placement affected by, 64
        restorative rehabilitation paradigm for, 58f, 59f
        sexual activity affected by, 62
        social relations affected by, 63–64
        travel affected by, 65

neurophysiology of, 20
parasympathetic nerve pathways and, 21–22
smooth muscles of, functions of, 21
as storage organ, 21
sympathetic system's effect on, 26–27
uninhibited overactive, defined, 267
Bladder control, supraspinal circuitry in, 4
Bladder dysfunction
    in diabetic patients, 343
    in multiple sclerosis patients, 298–306. *See also* Multiple sclerosis, bladder dysfunction in patients with
        with erectile dysfunction, 295
        impotence related to, 291, 292f
    in multiple system atrophy, 245–248. *See also* Multiple system atrophy, bladder dysfunction in
    neurogenic, in spinal cord–injured patients, 276
    in spina bifida, 354–357. *See also* Spina bifida, bladder dysfunction in
Bladder emptying
    incomplete. *See* Incomplete bladder emptying, treatment of
    in low-pressure areflexic bladder, 284
    in spina bifida, 361–362
    in spinal cord–injured patients, 279–282
        continuous catheter drainage for, 280
        external urethral sphincterotomy for, 281
        intermittent self-catheterization for, 279–280
        pharmacologic, 280
        shaped wheelchair cushion for, 279
        suprapubic diversion for, 281–282
        urethral stent for, 281
Bladder function
    cortical control of, 229–239
        after cerebrovascular accidents, 235–240, 237f, 237t. *See also* Cerebrovascular accidents
        functional brain-imaging techniques for evaluation of, 229–233, 230f–232f
        micturition, 238–239, 239f
        in patients with brain lesions, 233–235
    overactive, defined, 267
    pathophysiology of, associated with neurologic disease at different neuroanatomic sites, 30f
    in spina bifida, assessment of, 359–360

Bladder hyperreflexia, in multiple sclerosis
    patients, 300, 302t
Bladder retraining, in incomplete bladder
    emptying, 177
Blood flow, vaginal, 37–38
Borrelia burgdorferi, infection with, neu-
    ropathies associated with, 346
Bowel
    disabilities associated with, 60
    handicaps associated with, 61–62
    housework affected by, 62–63
    impairments of, 59–60
    neuroanatomic sites in modulation of,
        22, 23f
    neuroanatomic specialization of,
        20–24, 23f
    neuropathic
        behavioral reactions to, 66
        consequences of, 57–67
        dependence on health services due
            to, 65
        employment affected by, 64–65
        nutrition affected by, 62
        parenting affected by, 63
        psychological issues associated with,
            65–66
        residential placement affected by, 64
        restorative rehabilitation paradigm
            for, 58f, 59f
        sexual activity affected by, 62
        social relations affected by, 63–64
        in spina bifida, 362
        travel affected by, 65
    neurophysiology of, 19
Bowel control, supraspinal circuitry in, 4
Bowel dysfunction
    in diabetic patients, 344
    disorders of, in parkinsonism, 255–264
Bowel function
    distal, brain stem lesion effects on, 4
    pathophysiology of, associated with
        neurologic disease at different
        neuroanatomic sites, 30f
    in spinal cord–injured patients, 285–286
Bowel problems, 185–207
    effects of, 187
    investigation of, 187–188, 189t
    management of, 189–203
        anal plug for, 202–203
        anal sphincter repair for, 197
        antegrade continence enema for,
            197, 198f
        artificial bowel sphincter for,
            199, 200f

    biofeedback for, 193–194
    bowel training programs for,
        194–195, 194t
    drugs for, 189–193
    dynamic graciloplasty for, 199, 199f
    general measures and advice for,
        200–201
    manual evacuation for, 196–197
    odor control for, 203
    pads for, 202
    pants for, 202
    sacral nerve stimulation for, 197
    stomas for, 199–200
    surgery for, 197–200, 198f–200f
    toileting aids for, 201–202
    prevalence of, 186
Brain, in sexual desire and reactions, 33–34
Brain injury(ies), traumatic, partner with,
    sex with, 81–82
Brain lesion(s)
    cortical control of bladder in patients
        with, 233–235
    urinary retention in patients with,
        234–235
Brain stem
    in control of micturition, 238–239, 239f
    lesions in, affect on urogenital and dis-
        tal bowel function, 4
    in sexual desire and reactions, 34
Bulbocavernosus reflex, components of, 148
Bulbocavernosus reflex testing, in neuro-
    genic erectile failure,
        148–149, 148f
Bulbus urethrae, cavernous tissue of, 37

Campylobacter jejuni, infection with, neu-
    ropathies associated with,
        346–347
Capsaicin
    for detrusor hyperreflexia, 167–168, 167f
    intravesical instillation of
        for continence in spinal cord–injured
            patients, 283
        for tropical spastic paraparesis,
            320–321, 321t
        for urinary symptoms in multiple
            sclerosis patients, 305
Catheter(s)
    indwelling, in incomplete bladder emp-
        tying, 172–173
    intermittent, in incomplete bladder emp-
        tying, 170–172, 171f, 172f
    Intex, for detrusor hyperreflexia,
        171, 172f

Catheter(s) (*continued*)
    Nelaton, for detrusor hyperreflexia,
        171, 171f
    Scott, for detrusor hyperreflexia,
        171, 172f
    suprapubic, in incomplete bladder emp-
        tying, 173–174, 173f, 174f
Catheter valves, in incomplete bladder
        emptying, 175, 175f
Cauda equina, 325–337
    anatomy of, 325–328, 326f–331f
    damage to
        back pain and, 330–331
        causes of, 328–330, 332–333, 332t
            developmental, 330, 332t
            high-velocity impacts to lum-
                bosacral spine, 328–329
            metastases, 332
            prolapse of intervertebral disk, 330
            spinal arteriovenous malforma-
                tions, 332
        erectile dysfunction due to, 150
        investigation of, 333–335
            colorectal, 334
            cystometry, 333–334, 334f
            neurophysiologic, 335
            radiologic, 333
            sexual dysfunction, 334–335
            urologic, 333–334, 334f
        management of, 335–336
        presentation of, 328–330, 332–333, 332t
        stimulation of, 128–129, 129f
        thecal sac of, nerve roots within, imag-
            ing of, 327–328, 327f–331f
Cavernosography, 157
Cavernosometry, 157
Cavernous relaxation, neurotransmitters in,
        52–53
Cavernous smooth muscle activity, neural
        modulation of, 51–52
Central motor pathways, assessment of,
        129–130
Cephalalgia, orgasmic, benign and malig-
        nant, 44–45
Cerebral somatosensory evoked potential,
        131–132, 131f
Cerebrovascular accidents
    bladder control after, 235–240, 237f, 237t
    urinary incontinence after, epidemiologic
        studies of, 236–238
    urodynamic studies of patients after,
        235–236, 237f, 237t
Children, vesicourethral dysfunction in,
        spinal bifida and, 353

Chronic inflammatory demyelinating
        polyneuropathy, 347
Cisapride, in spinal cord–injured
        patients, 280
Clam ileocystoplasty, for detrusor hyper-
        reflexia, 169
Clean intermittent catheterization, in spina
        bifida, 362
Clinical neurophysiology, 109–143
    autonomic nervous system responses,
        measurement of, 135–138, 137f
    electromyography, 109–125
    nerve-conduction studies, 125–130
    sacral reflexes measurement, 132–135
    sacral sensory system neurophysiology,
        130–132
Clitoris
    cavernous tissue of, 37
    electrical stimulation of, sacral reflex in
        response to, 133–135, 134f
    innervation of, 35–36
    neurophysiology of, 36
    stimulation of, reflexes evoked by, 36
    unstimulated, size of, 36
Coccygeal dorsal spinal rami, 15
Coccygeal plexus, 14
Coccygeus muscle, 5, 6, 6f
Codeine phosphate, for constipation, 193
Cognition, disorders of, effects of on sex-
        ual response, 74
Color duplex ultrasonography, with intra-
        cavernosal injection, in vascu-
        logenic erectile failure
        evaluation, 155–156
Colorectal dysfunction, in multiple sclero-
        sis patients, symptoms of,
        310, 310t
Colorectum
    functions of, 20
    intrinsic nerve supply to, 21
    parasympathetic nerve pathways and,
        21–22
    smooth muscles of, functions of, 21
    as storage organ, 21
Compliance, defined, 102
Computed tomography, contrast-enhanced, of
        thecal sac of cauda equina, 327
Concentric needle electrode electromyog-
        raphy of pelvic floor,
        113–115, 113f–116f
Constipating agents, for diarrhea, 192–193
Constipation
    complications of, 19
    defined, 259

in multiple sclerosis patients, 310–311
in neurologic disease, 19
treatment of, 190–192, 190t, 191f
 bowel training programs,
  194–195, 194t
Continence
 control of anorectum during, 29f
 fecal, control of, 27–28, 29f
 in low-pressure areflexic bladder, 284
 in spinal cord–injured patients,
  282–284
  high bladder pressures in, 282–284
  management of
   bladder emptying, 284
   detrusor myectomy, 283
   enterocystoplasty, 283–284
   intravesical instillation of cap-
    saicin, 283
   for overdistention, 282–283
   pharmacologic, 282
   sacral deafferentation, 283
 urinary, control of, 24–27, 25f
Contraception, 89
Conus medullaris, 325
Corpora, 47
Corpus cavernosum electromyography, 138
 in neurogenic erectile failure, 152–154,
  152f, 153f
Counseling, psychological, for erectile dysfunction, 219
Credé's maneuver, in spina bifida, 361
Cystometry, 100–104, 101f–103f
 in cauda equina damage evaluation,
  333–334, 334f
 defined, 100
 medium-fill, 101
 rapid-fill, 101
 slow-fill, 101
Cystopathy, diabetic, 343–344
Cytoplasty, reduction, in incomplete bladder emptying, 178

Danazol, for tropical spastic paraparesis,
  321–322
Deafferentation, in spinal cord–injured
  patients, 284–285
Defecation
 control of, 27–28, 29f
 control of anorectum during, 29f
 cortical control of, 240
 normal, initiation of, 22–23
 process of, 28
Depression, erectile dysfunction with,
  sildenafil citrate for, 216

Desmopressin acetate, for detrusor hyperreflexia, 166–167
Detrusor hyperactivity with impaired contractile function, 266
 in the elderly, 271–272
Detrusor hyperreflexia, 266
 during cystometry, 163–164, 164f
 defined, 267
 in diabetic patients, 343
 spinal, 267
 treatment of, 164–169
  anticholinergics for, 164–166, 165f
  capsaicin for, 167–168, 167f
  clam ileocystoplasty for, 169
  desmopressin acetate for, 166–167
  detrusor myectomy for, 169
  drugs for, 164–168
  electrical stimulation for, 169
  magnetic stimulation for, 169
  oxybutynin chloride for, 165–166
  propantheline bromide for, 166
  resiniferatoxin for, 168
  subtrigonal phenol injection for,
   168–169
  surgery for, 169
Detrusor
 instability, defined, 267
 phasic, defined, 267
 leak-point pressure, 104–105
 myectomy
  for continence in spinal cord–injured
   patients, 283
  for detrusor hyperreflexia, 169
Detrusor sphincter dyssynergia, 111, 302
Diabetes mellitus
 detrusor hyperreflexia in, 343
 diarrhea in, 344
 neuropathies associated with, 215–216,
  343–345
  bowel dysfunction, 344
  cystopathy, 343–344
  erectile dysfunction, 215–216
  sexual dysfunction, 344–345
  type 1, autonomic neuropathy in, 343
Diabetic cystopathy, 343
Diarrhea, diabetic, 344
Disability(ies)
 acquired, sex with partner with, 80–84, 83f
 bladder, 60
 bowel, 60
 defined, 57
L-Dopa
 in parkinsonism, 255–264
 in Parkinson's disease, 248–249

Dorsal penile nerve, electroneurography of, 130
Dorsal sacral roots, electroneurography of, 130–131
Drainage bags, in incomplete bladder emptying, 174
DUO system, for erectile dysfunction, 211f
Dyadic, defined, 69
Dyadic relationship, neurologic disability effects on, 72–74, 73f
Dynamic graciloplasty, in bowel problem management, 199, 199f
Dysreflexia, autonomic, in spinal cord–injured patients, 277–278
Dyssynergia, detrusor sphincter, 111, 302

Ejaculation
    cervical spinal cord in, 34
    female, 41
    male, 51
    in multiple sclerosis patients, 295, 296f
    retrograde, in diabetic patients, 345
    in spinal cord–injured patients, 286–287
Elderly
    bladder problems in, causes of, 265
    frail, established urge incontinence in, cerebral causes of, 269, 270f
    urinary incontinence in, 265–273
        detrusor hyperactivity with impaired contractile function in, 271–272
        functional brain scanning results in young men, 271
        gender differences, 269–271
        postvoid residual urine in, 271–272
        research findings in, 267–271, 268f, 270f
        severity of, factors determining, 271
        types of, 266–267
        urodynamic findings in, 267–269, 268f
Electrical stimulation, for detrusor hyperreflexia, 169
Electroejaculation, rectal probe, for male infertility, 220
Electromyography
    of anal or urethral sphincter, in neurogenic erectile failure, 150
    corpus cavernosum, 138
        in neurogenic erectile failure, 152–154, 152f, 153f
    in nonpsychogenic urinary retention in young women, 368–370, 368f
    of pelvic floor, 109–125
        with concentric needle electrode, 113–115, 113f–116f
        in examination of motor unit details, 111–112
        findings due to denervation and reinnervation, 117–120, 118f–122f
        in genuine stress incontinence, 120–122
        kinesiologic, 109–111, 110f, 111f
        in primary muscle disease, 124
        with single fiber electrode, 115–116, 117f
        in women with urinary retention and obstructed voiding, 122–124, 123f
    sphincter, in multiple system atrophy diagnosis, 150–151, 151f, 247–248
Electroneurography, of sacral sensory system, 130
Electrosensitivity thresholds, in bowel problem evaluation, 188
Emission, male, 51
Emotion(s), disorders of, sexual response effects of, 74
Employment, effects of bladder and bowel problems on, 64–65
Encephalopathy(ies), myo-neuro-gastrointestinal, 348
Endothelium derived relaxing factor, 52
Enema(s), antegrade continence with, in bowel problem management, 197, 198f
Enterocystoplasty, for continence in spinal cord–injured patients, 283–284
Eperisone hydrochloride, for tropical spastic paraparesis, 322
Ephedrine hydrochloride, for bladder dysfunction in spina bifida patients, 362
Epilepsy
    sexual behavior in patients with, modification of, 44
    sexual issues in patients with, 42–44
Erectile dysfunction. *See* Male erectile dysfunction
Erection
    cortical control of, 241
    neurophysiology of, 49–51
        afferent pathways in, 50–51
        efferent pathways in, 49–50

physiology of, 48–49
in spinal cord–injured patients, 286
Erythromycin, for tropical spastic paraparesis, 322
Esophageal alterations, in Parkinson's disease, 255–256, 256t
Evacuating proctography, in bowel problem evaluation, 188
Evacuation, manual, for constipation,
196–197
Exercise(s), pelvic floor, in incomplete
bladder emptying, 176–177
Expectation(s), unrealistic, effects on sexual response, 76–78, 77t, 78t
External urethral sphincterotomy, in spinal
cord–injured patients, 281

Fecal continence, control of, 27–28, 29f
Fecal incontinence
factors affecting, 19
intractable, management of,
202–203, 203f
prevalence of, 186
Female sexual function
brain in, 33–34
brain stem in, 34
cavernous tissue of clitoris, bulbus urethrae, labia, and vagina, 37
ejaculation, 41
innervation of clitoris, 35–36
innervation of internal sex organs,
34–35
orgasm, 40–41
oxytocin secretion, 39
pelvic floor muscles in, 39–40
physiology of, 33–41
sexual response phases in, 33
spinal cord in, 34
uterine physiology during sexual
arousal and orgasm, 39
vaginal blood flow in, 37–38
vaginal changes during sexual arousal,
38–39
vaginal lubrication in, 38
Female sexuality, effect of neurologic diseases on, 41–42
Fertility, 88–89
Filum terminale, 325
Fosfomycin tromethamine, for tropical
spastic paraparesis, 322
Fowler's syndrome, 368
Frankenhäuser's ganglion, 35
Frontal lobe, influence on bladder, bowel,
and sexual function, 4

Ganglion(a)
Frankenhäuser's, 35
hypogastric, 35
Gastrointestinal dysfunction, in multiple
sclerosis patients, 309–313.
See also Multiple sclerosis,
gastrointestinal dysfunction in
Gender, as factor in urinary incontinence in
the elderly, 269–271
Genital nerves
female, 342
male, 341–342
Genitofemoral nerve, 12
Genitourinary tract
innervation of, 340–341
infections of, effect on male infertility, 221
Genuine stress incontinence, defined, 266
Graciloplasty, dynamic, in bowel problem
management, 199, 199f
Guillain-Barré syndrome, neuropathies
associated with, 346

Handicap(s)
bladder, 61–62
bowel, 61–62
defined, 58
Head injuries, sexual problems after,
241–242
Headache(s), benign orgasmic cephalalgia,
44–45
Health services, dependence on, bladder and
bowel problems effects on, 65
Heparin sodium, for tropical spastic para-
paresis, 322
Hereditary amyloid neuropathy, 347–348
Hereditary autonomic neuropathy, 348
Hereditary sensory neuropathies, 348
Hirschsprung's disease, 348
Human T-cell lymphotropic virus type
I–associated myelopathy/trop-
ical spastic paraparesis, 315
Human T-cell lymphotropic virus type I
infections, 315–324. *See also*
Tropical spastic paraparesis
incidence of, 315
seroprevalence of, 315
Hydrocortisone, for tropical spastic paraparesis, 322
Hyperreflexia
bladder, in multiple sclerosis patients,
300, 302t
detrusor, 266, 267
in diabetic patients, 343
treatment of, 164–169

Hypogastric ganglion, 35
Hypogastric plexus, 34–35
Hypogastric sheath, 340
Hypothalamus, in sexual desire and reactions, 33–34

Iliococcygeus muscle, 6, 6f
Iliohypogastric nerve, 11
Ilioinguinal nerve, 12
Iliosacralis, 6
Immune-mediated neuropathies, neuropathies associated with, 346
Immunomodulatory therapies, for tropical spastic paraparesis, 322
Impairment(s)
    bladder, 59–60
    bowel, 59–60
    defined, 57
Impotence
    erectile, in diabetic patients, 344
    in multiple sclerosis patients, 289–290, 290f
        prevalence of, 291
Incomplete bladder emptying, treatment of, 170–178
    behavioral retraining for, 177
    bladder retraining for, 177
    catheter valves for, 175, 175f
    drainage bags for, 174
    indwelling catheters for, 172–173
    intermittent catheters for, 170–172, 171f, 172f
    myoplasties for, 178
    nerve root stimulation for, 177–178
    pelvic floor exercises for, 176–177
    prostheses for, 178
    Queen Square bladder stimulator for, 176, 176f
    reduction cytoplasty for, 178
    suprapubic catheters for, 173–174, 173f, 174f
    surgery for, 177–178
    urinary diversion for, 178
    vesicoplication for, 178
    voiding techniques for, 170
Incontinence
    absorbent products for, 180, 180f
    appliances for, 178–180, 179f, 180f
        Conveen Continence Guard, 179
        Femassist, 179
        penile sheath, 179–180, 179f
        Reliance, 179
    fecal, 186
        factors affecting, 19

    intractable, management of, 202–203, 203f
    in multiple sclerosis patients, 311
    neurogenic, 185
    neurologic lesions and, 20
    practical management of, 170–178. *See also* Incomplete bladder emptying, treatment of
    stress, 20
    electromyographic changes in, 120–122
    genuine, defined, 266
    urinary, 20. *See* Urinary incontinence
Indwelling catheters, in incomplete bladder emptying, 172–173
Infection(s), neuropathies associated with, 346
Inferior hypogastric plexus, 34–35
Infertility
    female, treatment of, 222
    male
        genitourinary tract infections and, 221
        treatment of, 219–222
            rectal probe electroejaculation in, 220
            vibratory stimulation in, 220
Inherited neuropathies, 347–349
Interferon-α, for tropical spastic paraparesis, 322
Intermittent catheters, in incomplete bladder emptying, 170–172, 171f, 172f
Intermittent self-catheterization
    in spinal cord–injured patients, 279–280
    for tropical spastic paraparesis, 320
    for urinary symptoms in multiple sclerosis patients, 305
Internal sex organs, innervation of, 34–35
Intimate relationship, neurologic disability effects on, sexual expression within, 85–86
Intracavernosal injection, color duplex ultrasonography with, in vasculogenic erectile failure evaluation, 155–156
Intracavernosal pharmacotherapy, for erectile dysfunction, 209–213
Intracorporeal injection therapy, for neurogenic erectile dysfunction in multiple sclerosis patients, 297
Intractable fecal incontinence, management of, 202–203, 203f

Intraurethral prostaglandin E₁ pellet, in multiple sclerosis patients, 290
Intraurethral pharmacotherapy, for erectile dysfunction, 213–214, 214f

Kidney(s), damage to, in spinal cord–injured patients, 278–279
Kidney stones, in spinal cord–injured patients, 278

Labia, cavernous tissue of, 37
Large bowel, effect of Parkinson's disease on, 258–262
Laxative(s)
    for constipation, 190–192, 190t, 191f
    for patients with normal pelvic floor relaxation, 262
Leak-point pressure, 104–105
Lesion(s)
    brain. *See* Brain lesion(s)
    neurologic, incontinence due to, 20
Levator ani, 5, 6f
Libido, cortical control of, 240–242
Ligament(s), anococcygeal, 8
Limb-girdle plexuses, defined, 5
Loperamide hydrochloride, for diarrhea, 192–193
Loperamide oxide, for diarrhea, 192
Lower alimentary tract, innervation of, 342
Lubrication, in females, effect of neurologic diseases on, 42
Lumbar dorsal (posterior primary) rami, 15
Lumbar plexus, 9–12
    branches of, 11–12
    deviation from ventral rami, 9–10, 10f, 11f
Lumbar sympathetic system, 15
Lymphocytapheresis, for tropical spastic paraparesis, 322

Magnetic resonance imaging, T₂FSE, of thecal sac of cauda equina, 327–328, 327f–331f
Magnetic stimulation, for detrusor hyperreflexia, 169
Male erectile dysfunction, 145–160
    causes of, 145
    in diabetic patients, 344
    diagnosis of, tests in, 146t
    in multiple sclerosis patients, neurophysiologic tests for, 293–295, 293t, 294f
    neurogenic erectile failure. *See* Neurogenic erectile failure

neurophysiologic investigations in, nervous system parts tested in, 147f
nocturnal penile tumescence testing in, 145–146, 146t
pathophysiology of, 53–54, 54t
with preserved libido, 241
treatment of, 209–219
    alprostadil for, 210
    drug combinations for, 211–212, 211f, 212f
    intracavernosal pharmacotherapy for, 209–213
    intraurethral pharmacotherapy for, 213–214, 214f
    moxisylyte hydrochloride for, 210–211
    in multiple sclerosis patients, 290
    oral medication for, 214–216
    penile prosthesis implantation for, 218–219, 218f
    pharmacologic erection program for, 212–213
    psychological counseling for, 219
    rehabilitation for, 219
    vacuum constrictor devices for, 217–218, 217f
vasculogenic erectile failure, 154–157. *See also* Vasculogenic erectile failure
Male sexual function
    anatomy related to, 47–48, 48f
    neurophysiology of erection, 49–51
    phases of, 47
    physiology of, 47–56
        ejaculation, 51
        emission, 51
        erection, 48–49
        neural modulation of cavernous smooth muscle activity, 51–52
        neurotransmitters in cavernous relaxation, 52–53
        neurotransmitters in smooth muscle contraction, 53
        orgasm, 51
Manometry, anal, in bowel problem evaluation, 187
Manual evacuation, for constipation, 196–197
Mechanical stimulation, 132
    sacral reflex in response to, 135
Medicated urethral system for erection
    for erectile dysfunction, 213–214, 214f
    in multiple sclerosis patients, 290

Medium-fill cystometry, 101
Metabolic neuropathies, 343–345
  amyloidosis, 345
  diabetes mellitus, 343–345
Metastasis(es), cauda equina damage due
    to, 332
Methylprednisolone, for tropical spastic
    paraparesis, 322
Microenema(s), for constipation, 191–192
Micturition
  brain stem control of, 238–239, 239f
  normal, initiation of, 22–23
  regulation of, 4
Mitochondrial disorders, 348
Mizoribine, for tropical spastic parapare-
    sis, 322
Motor conduction studies, of pelvic floor,
    125–128, 125f–127f
Moxisylyte hydrochloride, for erectile dys-
    function, 210–211
Multiple endocrine neoplasia type 2B,
    348–349
Multiple sclerosis, 289–308
  bladder dysfunction in patients with,
    298–306
    impotence related to, 291, 292f
    lower urinary tract symptoms of,
      299–300, 299t, 301t
    neurologic features of, 303, 305f, 306f
    upper urinary tract symptoms of,
      303, 305
    urinary symptoms, 300, 301t
      management of, 305
    urodynamic studies of, 300, 302,
      302t, 303f, 304f
  colorectal dysfunction in, symptoms of,
    310, 310t
  gastrointestinal dysfunction in, 309–313
    constipation, 310–311
    incontinence, 311
    management of, 312
    pathophysiology of, 309–310, 310t
    prevalence of, 309
    studies of, 311–312
    symptoms of, 309
  sexual dysfunction in men with,
    289–298
    ejaculatory dysfunction, 295, 296f
    erectile dysfunction, 289–290, 290f
      bladder function and, 295
      management of, 297
      neurophysiologic tests for,
        293–295, 293t, 294f
    neurologic features of, 291–293, 292f

    sexual dysfunction in women with, 298
    urinary retention in patients with, 300
Multiple system atrophy
  bladder dysfunction in, 245–248
    clinical consequences of,
      246–247, 247t
    symptoms of, 246–247
    treatment of, 249–251
  diagnosis of, 245
    clinical urogenital criteria for,
      247, 247t
    sphincter electromyography in,
      247–248
  dysfunction in, presumptive pathophysi-
    ologic causes of, 246
  in neurogenic erectile failure, diagnosis
    of, sphincter electromyogra-
    phy in, 150–151, 151f
  sexual dysfunction in, 252–253
Muscle(s)
  diseases of, electromyographic changes
    in, 124
  of pelvic floor, 5–9, 39–40. *See also*
    specific muscle and Pelvic
    floor, muscles of
Muscle relaxants, striated, in spinal
    cord–injured patients, 280
Myectomy, detrusor
  for continence in spinal cord–injured
    patients, 283
  for detrusor hyperreflexia, 169
Myo-neuro-gastrointestinal encephalopa-
    thy, 348
Myoplasty(ies), in incomplete bladder
    emptying, 178

Nephropathy, reflux, in spinal cord–injured
    patients, 278–279
Nerve(s)
  genitofemoral, 12
  iliohypogastric, 11
  ilioinguinal, 12
  pudendal, 13–14, 14f
Nerve root stimulation, in incomplete blad-
    der emptying, 177–178
Nerve-conduction studies
  anterior sacral root stimulation,
    128–129, 129f
  central motor pathway assessment,
    129–130
  motor conduction studies, 125–128,
    125f–127f
  of pelvic floor, 125–130
Nervus furcalis, 10

Neurogenic bladder
  components of, 163
  dysfunction of
    assessment of, initial, 163–164
    classification of, 276, 277t
    detrusor hyperreflexia, treatment of,
      164–169. *See also* Detrusor
      hyperreflexia
    in spinal cord–injured patients,
      276, 277t
    treatment of, 163–184
    tropical spastic paraparesis and,
      geographic distribution of,
      316, 316f
Neurogenic erectile failure, 147–154
  autonomic function testing in, 151–152
  corpus cavernosum electromyography
    in, 152–154, 152f, 153f
  electromyography of anal or urethral
    sphincter in, 150
  pudendal evoked responses in,
    149–150, 149f
  sacral reflex testing in, 147–149, 148f
  sphincter electromyography in multiple
    system atrophy diagnosis,
    150–151, 151f
  sympathetic skin response(s) in, 151,
    152–154, 152f, 153f
Neurogenic incontinence, 185
Neurologic lesions, incontinence due to, 20
Neuromodulation, sacral nerve root,
    177–178. *See also* Sacral
    nerve stimulation, in bowel
    problem management
Neuropathic bowel. *See* Bowel, neuro-
    pathic
Neuropathy(ies)
  amyloid, hereditary, 347–348
  autonomic, hereditary, 348
  hereditary, 347–349
  metabolic, 343–345
    amyloidosis, 345
    diabetes mellitus, 343–345
  nutritional, 345–346
  peripheral, 339–352. *See also* Periph-
    eral neuropathy
  pudendal, 128
  sensory, hereditary, 348
  toxic, 345–346
Neurotransmitter(s)
  in cavernous relaxation, 52–53
  nonadrenergic noncholinergic, in cav-
    ernous relaxation, 52
  in smooth muscle contraction, 53

Nocturnal penile tumescence testing, for
    male erectile dysfunction,
    145–146, 146t
Nonadrenergic noncholinergic neurotrans-
    mitters, in cavernous relax-
    ation, 52
Nonpsychogenic urinary retention, in
    young women, 367–371. *See
    also* Urinary retention,
    nonpsychogenic, in young
    women
Nucleus(i), 246
  Onuf's, 13, 34, 246
Nutrition, and bowel and bladder func-
    tions, 62
Nutritional neuropathies, 345–346

Obstructive uropathy, in spinal
    cord–injured patients, 279
Odor control, in bowel problem manage-
    ment, 203
Onuf's nucleus, 13, 34, 246
Orgasm
  capacity of, effect of neurologic dis-
    eases on, 42
  cervical spinal cord in, 34
  female, 40–41
  male, 51
    components of, 51
  physiology of uterus during, 39
  quality of, effect of neurologic diseases
    on, 42
Overactive bladder function, defined, 267
Oxybutynin chloride
  for bladder dysfunction in spina bifida
    patients, 362
  for detrusor hyperreflexia, 165–166
  for tropical spastic paraparesis, 320
  for urinary symptoms in multiple scle-
    rosis patients, 305
Oxytocin secretion, in female sexual func-
    tion, 39

Pad(s), for urinary incontinence, 202
Pain, disorders of, effects of on sexual
    response, 76
Parenting, effects of bladder and bowel
    problems, 63
Parkinsonism. *See also* Parkinson's
    disease
  diagnosis of, onset of urinary symptoms
    in, 246
Parkinson's disease
  bowel function disorders in, 255–264

Parkinson's disease (*continued*)
  constipation in, 259
  esophageal alterations associated with, 255–256, 256t
  idiopathic
    bladder dysfunction in, 248–249
      clinical consequences of, 249, 250f
      treatment of, 250–251, 251f, 252f
    L-dopa in, 248–249
    sexual dysfunction in, 252–253
  intestinal dysfunction associated with, 255
  large bowel effects of, 258–262
  MPTP (1-methyl-4-phenyl-1,2,3,6-tetrahydropyridine)-induced, 248
  partner with, sex with, 82–84, 83f
  small bowel effects of, 257–258
  stomach effects of, 256–257, 258f
  swallowing abnormalities associated with, 255–256, 256t
Past experiences, disorders of, effects on sexual response, 78
Pelvic floor
  comparative anatomy of, 16–17
  electromyography of, 109–125. *See also* Electromyography, of pelvic floor
  muscles of, 5–9, 39–40
    anal, 6f, 8
    coccygeus, 5, 6, 6f
    iliococcygeus, 6, 6f
    levator ani, 5, 6f
    perineal, 7–8, 7f
    pubococcygeus, 5–6, 6f
    sacrococcygeal, 6
    urogenital, 7f, 9
Pelvic floor exercises, in incomplete bladder emptying, 176–177
Pelvic nerves, injuries to, 349–350
Pelvic organ(s),
  dysfunctions of
    after spinal cord lesions, 4
    neurologic aspects of
      disinterest in, reasons for, 3
      interest in, reasons for, 3
  function of, 3–4
Pelvic plexus, 34–35
Pelvic sympathetic system, 16
Penile nerve, dorsal, electroneurography of, 130
Penile prosthesis implantation, for erectile dysfunction, 218–219, 218f
Penile sheath, for incontinence, 179–180, 179f

Penile/brachial index, in vasculogenic erectile failure evaluation, 154–155
Penis
  anatomy of, 47–48, 48f
  arterial supply of, 47–48, 48f
  electrical stimulation of, sacral reflex in response to, 133–135, 134f
  vasculature of, 47–48, 48f
Perineum, male, musculature of, 7–8, 7f
Peripheral nervous system, components of, 339
Peripheral neuropathy, 339–352
  in diabetic patients, 343–345. *See also* Diabetes mellitus, neuropathies associated with
  hereditary amyloid, 347–348
  immune-mediated, 346–347
  infective, 346
  inherited, 347–349
    hereditary amyloid neuropathy, 347–348
    hereditary sensory neuropathies, 348
    Hirschsprung's disease, 348
    mitochondrial disorders, 348
    multiple endocrine neoplasia type 2B, 348–349
    porphyria, 347
  metabolic, 343–345
    amyloidosis, 345
    diabetes mellitus, 343–345
  nutritional, 345–346
  pelvic nerve injuries, 349–350
  toxic, 345–346
Pharmacologic erection program, for erectile dysfunction, 212–213
Phasic detrusor instability, defined, 267
Pontine detrusor nucleus of Barrington, 238
Porphyria, 347
Prostaglandin(s), in cavernous relaxation, 53
Prednisolone, for tropical spastic paraparesis, 322
Pressure/flow plot, 104
Priapism, defined, 212
Probanthine, for tropical spastic paraparesis, 320
Proctography, evacuating, in bowel problem evaluation, 188
Profilometry, urethral pressure, 105–106, 106f
Propantheline bromide
  for bladder dysfunction in spina bifida patients, 362
  for detrusor hyperreflexia, 166

Prostaglandin E₁, for intracorporeal injection therapy, in multiple sclerosis patients, 290

Prostatectomy, radical, erectile dysfunction after, sildenafil citrate for, 216

Prosthesis(es), in incomplete bladder emptying, 178

Psychological counseling, for erectile dysfunction, 219

Psychological issues, effects of bladder and bowel problems, 65–66

Puboanalis, 5

Pubococcygeus muscle, 5–6, 6f

Pubovaginalis, 5

Pudendal-evoked responses, in neurogenic erectile failure, 149–150, 149f

Pudendal nerve, 13–14, 14f

Pudendal neuropathy, 128

Radical prostatectomy, erectile dysfunction after, sildenafil citrate for, 216

Radiography
in bowel problem evaluation, 188
in cauda equina damage evaluation, 333

Ramus(i)
coccygeal dorsal spinal, 15
lumbar dorsal, 15
sacral dorsal spinal, 15
ventral primary, 9–10, 10f, 11f

Rapid-fill cystometry, 101

Reconstructive bladder surgery using bowel, for bladder dysfunction in spina bifida patients, 363

Rectal probe electroejaculation, for male infertility, 220

Rectoanal inhibitory reflex, in bowel problem evaluation, 188

Reduction cytoplasty, in incomplete bladder emptying, 178

Reflux nephropathy, in spinal cord–injured patients, 278–279

Rehabilitation, for erectile dysfunction, 219

Relationship(s), intimate, neurologic disability effects on, 85–86

Reliance, for incontinence, 179

Renal function, in spina bifida, assessment of, 359

Residential placement, bladder and bowel problems effects on, 64

Resiniferatoxin, for detrusor hyperreflexia, 168

Retraining
behavioral, in incomplete bladder emptying, 177

bladder, in incomplete bladder emptying, 177

Retrograde ejaculation, in diabetic patients, 345

Rhabdosphincter, 21

Rhinencephalon, in sexual desire and reactions, 34

Sacral anterior root stimulation, in spinal cord–injured patients, 284–285

Sacral deafferentation, for continence in spinal cord–injured patients, 283

Sacral dorsal spinal rami, 15

Sacral nerve stimulation, in bowel problem management, 197

Sacral plexus, 12–14, 14f

Sacral reflex(es)
measurement of, 132–135
methods of, 132–133
in neurogenic erectile failure, defined, 147–148
physiologic background of, 132–133
in response to electrical stimulation of penis or clitoris, 133–135, 134f
in response to mechanical stimulation, 135
terminology related to, 132–133
testing of, in neurogenic erectile failure, 147–149, 148f

Sacral roots, dorsal, electroneurography of, 130–131

Sacral sensory system, neurophysiology of, 130–132

Sacrococcygeal muscles, anterior and posterior, 6

Salazosulfapyridine, for tropical spastic paraparesis, 322

Seizure(s), epileptic
focal sexual, 42–43
sexual activity and, 44

Selective pudendal arteriography, in vasculogenic erectile failure evaluation, 156

Self-catheterization
clean intermittent, in spina bifida, 362
intermittent
in spinal cord–injured patients, 279–280
for tropical spastic paraparesis, 320
for urinary symptoms in multiple sclerosis patients, 305

Sensory neuropathies, hereditary, 348

Sex, neurologic disability effects on, 69–94
  in adolescents, 79–80
  different perceptions of men and
        women, 86–87
  intimate relationships, 85–86
  management of, 87–89, 89f
    contraception, 89
    fertility, 88–89
    intensive therapy, 88
    limited information in, 88
    permission in, 87
    P-LI-SS-IT model in, 87
    suggestions for, 88
  nondisabled partners, 84–85
  Parkinson's disease, 82–84, 83f
  in partner with acquired disability,
        80–84, 83f
  persons without sexual partner, 86
  psychosomatic circle of, 75f
  spinal injuries, 80–81
  traumatic brain injuries, 81–82
Sex organs, internal, innervation of, 34–35
Sexual activity
  and bowel and bladder functions, 62
  epileptic seizures due to, 44
Sexual arousal
  neurologic disability effects on,
        70–71, 72f
  physiology of uterus during, 39
  vaginal changes during, 38–39
Sexual desire
  cortical control of, 240–242
  female
    brain in, 33–34
    effect of neurologic diseases on,
          41–42
Sexual development, phases in, 69
Sexual dysfunction
  cauda equina damage and, investigation
        of, 334–335
  in diabetic patients, 344–345
  female, 43t
    treatment of, 222
  male, 43t
  in multiple sclerosis patients, 289–298.
        See also Multiple sclerosis,
        sexual dysfunction in men
        with; Multiple sclerosis, sex-
        ual dysfunction in women with
  in Parkinson's disease, 252–253
    in multiple system atrophy, 252–253
  treatment of, 209–225. *See also* Male
        erectile dysfunction
    erectile dysfunction, 209–219

female infertility, 222
  infertility, male, 219–222
Sexual expression
  in adult life, 70–79
    attitudes and, 78–79
    behavioral disorders and, 74
    cognitive disorders and, 74
    dyadic relationship, 72–74, 73f
    emotional disturbances and, 74
    fear of precipitating major illness
          and, 76
    pain and, 76
    past experience and, 78
    sexual arousal, 70–71, 72f
    sexual expression, 74
    sexual response, 70, 71f
    unrealistic expectations and, 76–78,
          77t, 78t
  factors affecting, 69
  myths in, 77t
  neurologic disability effects on, 74
Sexual function
  cortical control of, 240–242
  female. *See* Female sexual function
  male. *See* Male sexual function
  spinal and supraspinal neural mecha-
        nisms in, 4
  in spinal cord–injured patients,
        286–287
Sexual issues, in epileptic patients, 42–44
Sexual partner, individuals without, neuro-
        logic disability effects on, 86
Sexual problems, after head injuries,
        241–242
Sexual reactions, female, role of brain in,
        33–34
Sexual response
  female, phases of, 33
  neurologic disability effects on, 70, 71f
Sexuality, female
  effect of neurologic diseases on, 41–42
  with spinal cord injuries, 287
Shock, spinal, bladder management after,
        276–277
Sildenafil citrate, for erectile dysfunction,
        214–216
  in depressed patients, 216
  in diabetic patients, 215–216
  after radical prostatectomy, 216
  side effects of, 214–216
  in spinal cord–injured patients, 216
  studies of, 214–216
Single fiber electrode electromyography, of
        pelvic floor, 115–116, 117f

Skin responses, sympathetic, in neurogenic erectile failure, 152–154, 152f, 153f

Slow-fill cystometry, 101

Small bowel, Parkinson's disease effect on, 257–258

Smooth muscle activity, cavernous, neural modulations of, in male sexual function, 51–52

Smooth muscle contraction, neurotransmitters in, 53

Social relations, bladder and bowel problems effects on, 63–64

Sphincter, neuroanatomic sites in modulation of, 22, 23f

Sphincterotomy
for bladder dysfunction in spina bifida patients, 363
external urethral, in spinal cord–injured patients, 281

Spina bifida, 353–365
bladder dysfunction in, 354
assessment of, 359–360
classification of, 358
management of, 361–363
Credé's maneuver in, 361
nonsurgical, 361–362
surgical, 362–363
studies of, 359–361
videourodynamic study of, information obtained on, 360–361
bladder emptying in, 361–362
case studies, 354–353–357
closed, 354, 355f, 356f
defined, 353
incidence of, 353
neuropathic bowel in patients with, 364
open, 354
renal function in, assessment of, 359
urethral function in, assessment of, 359–360

Spina bifida occulta, 354

Spinal cord
anatomy of, 325–328, 326f–331f
in sexual desire and reactions, 34

Spinal cord injuries, 275–288
autonomic dysreflexia due to, 277–278
bowel function in patients with, 285–286
deafferentation in patients with, 284–285
ejaculation in patients with, 286–287
erectile dysfunction in, sildenafil citrate for, 216
erection in patients with, 286
kidney stones in patients with, 278

logistics associated with, 287
neurogenic bladder dysfunction associated with, management of, 279–284
bladder emptying, 279–282. *See also* Bladder emptying, in spinal cord–injured patients
continence in, 282–284
obstructive uropathy in patients with, 279
partner with, sex with, 80–81
reflux nephropathy in patients with, 278–279
renal damage in patients with, 278–279
sacral anterior root stimulation in patients with, 284–285
sexual function in patients with, 286–287
sexuality in women with, 287
urologic follow-up in patients with, 287
women with, sexuality in, 287

Spinal detrusor hyperreflexia, 267

Spinal shock
bladder management after, 276–277
defined, 276

St. Mark's stimulator, 126, 126f, 127f

Stent(s), urethral, in spinal cord–injured patients, 281

Stigma: The Management of Spoiled Identity, 78–79

Stoma(s), in bowel problem management, 199–200

Stomach, effect of Parkinson's disease on, 256–257, 258f

Stress incontinence, 20
electromyographic changes in, 120–122
genuine, defined, 266

Subtrigonal phenol injection, for detrusor hyperreflexia, 168–169

Suprapubic diversion, in spinal cord–injured patients, 281–282

Swallowing abnormalities, in Parkinson's disease, 255–256, 256t

Sympathetic skin response, 136, 137f
in neurogenic erectile failure, 151, 152–154, 152f, 153f

Thyrotropin-releasing hormone, for tropical spastic paraparesis, 322

Toxic neuropathies, 345–346

Transit studies, in bowel problem evaluation, 188

Traumatic brain injuries, partner with, sex with, 81–82

Travel, bladder and bowel problems and, 65
Treponema pallidum, infection with, neu-
    ropathies associated with, 346
Tropical spastic paraparesis, 315–324
    clinical features of, 318
    management of, 320–322, 320t
        clean intermittent self-catheteriza-
            tion in, 320
        danazol in, 321–322
        immunomodulatory therapies
            in, 322
        intravesical instillation of capsaicin
            in, 320–321, 321t
        lymphocytapheresis in, 322
        oral anticholinergics in, 320
    neurogenic bladder due to, geographic
        distribution of, 316, 316f
    pathophysiology of, 316–317
    studies of, 318–319
    vesical pathology in, 317, 318f

Ultrasonography
    anal, in bowel problem evaluation, 188
    color duplex, with intracavernosal injec-
        tion, in vasculogenic erectile
        failure evaluation, 155–156
Uninhibited overactive bladder, 267
Upper motor neuron lesions, 20
Urethra, electrical stimulation of, 132
Urethral function, in spina bifida, assess-
    ment of, 359–360
Urethral pressure profile, 105, 106f
Urethral pressure profilometry,
    105–106, 106f
Urethral sphincter, damage to, electromyog-
    raphy of, 150
Urethral stent, in spinal cord–injured
    patients, 281
Urge incontinence, in frail elderly, evi-
    dence for cerebral causes,
    269, 270f
Urinary continence, control of, 24–27, 25f
Urinary diversion, in incomplete bladder
    emptying, 178
Urinary incontinence, 20
    defined, 265
    in the elderly, 265–273. *See also* Elderly,
        urinary incontinence in
    after cerebrovascular accidents,
        236–238
    types of, 266–267
Urinary retention
    in multiple sclerosis patients, 300

nonpsychogenic, in young women,
    367–371
    causes of, 367, 371
    electromyography in, 368–370, 368f
    ephaptic transmission occurring in
        striated urethral sphincter,
        diagrammatic representation
        of, 369f
    historical background of, 367–368
    natural history of, 369–370
    treatment of, 370
in patients with brain lesions, 234–235
women with, 367–371
    electromyographic changes in,
        122–124, 123f
Urinary tract
    lower
        effects of bladder dysfunction in
            multiple sclerosis patients on,
            299–300, 299t, 301t
        innervation of, 340–341
    upper, effects of bladder dysfunction in
        multiple sclerosis patients on,
        303, 305
Urine
    postvoid residual, in the elderly,
        271–272
    retention of, 20
Urodynamics, 97–107
    ambulatory, 102
    cystometry, 100–104, 101f–103f
    defined, 97
    leak-point pressure, 104–105
    urethral pressure profilometry,
        105–106, 106f
    uroflowmetry, 97–100, 98f, 99f
    videocystometrography, 104
Urogenital disorders
    in multiple system atrophy, 245–248.
        See also Multiple system atro-
        phy, bladder dysfunction in
    in Parkinson's disease, 248–249
Urogenital muscles
    female, 9
    male, 7f, 9
Urogenital triangle, 8
Uropathy, obstructive, in spinal
    cord–injured patients, 279
Uterus, physiology of during sexual arousal
    and orgasm, 39

Vacuum therapy, for erectile dysfunction,
    217–218, 217f

Vagina
blood flow to, 37–38
cavernous tissue of, 37
innervation of, 35
lubrication of, 38
sexual arousal effects on, 38–39
Valsalva leak-point pressure, 104–105
Vanilloid receptor subtype, 167
Vasculogenic erectile failure
arterial inflow evaluation in,
154–156
evaluation of
color duplex ultrasonography with
intracavernosal injection in,
155–156
intracavernosal injection test in, 155
penile/brachial index in, 154–155
selective pudendal arteriography
in, 156
venous leakage in, evaluation of,
156–157, 156t
Vasoactive intestinal polypeptide, in cavernous relaxation, 53

Venous leakage, evaluation of, in vasculogenic erectile failure evalua-
tion, 156–157, 156t
Ventral primary rami, 9–10, 10f, 11f
Vesicoplication, in incomplete bladder
emptying, 178
Vesicostomy, for bladder dysfunction in
spina bifida patients, 363
Vesicourethral dysfunction, in children,
spinal bifida and, 353
Viagra. *See also* Sildenafil citrate, for erectile dysfunction
Vibratory stimulation, for male infertility, 220
Videocystometrography, 104
Vitamin C, for tropical spastic paraparesis, 322
Voiding
control of, 24–27, 25f
normal, 24, 25f
obstructed, women with, electromyographic changes in,
122–124, 123f